NURSING CARE EVALUATION

Concurrent and retrospective review criteria

SENIOR AUTHOR

Sharon Van Sell Davidson, R.N., B.S.N., M.Ed.
President, C.P.E., Inc.,
Colorado Springs, Colorado

COORDINATING AUTHORS

Bette Clark Burleson, R.N., B.S.N., M.N.
Clinical Supervisor,
New Cumberland, Pennsylvania

Jean Ellen Scheel Crawford, R.N., B.S.N., M.N.
Director of Nursing,
The Orthopaedic Hospital of Charlotte,
Charlotte, North Carolina

Sue Christofferson, R.N.
Review Coordinator Director,
Foundation for Health Care Evaluation,
Minneapolis, Minnesota

The C. V. Mosby Company

Saint Louis   1977

The C.V. Mosby Company
11830 Westline Industrial Drive, St. Louis, Missouri 63141

Library of Congress Cataloging in Publication Data

Davidson, Sharon Van Sell, 1944-
  Nursing care evaluation.

  Bibliography: p.
  Includes index.
  1. Nursing audit. 2. Professional standards
review organizations (Medicine). I. Title.
[DNLM: 1. Evaluation studies. 2. Nursing audit.
3. Nursing care—Standards. WY16 D253n]
RT85.5.D38   610.73   77-5069
ISBN 0-8016-1210-1

TS/VH/VH 9 8 7 6 5 4 3 2 1

RESEARCH ASSISTANTS

Nancy L. Irwin, B.S., M.Ed.
Research Assistant,
Washington, D.C.

Arra Johnson
Research Assistant,
Colorado Springs, Colorado

CONTRIBUTORS

Gailene Alteman, R.N., B.S.N., M.S.
Instructor, School of Nursing,
University of Washington,
Seattle, Washington

Lucille Ashley, R.N., M.S.N.
Director of Nursing,
Metropolitan Washington Regional Medical
Program,
Washington, D.C.

Diane Baker, R.N., B.S.N., M.G.C.
Associate Director of Nursing Service;
Baptist Memorial Hospital,
Memphis, Tennessee

Amy A. Chow, R.N., B.S., M.A.
Clinical Nurse Specialist,
New York, New York

Sharon Hulow Cox, R.N., B.S.N., M.S.N.
Instructor of Management of Patient Care,
University of North Carolina at Charlotte,
Charlotte, North Carolina

Donald Albert Dennis, Ph.D.
Director of Medical Education,
Daniel Freidman Hospital,
Inglewood, California

Suzanne S. Dziak, R.N., B.S.N., M.N.
Chief Nurse,
Veterans Hospital,
Washington, D.C.

Holly Emrich, R.N., B.S.N., M.S.
Maternal-Child Health Consultant,
Denver, Colorado

Diane Wall Gainey, R.N.
Coordinator, Pediatric Intensive Care,
Presbyterian Hospital,
Charlotte, North Carolina

Mary Ellen Gill, R.N., B.S.
Senior Staff Nurse,
New York Hospital,
Cornell Medical Center,
New York, New York

PREFACE

With the enactment of Public Law 92-603, the Professional Standards Review Organization (PSRO) was established, with its primary purpose being to provide quality assurance programs that will attain the highest degree of excellence in the delivery of health care. The PSROs membership is comprised of doctors of medicine and osteopathy, and the organizational direction is toward medical quality assurance. The major program components include admission certification, continued stay review, medical care evaluation studies, and profile analysis. A great deal of time and financial assistance were expended to develop medical screening criteria to assist in the program's implementation.

It is unrealistic to believe that a legally mandated quality assurance program would not have a far-reaching effect on other members of the health team and particularly on the practice of nursing. However, the profession of nursing has addressed the current modifications in practice in a positive manner, without benefit of funding sources, without mass education of its practitioners in the implementation and regulations of PSRO, and without adequate nursing research. There has been some confusion throughout the country concerning nursing quality assurance programs because of a lack of understanding about PSRO regulations and the Joint Commission on the Accreditation of Hospitals (JCAH) audit requirements, a lack in uniformity of approaches, a lack of common nomenclature, and, most importantly, a lack of substantial norms, standards, and criteria guides. *Nursing Care Evaluation: Concurrent and Retrospective Review Criteria* addresses these concerns and provides guidelines by which the profession of nursing can move forward in its involvement with PSRO activities.

The introductory section discusses the implications of PSROs in the health care setting and explores the expected role of the nurse in the organizational framework. A comprehensive overview of quality assurance is included, which emphasizes nursing care evaluation and its major components. The purposes and objectives of concurrent and retrospective review are defined, and the methodology for criteria development is analyzed. Examples of nursing care evaluation formats are presented with explanations for their modification and implementation.

The model nursing criteria sets are arranged in alphabetical order for quick reference. The nursing criteria amplify and extend physician's criteria by providing for psychosocial needs, patient education, discharge planning, adaptation to health status, retrospective criteria, and critical nursing management for complications, which is frequently initiated before medical management of complications. Both concurrent and retrospective review criteria have been developed for over 250 major diseases and medical conditions, and the criteria sets are referenced to established systems of coding (HICDA, Hospital International Classification of Diseases adapted for use; ICDA-8, International Classification of Diseases Adapted for Use; and DSM-II, Diagnostic and Statistical Manual of Mental Disorders, Vol. 2). Numerical designations are included to indicate which diagnoses apply to a particular criteria set. Coding each criteria set in this manner will be useful in coordinating the model nursing criteria with the medical criteria and in identifying exactly which criteria sets apply to which diagnostic entities.

In addition, a glossary of pertinent terms specifically pertaining to PSRO is included in Appendix B.

This book is written primarily for those nurses and nurse administrators who are involved in PSRO, by providing guidelines for the development and implementation of audit criteria. However, these comprehensive criteria can also be used by staff nurses making clinical assessments, as a guideline in identifying a patient's physical or psychological needs and concerns; and by team leaders and primary nurses, as a learning tool for making clinical observations, writing nursing care plans, and evaluating their own performances.

The audit methods presented in this book are not to be considered the "last word" in or the "best methods" of nursing care evaluation but rather are to serve as an alternative approach to present nursing care evaluation programs or to be modified and revised to meet the needs of each individual hospital, health care institution, or PSRO organization. It is hoped that this book will stimulate the evaluation of existing programs and will move the profession of nursing forward in the evolutionary process of determining appropriate, cost effective, efficient quality assurance for nursing that is compatible with the Professional Standards Review Organizations and improved nursing care.

We would like to acknowledge the efforts of many nurses throughout the country who assisted us in determining and analyzing the "state of the art" in their individual hospitals. In particular, we would like to extend our sincere thanks to Lucille Ashley, Diane Baker, Suzanne Dziak, and Dianne Goodspeed, whose assistance in planning the methods developed in this book have been invaluable.

Sharon Van Sell Davidson
P.O. Box 9915
Colorado Springs, Colorado 80932
Bette Clark Burleson
Jean Ellen Scheel Crawford
Sue Christofferson

CONTENTS

SECTION THREE

Complications, 329

SECTION ONE

Introduction

PROFESSIONAL STANDARDS REVIEW ORGANIZATIONS
Overview

Many forces have influenced the current thrust for quality assurance within the total spectrum of the health care delivery system. Court decisions charging physicians, hospitals, nurses, or nursing services with inadequate care, negligence, and even malpractice have reached alarming proportions. The voice of the consumer, once a murmur, is growing stronger in expressing dissatisfaction with the health care system. Within the nursing profession, organizations such as the American Nurses' Association have made recurring statements attempting to identify the nurses' responsibilities for monitoring the quality of care and services. The release of standards for practice in the major clinical areas attests to the profession's recognition of its responsibility to society. The most recent revisions of standards for accreditation by the Joint Commission on Accreditation of Hospitals (JCAH) requires that hospitals demonstrate an effective method for assessing the quality of care provided to patients. Certainly, the major force for quality care has been the formalization of quality assurance programs in health care, mandated in Public Law 92-603— the 1972 amendments to the Social Security Act—which provided for the creation of Professional Standards Review Organizations (PSROs).

The PSRO is a program organized, administered, and controlled by local physicians and osteopaths to evaluate the necessity for and quality of medical care delivered in their designated areas under Medicare, Medicaid, and Maternal Child Health Programs. The organization of PSROs is based on the "concept that health professionals are the most appropriate individuals to evaluate the quality of medical services and that effective peer review at the local level is the soundest method for assuring the appropriate use of health care resources and facilities."[*]

PSRO legislation was enacted because there were compelling arguments for such a law. As one physician spokesman stated, "PSRO is here because of failures in the system in the past. Those failures are the major reasons why quality of care in this country is spotty and why, in the Medicare and Medicaid programs, much abuse and misutilization occurred, with its resultant, serious inflation of health care costs."[†]

A PSRO manual containing the initial information and procedural materials needed for implementation of the provisions of the law relating to professional standards review has been prepared by the staff of the Bureau of Quality Assurance. It has been designed to accommodate new or supplemental material as further interpretations of the law and changes in procedures are made.

PSROs utilize the guidelines included in this manual as the base for their programs. A summary of PSRO review responsibilities appearing in the manual includes:

1. Professional Standards Review Organizations will review the health care provided under Medicare, Medicaid and Maternal and Child Health Programs and make judgements on the medical necessity and quality of care. In addition, PSROs will determine whether care is proposed to be provided or has been provided at a level of care that is most economical and consistent with the patient's medical care needs.
2. PSROs are required over a period of time, to perform review of the care provided in institutions (for example, short-stay general hospitals, tuberculosis hospitals, mental health hospitals, skilled nursing facilities, and intermediate care facilities). A PSRO may review non-insti-

---

[*]*Report of the Committee on Finance United States Senate*, U.S. Government Printing Office, Washington, D.C., Sept. 26, 1972, p. 265.
[†]Simmons, Henry, Nov. 7, 1973.

tutional care if it requests to do so and if the Secretary of the Department of Health, Education, and Welfare approves such a request.

3. Initially, PSROs should, at a minimum, establish a system for review of care provided to inpatients in short-stay general hospitals and develop a phased plan for the performance review in long-term care facilities. If it demonstrates capability in these areas, the PSRO may develop review systems for care provided in other institutions and for non-institutional care.

4. For review in short-stay hospitals, the PSRO will be required at a minimum to perform (A) admission certification concurrent with the patient's admission, (B) continued stay review, and (C) medical care evaluation studies. As the capability progresses in its area to develop profiles, the PSRO will be required to review these. The PSRO will develop criteria and standards and select norms for each type of review which it performs . . . (note: alternate approaches developed by applicant PSROs will be reviewed and may be found acceptable providing they have the potential to result in the establishment and operation of an equally or more effective review system than that outlined in the manual).

5. PSROs are required to utilize the services and adopt the findings of review committee(s) of hospitals which in the judgment of the PSRO, are capable of performing review effectively . . .

6. The PSRO will work closely with Medicare, Medicaid and Maternal and Child Health Administrative and fiscal agents in the development, implementation and operation of its review program . . .*

The nurse's role in the PSRO

Nurses are included in the PSRO as non-physician health care practitioners. The PSRO Program Manual emphasizes that the Professional Standards Review Organizations are expected, over a period of time, to provide evidence that non-phy-

*P.S.R.O. program manual, Office of Professional Standards Review, U.S. Department of Health, Education, and Welfare, Mar. 1974, pp. 1-3.

sician health care practitioners are involved in the following activities:

1. Development and ongoing modification of norms, criteria, and standards for their areas of practice

2. Development of review mechanisms to be used for peer assessment of the performance of non-physician health care practitioners

3. Conduct of health care review of non-physician health care practitioners by their peers

4. Working with established continuing education programs to assure utilization of results of review in educational efforts

5. Where appropriate, participation by both physicians and non-physician health care practitioners in review committee activities

Professional nurses also have other mechanisms for input into the organization. The guidelines permit inclusion of non-physicians on the governing body of the PSRO, but they are not eligible to vote on issues relating to the physician practice of medicine and osteopathy. Advisory groups are to be established to assist each state Professional Standards Review Council or PSRO in states without councils. The advisory groups are to include representatives from the non-physician health care professions within the PSRO area.

In evaluating the status of PSRO organizations, it was determined that little or no activity was being directed toward the non-physician health care practitioners (especially nurses). Local nursing groups have experienced difficulty in implementing programs that comply with the regulations set forth by the PSROs. Factors impeding progress in this area are a lack of financial resources, limited knowledge of legislative regulations, non-availability of reference materials for education, and inadequate nursing research in quality assurance. As a result, local nursing groups have been left with a piecemeal grouping of norms, standards, and criteria and the development, in various parts of the country, of specialized, limited approaches that are not comprehensive enough to meet the needs of individual health care institutions and PSRO programs.

In order to comply with the PSRO regulations, local nursing groups will have to develop norms, criteria, and standards for their areas of practice and must agree on the definitions of these terms. For the purpose of this discussion, norms, standards, and criteria are defined as follows: (1) norms are numerical or statistical measures of usual observed performances; (2) standards are professionally developed expressions of the range of acceptable variation from a norm or criteria; (3) criteria are predetermined elements against which aspects of the quality of a medical service or nursing service can be measured.

Confusion during physician and nurse review activities will be minimized when both groups adopt the same terminology.

NURSING QUALITY ASSURANCE

Nursing quality assurance can be defined as a commitment to excellence in the delivery of health care. It is a program designed to determine the extent to which a specific nursing practice achieves selected objectives (criteria) based on specified values (norms). These specified values are then measured in terms of predetermined standards. Analysis of data collected exposes deficiencies or variations in nursing care. Continuing education programs can then be implemented to correct these variations and upgrade professional performance. Re-evaluation will reveal the change in professional behavior instituted through nonpunitive, educational measures. The overall effectiveness of the nursing quality assurance program and the identification of review priorities will be realized through profile analysis.

With the current legislative interest and an increase in available literature about nursing quality assurance, one might think that this is a new concept. However, the concept of quality control in nursing care is not new to nurses. When it is analyzed, the Nightingale Pledge attests to quality—and most professional nurses have made public proclamation to support the pledge. Among the earliest efforts to assess adequacy of medical and nursing care and its impact on recipients can be found in *Notes on Matters Affecting the Health, Efficiency and Hospital Administration of the British Army* by Florence Nightingale. Published in 1858, this work included comparing mortality experience in the British armed forces during the Crimean War with experience in civilian populations. This work forcefully brought to the attention of the government and the public the atrocious standards of care for military personnel. Although by today's standards the data are crude, the report was, nevertheless, instrumental in bringing about basic reforms in living standards and health services for the British armed forces.

In the past, quality assurance consisted primarily of hospital environmental and organizational standards. It was also assumed that if a nurse met certain educational requirements for licensure quality nursing care would naturally follow. Today, quality assurance considers not only environmental, organizational, and educational factors, but also focuses attention on the impact of nursing care on the patient. At one time or another all nurses have been involved in a "checklist" that evaluates room temperature, cleanliness, safety, medication given promptly, and the utilization of the nursing staff. These situations deal with certainties—either one did or did not perform. Nursing has the current responsibility of teaching nurses, especially staff nurses, to deal with probabilities or outcomes, nursing priorities on a concurrent basis, identification of patterns of nursing care based upon validated criteria, and the utilization of concurrent criteria to improve patient care while a patient is hospitalized. Therefore, the purpose of nursing quality assurance is to provide for a systematic approach to nursing care, which not only will be compatible with the goals of the PSRO but also will be of benefit to the patients.

A comprehensive system of nursing quality assurance incorporates the following components:

Nursing care evaluation (NCE)—the combined analysis of concurrent and retrospective nursing review

Concurrent nursing care review or concurrent nursing audit—the evaluation of nursing care of a patient while that care is being rendered

Retrospective nursing care review or retrospective nursing audit—the evaluation, after the discharge of the patient, of the quality of nursing care that was rendered

Continuing education—an educational program for members of the nursing staff, presented to improve the quality of patient care, based on the problems or deficiencies identified during the review process

Profile analysis—the evaluation of the effectiveness of nursing review components, the identification of review priorities, and comparison with other local nursing groups

NURSING CARE EVALUATION
Concurrent nursing care review

The purpose of concurrent nursing care review in nursing care evaluation is to assure the identification of nursing care priorities and to provide optimum nursing care while the patient is still hospitalized. Concurrent nursing audit is an "open chart" review for the evaluation of the quality of nursing care being given to the patient. It is a vehicle by which variations from the standard criteria in individual and group practice can be identified in time to realize a qualitative improvement in the ongoing care of the

audited patient. Frequently, the criteria used in concurrent audit are those that were developed for use in the retrospective audit of outcomes and that simply are applied earlier in the sequence. However, the concurrent review methodology proposed in this book requires the development, ratification, and modification of concurrent review criteria appropriate for application during a patient's hospitalization rather than adaptation of retrospective criteria for concurrent review.

Concurrent nursing audit has existed formally and informally for some time. Making rounds to each patient on a given unit is an audit, although a potentially ineffective one when not done with specific purpose. To avoid a mere bed check or head count, various assessment tools have been developed, with an emphasis on safety, cleanliness, nutrition, elimination, and comfort. Such tools, developed within individual hospitals, vary greatly in depth and precision but do represent an organized attempt at quality measurement. Frequently these tools have been designed and used by nursing supervisors in a punitive way. This approach destroys the commitment advantage inherent in a peer-developed approach. Concurrent nursing care review in nursing care evaluation offers an objective means to evaluate care and implement immediate corrective nursing action that will benefit a patient during hospitalization.

Other modes of concurrent nursing care review include the daily review of nursing notes by team leaders and head nurses and the patient-centered care conference in which patient progress is compared with the goal of care. In both the nursing actions and interventions are reexamined, and modifications in the nursing care plan are implemented. The focus is narrowed to one patient, the criteria used are usually unique to that patient, and variations or deficits in care approaches are identified in isolation.

The problem is that the outcome of these conferences, although generally of benefit to the patient, is not communicated to other nursing units, thus preventing easy identification of patterns of care. Consequently, the same deficit may occur in the care of several patients on different units in the same hospital, and the deficiency must be rediscovered in each case.

With concurrent review criteria in use on each nursing unit, objective evaluation can identify deficiencies and motivate immediate corrective action. Following appropriate corrective action, failure to return to the standard should be recorded. Failure of nurses to conduct concurrent audits and to take corrective action is in itself a process deficit that will be discovered when the undesirable outcome is audited retrospectively.

Retrospective nursing care review

The purpose of retrospective nursing care review in nursing care evaluation is to identify deficiencies in the organization and administration of nursing care; to correct such deficiencies through education and administrative change; and, periodically, to reassess performance to assure that improvements have been maintained. It is an organized and systematic process designed to provide a means of determining the effectiveness of the concurrent review component and to identify patterns of nursing care requiring evaluation. This process also assists in validating criteria, norms, and standards and provides evidence helpful in their revision.

The retrospective audit is an evaluation of the quality of nursing care of patients that is made after the patients have already been discharged. It is a "closed chart" review of predetermined outcomes for the purpose of identifying variations in care, patterns of nursing care, or nursing care under a set of specific conditions. The well-developed retrospective audit system generates valid statistics on

norms and trends and becomes the basis for future criteria development. Retrospective audit depends on documentation of care. If the chart does not reveal a care component, then it must be assumed the component was missing. A need for more diligent documentation is recognized immediately, as well as a need for an efficient data retrieval system. The mere existence of a retrospective audit system can improve the documentation of nursing care.

Retrospective review of nursing care includes several components: process audit, structure audit, and behavioral outcome audit. One of the most prevalent misconceptions about a process audit is that it is the same procedure as concurrent audit. Actually, they are different review procedures. Process nursing audit incorporates a step by step evaluation of a problem or complication that has been identified through retrospective review of nursing care. For example, if the retrospective review of newly delivered mothers revealed that a high percentage of the patients developed urinary tract infections as a result of being catheterized in the delivery room, these results would lend themselves to the development of a process nursing audit to evaluate the method of catheterization by each delivery room nurse. Even though the process audit may be administered as the care is being rendered, it is not a true concurrent review mechanism because the process audit is really an in-depth study of a problem or complication that has been identified during a retrospective audit. A structure audit is one that evaluates the physical, fiscal, and organizational characteristics of an agency, unit, or service. A behavioral outcome audit reviews the end result of the patient's health. It asks what happened to the patient as a result of nursing intervention and at what points different aspects of care should be administered. Each of these types of audit looks at "patterns of care" over a given period of time.

7

Comments

The Joint Commission on Accreditation of Hospitals has developed the retrospective review methodology and has successfully educated the masses of professional personnel about it. Because of their position as the accrediting agency, they have been able to require retrospective medical and nursing review as a condition for accreditation. This type of ruling has had positive effects in mandating the direction of review activities. The retrospective review of medical care does appear the most effective system for identifying patterns of medical care that can be related to individual practitioners, if indicated. The difficulty is that nursing, at this time, does not have individual nurses responsible for a given patient's care. Therefore the profession of nursing may be more effectively reviewed on a concurrent basis, and the development of concurrent methodology has been stymied as a result of the great emphasis on retrospective review.

The primary reason for instituting concurrent review of nursing care is for the improvement of patient care while the patient is still hospitalized. For example, the patient who is allowed to develop a pressure sore (decubitus ulcer) because skin integrity is not maintained on his paralyzed side is not likely to be enthusiastic when, 6 months after his discharge, the hospital determines through a retrospective nursing audit that all patients on Unit 7B developed pressure sores. The discharged patients already suffered the extended hospitalizations and the retarding of rehabilitation services as the result of pressure sores. However, if a concurrent review of nursing care had identified and corrected the situation before the problem developed for the patients, the overall desired medical and nursing outcomes would have been improved, and the hospitalizations would not have been extended because of preventable complication. In conclusion, a nursing quality assurance system should incorporate a nursing care evaluation system that includes concurrent and retrospective review components, continuing education, and profile analysis.

THE NURSING CARE EVALUATION PROCESS

Nursing care evaluation studies cannot be instituted until the nursing staff has developed and ratified criteria to be used in evaluating the nursing care on a concurrent and retrospective basis. Criteria can be developed along the lines of medical diagnosis or nursing problems. This book uses the medical diagnosis model for examples, since the majority of criteria are related to medical diagnosis. The use of medical diagnosis allows for each model criteria set to be referenced by an established system of numerical coding, that is the Hospital Adaption of International Classification of Diseases (HICDA), the International Classification of Diseases Adapted for Use (ICDA-8), or the Diagnostic and Statistical Manual of Mental Disorders, Vol. 2 (DSM-II). This coding will be useful to local nursing groups in adapting or establishing new criteria sets because it is important to know exactly which criteria sets apply to which diagnostic entities.

The concurrent review of nursing care should be conducted at 48 hours from admission and at the twenty-fifth and fiftieth percentile of the expected length of stay. This review could be completed by a PSRO utilization review coordinator or a PSRO-trained nurse on the unit. Adverse determinations from the concurrent review would be referred to a nurse advisor for evaluation. The PSRO utilization review coordinator would only render positive judgments about the provision of nursing care. Failure of nurses to implement the major items identified in the concurrent review format would probably lead to an extended hospital stay and less than desirable health outcomes for the patient.

The retrospective review of nursing care should be consistent with the yearly determination of the number of medical care evaluation studies required by the Bureau of Quality Assurance in the Department of Health, Education, and Welfare. The proposed number is calculated from admission rates and is identical with the Joint Commission on the Accreditation of Hospitals (JCAH) numbers, which are as follows: less than 2,500 total admissions—four studies; 2,500 to 4,999 admissions—six studies; 5,000 to 9,999—eight studies; 10,000 to 19,999—ten studies; and more than 20,000—twelve studies. Retrospective studies can be spaced throughout a calendar year and can be used to evaluate care provided prior to the current year.

The actual retrieval of data for both the concurrent and the retrospective review aspects should be accomplished by medical records data analysts. The results of nursing care evaluation studies are evaluated by a nursing audit committee with results being reported to the nursing administrator, the hospital administrator, the hospital board of trustees, and the PSRO organization.

Variations in nursing practices identified through concurrent or retrospective reviews would be linked to hospital inservice programs as well as to professional organization's education programs or continuing education programs of the local universities. The reauditing, at a predetermined future date, would assess changes in professional behavior. The thrust of the review activities is not intended to be punitive but rather is to improve the quality of nursing care through the education of the nursing practitioner.

Because the profession of nursing is only one of the many professions involved in the health care setting, the most logical progression for evaluation of patient care is toward an interdisciplinary health care evaluation system. One step toward the interdisciplinary process is the inclusion of nurses on medical audit or utilization review committees. Before nurses can actively participate, they must understand the elements and data required for the assessment of quality nursing care both concurrently and retrospectively.

NURSING CARE EVALUATION FORMAT

Even though the NCE format was developed primarily with the acute care facility in mind, the format has been adapted for public health nursing and long-term care areas. The inclusion of criteria sets should stimulate thought and assist local nursing groups in developing and refining review criteria. The criteria sets *must* be ratified by the nursing groups implementing them, which means modification and revision before adoption of concurrent and retrospective review criteria. The following is an example format of a nursing care evaluation.

NURSING CARE EVALUATION

Topic:_____ Code:_____

CONCURRENT REVIEW CRITERIA

I. Identification of patient's physical and psychological needs and/or concerns (limited to five or fewer entries)*

II. Recommended nursing action consistent with diagnosis
   A. Nursing services (limited to five or fewer entries)
   B. Health education (limited to five or fewer entries)

III. Indicators for discharge
   A. Adaptation of health status (limited to five or fewer entries)
   B. Examples of community resources (limited to three or fewer entries)

RETROSPECTIVE REVIEW CRITERIA

I. Health
II. Activity
III. Knowledge

COMPLICATIONS

---

*These are suggested numbers of entries. There may be variations.

The nursing care evaluation format is not meant to become a laundry list for the provision of nursing care, but should assist in identifying nursing priorities necessary for the achievement of desired nursing outcomes (refer to the Nursing Care Evaluation format). The title of the format refers to the medical diagnosis or nursing problem for which criteria is being developed. The code number refers to the HICDA, ICDA-8, or DSM-II system of coding, and the medical records administrator can assist in the determination of appropriate codes. These code numbers will assist in the retrieval of data and development of statistical reports that may, at some time, be compared between health institutions.

Concurrent review criteria

Part one of the concurrent review criteria seeks the *identification of patient's physical and psychosocial needs and/or concerns.* This is limited to five or fewer entries* and should contain the major patient needs, which must be identified for nursing action implementation in order to ensure that the patient outcome is consistent with the desired nursing goals.

Part two pertains to recommended nursing action consistent with diagnosis. The nursing services to be provided are limited to five or fewer entries and should contain nursing actions and nursing prescriptions. The health education section is limited to five or fewer entries and requires identification of the major areas for patient and/or family education. The section on recommended nursing action consistent with diagnosis will be extremely useful to the staff nurse (or the primary care nurse) in planning care or evaluating the care being rendered. The nurse will be able to ensure that services required have been provided and that the patient has been taught as indicated. The

supervisor (or head nurse) will find this area helpful in determining the staffing and the qualifications needed for personnel on each shift. For example, if a patient requires a colostomy irrigation every 8 hours, the supervising nurse can review the staffing to be sure that at least one nurse per shift understands and can administer a colostomy irrigation.

Part three refers to indicators for discharge, which includes information on the adaptation of health status and examples of community resources appropriate for discharge planning. The adaptation of health status identifies the modification of a patient's health status in order to be considered for discharge from the acute care institution. This section also helps to focus on major nursing priorities during hospitalization. Examples of community resources provide suggestions for appropriate types of community agencies to which patients may be referred for continuity of nursing care following hospital discharge.

Retrospective review criteria

The section on retrospective review criteria is divided into three sections: health, activity, and knowledge. These elements describe the patient's *expected status* at the time of discharge. Health refers to the desired discharge health status and includes the resolution, modification, or adaptation of the admitting condition. Activity refers to the physical and mental activity that a patient should exhibit on discharge. For example, a myocardial infarction patient should be able to walk 50 feet without experiencing chest pain. Knowledge refers to demonstrated comprehension of elements necessary for continued improvement or a return to a previous health level. For example, a diabetic patient should be able to demonstrate knowledge of sterile technique necessary for the administration of insulin. These categories are the same as those required by the JCAH retrospective nursing audit.

---

*These are suggested numbers of entries. There may be variations.

The section on complications lists the medical complications usually considered in the treatment of a specific diagnosis. Because of the repetition of complications, critical nursing management, health education, and special instructions for data retrieval, the complications are listed alphabetically in Section three of this book (beginning on p. 329).

The complications section is used in the retrospective review of nursing care and can serve as a review for the practicing nurse who must assess complications and frequently must implement critical nursing management while the physician is being notified or the physician's orders are being obtained.

Standards should be developed for all criteria, whether concurrent or retrospective. These standards must be determined by the group ratifying the criteria. The JCAH has suggested 100% achievement for criteria other than complications and 0% appearance of complications. Other groups have proposed criteria that reflect local professional consideration of acceptable levels of practice within a given area. The standard of practice should be high enough to represent a goal for attainment and should be revised as the standard is met. The model criteria sets do not include a standard because of the great variation across the nation. The ratifying groups should add a standard to each criteria set.

For ease in data retrieval by nonnursing personnel, the inclusion of exceptions to the criteria and special instructions for data retrieval should be provided. Again, because of the great variation across the nation, the exceptions and special instructions should be determined by the local nursing groups. An example of a modified nursing care evaluation form (pp. 12-13) and a completed form (pp. 14-19) is provided as an example for use by the local nursing groups. The format provides parallels and is adapted from the format suggested by the JCAH.

Schematic of Nursing Care Evaluation studies

The following method for NCE studies provides a systematic patient care evaluation procedure that changes the focus of review from the more traditional chart or subjective techniques toward objective concurrent review and identification of patterns of care in a retrospective review technique. This enables the reviewers to evaluate and implement nursing care, to implement corrective action while a patient is still hospitalized, and to evaluate patterns of patient care rather than to devote an inordinate amount of time and energy to the review of isolated incidents of nursing care.

This method produces a relatively large return through the evaluation of aggregate data about nursing care, objectively based on criteria, utilizing limited investment of the health professional's time and shifting the social and psychological criteria burden from the individual reviewers to the system.

Of extreme importance is that this systematic method of performing NCE studies directs itself to continually improving nursing care through a planned and positive change program with active involvement of the nursing professionals.

General aspects of Nursing Care Evaluation studies
Definition

NCE studies are a type of health care review performed for the purpose of improving patient care through systematic and objective evaluation of the nursing care being rendered and through education and/or action-change programs designed to meet specific identified needs.

Objectives of NCE studies

1. To assure that nursing care services are appropriate to the needs of the patient

Text continued on p. 20.

NURSING CARE EVALUATION: Modified form

Topic: _____ Code: _____ Date: _____

Criteria	Standard			Exceptions	Special instructions for data retrieval
	100%	Expected %	Actual %		
Concurrent *Identification of patient's physical and psychosocial needs and/or concerns*					
Recommended nursing action consistent with diagnosis Nursing service					
Health education					
Indicators for discharge *Adaptation to health status*					
Examples of community resources					

Recommended nursing action consistent with diagnosis

Nursing services

Perform nursing measures to ensure adequate hydration, nutrition, an elimination; observe type and amount of food intake; implement carbohydrate restriction; observe therapeutic action of patient's diet in terms of growth needs, activity, and diabetic control; report any adverse effects; encourage patient to adhere to ordered diet by making appropriate substitutions from exchange list when necessary to include food preferences; and incorporate child's normal dietary habits to facilitate diet adherence	x	95	89	None	See nursing assessment, nurse's notes, intake and output record, dietary flow sheet, and referral to dietary consultant
Survey patient's response to medical management, including test for fasting blood sugars; coordinate all diagnostic test to prevent prolonged period of fasting from interfering with insulin administration and diet control of disease	x	95	91	None	See Clinitest and acetone record, diabetic flow sheet, nurse's notes, and laboratory reports
Administer insulin according to orders with close observation for insulin shock or coma and prompt nursing intervention should either occur	x	95	95	None	See medication record, diabetic flow sheet, and nurse's notes
Maintain activity requirements and prevent infection	x	95	89	None	See nurse's notes or activity record and diabetic flow sheet
Give emotional support to family/patient necessary for acceptance of diagnosis and treatment regimen	x	95	93	None°	See nurse's notes

Health education

Instruct on signs and symptoms of insulin shock, diabetic acidosis, and appropriate actions to take should either occur	x	95	94	None	See diabetic teaching sheet and nurse's notes
Instruct on diet and dietary restrictions	x	95	95	None°	See diabetic teaching sheet, dietary flow sheet, and nurse's notes

° If patient is unteachable and there is no family, the responsible party assuming health care supervision is required to know the criteria, and this must be documented on the nurse's notes.

Continued.

15

NURSING CARE EVALUATION: Completed format

Topic: Diabetes mellitus, juvenile   **Codes:** 250, 250.3, 250.4   **Date:** August 30, 1977

Criteria	Standard			Exceptions	Special instructions for data retrieval
	100%	Expected %	Actual %		
Instruct on methods of preventing skin irritation and infections and skin hygiene; stress immunizations and dental care	x	95	94	None*	See diabetic teaching sheet and nurse's notes
Instruct on sterilization of insulin injection equipment, technique for drawing up proper dosage, proper technique for administering insulin, name of insulin, dosage, frequency, importance of rotating sites of injection, and relationship of activity to diet to insulin in diabetic control	x	95	92	None*	See diabetic teaching sheet, nurse's notes, and medication record for self-administration
Stress importance of continual medical care follow-up	x	95	95	None	See diabetic teaching sheet and nurse's notes
Indicators for discharge *Adaptation to health status* Condition stable	x	95	93	None	See nurse's notes, diabetic flow sheet, and laboratory report (fasting blood sugar within normal limits)
No complications evident	x	95	91	None	See nurse's notes
Health teaching complete	x	95	94	None	See diabetic teaching sheet and nurse's notes
Referrals made	x	95	94	None	See nurse's notes for referrals to appropriate community agencies

Complications*	Standard			Critical nursing management	Health education	Special instructions for data retrieval
	Expected %	Actual %	0%			
Dehydration	8	4	x	Observe, record, and report presence of thirst, flushed dry skin, skin turgor, dry coated tongue, atonic muscles, elevated blood urea nitrogen, or dyspepsia	Instruct family that only fluids taken are recorded; any fluids they give are to be put on intake—output record	See nurse's notes for description of increased thirst, flushed dry skin, decreased skin turgor, dry coated tongue, atonic muscles, anorexia, or dyspepsia
				Maintain intake and output record; schedule oral fluids, taken from 7 a.m. to 12 p.m.; 950 ml between 5 p.m. to 10 p.m. or so that 2,800 ml are taken in within 24 hours	Instruct family about the importance of a fluid intake 2, 800 ml per 24 hours	Schedule fluid oral intake to reach 2,800 ml per 24 hours. Instruct family to record fluids taken on the intake record
				Encourage intake of fluids easily tolerated—tea, jello, ice cream, carbonated beverages, bland juices, soups, and milk—at times in above schedule		Maintain intake and output record for intake of at least 2, 800 ml per 24 hours. Identify on dietary sheet patient's preference for fluids, such as ice cream rather than bland juices
				If an antiemtic has been prescribed, give it ½ hour before breakfast, lunch, supper, and late snack, if not contraindicated		Check laboratory report for increase in blood urea nitrogen
				If nothing by mouth ordered and on parental fluids, maintain rate of infusion per order amount per 24-hour period per order. Should infusion rate get behind, increase rate of flow by no more than 50-75 ml per hour until caught up		Compare doctor's orders for parental fluids with intravenous infusion record for accuracy in administration

*Additional complications would also be listed here; see p. 123, Diabetes mellitus, juvenile, complications.

2. To assure that nursing services are acceptable in quality
3. To assure that nursing care organizations and administrations support the timely provision of quality care

General characteristics of NCE studies

1. NCE studies are specifically designed, in-depth studies focusing particularly on potential problem areas.
2. They are usually of short duration.
3. They may be performed by a single institution, by a group of institutions in a coordinated effort, or by the Professional Standards Review Organizations.
4. Concurrently, they deal, for the most part, with identification of deficiencies in nursing care that can be corrected to enhance the desired outcome of a patient.
5. Retrospectively, they do not deal, for the most part, with an individual patient or practitioner but will require information related to the care provided by a number of practitioners to a number of patients.
6. They constitute an important link in continuing professional nursing education; the results of NCE studies should be used by the nursing organizations or the Professional Standards Review Organizations in directing the development of curriculum for and in monitoring the effectiveness of its continuing education efforts.
7. The results of NCE studies can be used to monitor the effectiveness of nursing quality assurance systems and to identify areas (such as diagnosis, problems, or nursing units) where additional review should be instituted or intensified.
8. The results of NCE studies will often identify needed changes in the organization and administra-

tion of nursing care delivery; when such is the case, the nursing organization should provide this information to those responsible for making such changes and help to assure that necessary action is taken.
9. Data necessary for NCE studies may be collected either concurrently or retrospectively by medical records personnel and by the review coordinators; analysis of the data is done retrospectively.
10. Where review of care is provided by nonphysician health care practitioners, the appropriate non-physician health care practitioners should participate in the NCE studies process.

Critical requirements of an NCE study

1. Objective criteria against which the actual performance is measured must be established.
2. For efficient and effective use of the professional nurse's time, nonnursing personnel should be appropriately utilized for time-consuming tasks that do not require clinical judgments.
3. There must be full documentation and recording of the topic, methodology, and results of the NCE study.
4. The clinical criteria and standards must be ratified by the nursing staff for clinical soundness and acceptance.
5. The criteria must be flexible to prevent stifling individual initiative and clinical advancement.
6. The NCE study must lead to a logical course of action, suited to any needs identified through the study.

Criteria, standards, and norms for NCE studies

1. Nursing care evaluation studies vary widely in their application and

reflect ratification of local criteria, standards, and norms.
2. Criteria, standards, and norms relate directly to the topic and objective of the study.

Data needs for NCE studies

The data needed to conduct NCE studies will vary depending on the nature of the study. Data will relate directly to the problem under study and to the criteria that have been developed.

General format for performing an NCE study

The following are the major steps for performing an NCE study (Fig. 1):
1. Identify the study topic.
2. Design the study, including setting objectives and developing draft criteria.
3. Ratify the criteria.
4. Perform data retrieval and display.
5. Analyze the results.
6. Analyze identified problem(s).
7. Develop corrective action.
8. Implement corrective action.
9. Evaluate corrective action.

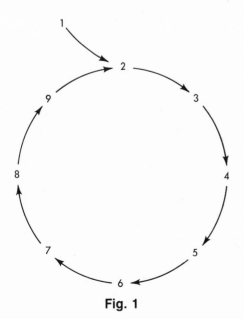

Fig. 1

Description of individual elements of an NCE study

I. Identifying study topic
  A. Resources that may yield topics
    1. Need perceived by NCE committee
    2. Findings from concurrent review component
    3. Suggestions resulting from other NCE studies
    4. Profile analysis
    5. Prearranged plan
    6. Recommendations from other sources
  B. Conditions that should be satisfied by topic selection
    1. High frequency (commonly seen in local area or institution)
    2. Severe problem in absence of nursing intervention
    3. Amenable to proper nursing intervention
    4. Generally noncontroversial (idea of NCE is to check application of previously verified practices to individual care setting, not to carry out basic clinical research)
  C. Areas that may be included
    1. Clinical topics
      a. Related to diagnosis
        (1) Outcome or results of nursing care
        (2) Validity or accuracy of nursing process
        (3) Quality of services (nursing management process)
      b. Related to nursing problems
        (1) Nursing priorities
        (2) Nursing interventions
        (3) Nursing prescriptions
      c. Related to nursing procedure
      d. Related to a therapeutic measure (vital signs monitoring, nursing observations)

e. Related to a social-psychological problem
f. Other nonclinical topics
(1) Administrative
(2) Housekeeping and related areas
II. Designing study, including development of draft criteria
A. Objectives set for the NCE study (see NCE study format below)
B. Parameters established to clearly define population for which criteria are being established
1. Age
2. Gender
3. Inclusions
4. Exclusions
5. Population, sample size, time period
6. Method to select the data source
C. Criteria selected
1. Setting of criteria
a. NCE committees
(1) Nursing specialty groups
(2) Interdisciplinary

NURSING CARE EVALUATION: Study format

I. Topic: _____ HICDA codes: _____
_____ _____

II. Objective of the study: _____
_____

III. Patient population: _____
_____

IV. Include: _____
_____

V. Exclude: _____
_____

VI. Study size and type of sample: _____
_____

VII. Study period: _____
_____

Criteria	Standards		
	% Screen	% Expected	% Actual

groups (such as M.D.,
R.N., O.T., or P.T.)
b. Hospitals, its committee
or department
c. Professional Standards
Review Organizations (local or other)
2. Included in criteria
a. Outcomes (end results of
nursing care in terms of
health satisfaction)
b. Processes (activities of
nursing care professionals
in the management of patients)
c. Structure (settings and instrumentalities available
and used for provision of
care)
d. Concurrent records (nursing criteria for open chart
evaluation of care provided concurrently)
3. Qualities of criteria
a. Explicit (capable of being
written down as opposed
to being implicit and subjective)
b. Critical (specific and
highly correlated with
good care)
c. Directly related to NCE
study objective
d. Concise (a few—4 to 8—
key elements for each
NCE format area)
e. Clear and specific enough
to be abstractable without
being subject to individual interpretation
D. Expected, acceptable performance levels (standards) established in terms of percentage,
that are thresholds for action
E. Commitment to taking action to
correct the deficiency made, if
the actual performance level for
a criterion falls below that
which is expected
III. Ratifying criteria and standards

A. Ratification by all nurses whose
performances are part of the
concurrent or retrospective review of care
B. Opportunity of each provider to
concur or amend
C. Purposes of ratification
1. To obtain a commitment to
acknowledge the existence of
a problem when presented
with data and to support its
solution
2. To obtain better ideas
3. To clarify any unnoticed ambiguities in criteria
4. To identify educational
needs
5. To be open and fair and to
avoid using unfamiliar or
unaccepted criteria and standards
IV. Performing data retrieval and display
A. Selection of data abstracting
method (see study abstract
sheet, p. 24)
B. Application of ratified criteria
(those criteria agreed upon by
providers whose performance
will be included in the NCE
study) to data source
C. Sources of data
1. Medical records
2. Nursing care plans
3. Others
D. Data retrieval by
1. Review coordinator (for concurrent review)
2. Medical records staff (for
concurrent or retrospective
review)
3. Other persons
E. Review, tabulation, and display
of data
V. Analyzing results
A. Comparing expected to actual
compliance percentages
B. Identifying areas of performance discrepancy—any NCE
study result that does not match

NURSING CARE EVALUATION STUDY ABSTRACT SHEET

Topic _____ Date _____

Committee _____ Abstractor _____

CODE:
1 = Yes
2 = No
3 = Not Recorded
4 = Not Applicable

Case No.	1	2	3	4	5	6	7	8	9	10	11	12	13	14	15
% of 1															
% of 2															
% of 3															
% of 4															

the expected performance level standard

C. Defining problems—those performance discrepancies that are identified as significant performance deficiencies—as any performance discrepancy that *can-*

not be explained by questions such as the following:

1. Were uncontrolled variables operating causing the performance to look worse than it really was?

2. Were there defects in the

COST RECORD

NCE topic_____

Department_____

Date completed____/____/____

Tasks—by person-hours	Director of nursing	Director of medical education	Medical records	Nursing secretary	Physician	Nursing	O.T.	P.T.	Respiratory therapy	Dietary	Computer time	Other	TOTAL person-hours	TOTAL cost
Notify about meeting														
Select audit topic														
Brainstorm criteria														
Set criteria														
Ratify/revise criteria														
Type criteria														
Develop code sheet														
Conduct pilot audit														
Conduct audit/reaudit (circle one)														
Pull sample/pull charts														
Apply criteria (abstracting)														
Set up for keypunching														
Keypunch														
Send to computer—machine operator														
Analyze														
Compile statistics														
Pull charts not complying to study														
Prepare display of material														
Present to audit committee														
Analyze problems														
Revise data														
Design remedial action/education program														
Pull charts for review														
Prepare data for department														
Present to department														
Prepare tickler file														
Draft minutes														
Draft summary of study														
Duplicate materials														
Other:														
TOTAL														

criterion—that is, it was not measurable or clear enough to allow for reliable extraction?

3. Were there major developments in the body of nursing knowledge causing a criterion formerly considered to be valid to be no longer considered so?

4. Was the expected performance level unrealistic given the institution's capabilities, and will lowering the performance level not in any way interfere with desirable nursing outcomes?

D. Analyzing study design for effectiveness and efficiency, including costs (see cost record, p. 25)

E. Presenting data and analysis to appropriate institution committees and departments

VI. Analyzing problems

A. Role of the NCE study committee

1. Developing a list of possible explanations for each performance deficiency by denoting which nursing care areas may be involved in inadequate performances

2. Deciding what additional data may be needed to substantiate whether or not these possible explanations for the performance deficiency are truly good explanations

3. Determining how to go about collecting the additional data

4. Presenting the data and problem analysis to appropriate Professional Standards Review Organization Committee, institution committee, and departments for discussion

VII. Taking corrective action by

A. Developing a series of *corrective objectives* that *describe* the type of performance and/or systems changes needed to correct the performance deficiency

B. Generating several remedial strategies for achieving the corrective objectives

C. Evaluating strategies by questioning

1. Is this strategy the *simplest* to implement?

2. Is this strategy likely to achieve the results the *fastest*?

3. Is this strategy relatively *inexpensive* to mount?

4. Is this strategy the *most effective* for achieving long-term results?

D. Establishing problem-specific corrective actions

1. Continuing education

2. Counseling

3. Nursing staff and institutional policy changes

4. Administrative changes

5. Reallocation of resources

6. Modification of focus of concurrent review

7. Intervention

8. Others appropriate to given problems

VIII. Implementing the corrective action

A. Should be based on the problem and corrective analysis

B. Should be documented (see Procedural checklist for audit studies, p. 27, and NCE study summary, p. 28)

1. When was action implemented?

2. How was it monitored and by whom?

3. When are results of the corrective action to be evaluated?

4. When are results to be reported to committee?

IX. Evaluating corrective action
   A. Monitoring and evaluating at an appropriate time to determine if the remedial action program achieved its objective (the type of performance needed to correct the performance deficiency), thereby improving the quality of care
      1. Reaudit of the problem at a predetermined time after implementation of the corrective strategy
      2. Concurrent review using statistical techniques, such as sequential analysis or probability curves, for each criterion
X. Establishing a profile for analysis
   A. Analysis of audit results as compared to other institutions
   B. Identification of patterns across several different audit topics
   C. Interface with PSRO profiles of institution, practitioner, local area, and nation.

PROCEDURAL CHECKLIST FOR AUDIT STUDIES

Study name _____

Assigned to _____

_____ Nursing audit committee _____

_____ Initial criteria developed: ___/___/___   Typed: ___/___/___

_____ Criteria developed: ___/___/___   Typed: ___/___/___

_____ Criteria ratified by audit committee: ___/___/___

_____ Abstract form developed: ___/___/___   Typed: ___/___/___

_____ Abstract form printed: ___/___/___

_____ Sent for keypunching: ___/___/___   Return: ___/___/___

_____ Data sent to computer center: ___/___/___

          Special instruction: _____
          _____

_____ Printouts received back: ___/___/___

_____ Data display given to MSS: ___/___/___

_____ Data presented to audit committee: ___/___/___

_____ Recommendations made: ___/___/___

_____ Data presented to department or subsection: ___/___/___

_____ Recommendations made: ___/___/___

_____ Study complete: ___/___/___

_____ Study to be redone: ___/___/___

_____ Revised concurrent review criteria forwarded to U.R.
          coordinator: ___/___/___

Recommendations—nursing audit committee _____
_____
_____

Recommendations—department or subsection _____
_____
_____

NURSING CARE EVALUATION STUDY SUMMARY

Nursing care evaluation study topic _____ **Date** _____

Summary of study and findings

Comments and recommendations	Action and responsibility

Signatures: _____   Date: _____
Nursing audit committee chairman

_____   _____
Nursing supervisor

_____   _____
Quality of patient care committee chairman

_____   _____
Director of nursing

_____   _____
Administrator

_____   _____
Governing board president

Application of concurrent or retrospective review

The ten steps described in the individual elements of the NCE study apply whether a concurrent or retrospective review is desired. Hopefully, during critera-setting sessions, both concurrent and retrospective criteria will be developed for a given topic.

Other forms for use with NCE

Many different groups are providing different types of forms to be used with audit procedures. An institution should adopt a form that reflects effectiveness and ease of implementation. If a nursing group experiences difficulty in applying forms, then they should modify or design a form appropriate to their needs. The forms available from the JCAH are included in Appendix.

Model criteria sets

The model criteria sets presented in this book should be used by local nursing groups to assist in the development, modification, and ratification of criteria for concurrent and retrospective review of nursing care.

PSRO INTERFACE

Professional nurses on the local level must develop an understanding of the components of the Professional Standards Review Organizations and design a methodology for nursing's inclusion in PSROs. The following activities should be initiated by the professional nursing group:

1. Educate all nurses within the state about the PSRO and utilize the PSRO staff for technical support in providing educational programs.
2. Seek implementation of a regulation by the Department of Health, Education, and Welfare that states that only professional nurses will be eligible to vote on issues relating to the practice of nursing, including all final determinations on reconsideration of adverse determinations rendered on the practice of nursing or resulting from a nursing care evaluation study.
3. Utilize the model criteria sets to develop and adapt criteria, standards, and norms appropriate for the local area and acceptable to the profession of nursing.
4. Accept and adopt NCE concurrent and retrospective review mechanisms for peer assessment of performance within the PSRO area.
5. Implement a mechanism to assure that the results of nursing care evaluation studies will be connected to continuing nursing education programs.
6. Conduct nursing care evaluation studies according to PSRO numerical guidelines.
7. Select nurses to represent the profession on PSRO advisory groups.
8. Complete a working document, which explains the criteria, standards, norms, nursing peer review mechanism, and key elements for nursing profile analysis, that is acceptable to the profession of nursing within the local area. This working document would be presented to the PSRO board of directors through the advisory group.
9. Insist that the PSRO obtain budget support for implementation of the nursing peer review mechanism under the PSRO program. A timetable for implementation should be developed in concert with the PSRO staff.
10. Do not accept "no" for an answer when requesting participation in the PSRO program. Frequently it is the squeaky wheel that receives attention; therefore, let the local nursing groups apply the pressure for participation.

The PSROs are accountable in their contracts with the Department of Health,

Education, and Welfare to show that nonphysician health care practitioners are developing standards, criteria, norms, peer review mechanisms, continuing education programs, and profile analysis. Since some type of activity must be implemented to comply with the contract items, the local nursing groups should initiate a program to define the direction, select the path, design the vehicle, and apply for fuel allocations (money) from the PSRO before rigid time frames are set and the possibility of federal control over quality assurance in the nursing profession is realized.

REFERENCES

1. Bennis, Warren G., Benne, Kenneth D., and Chris, Robert, editors: The planning of change, ed. 2, New York, 1969, Holt, Rinehart and Winston, Inc.
2. Brown, Clement R., and Uhl, Henry S. M.: Mandatory continuing education, sense or nonsense? J.A.M.A. 213(10):1660-1668, Sept. 7, 1970.
3. California Medical Association/California Hospital Association: Educational Patient Care Audit Program materials.
4. Cochran, William G.: Sampling techniques, ed. 2, New York, 1963, John Wiley and Sons, Inc.
5. Davidson, Sharon V., editor: PSRO: utilization and audit in patient care, St. Louis, 1976, The C. V. Mosby Co.
6. Dixon, Wilfrid J., and Massey, Frank J., Jr.: Introduction to statistical analysis, 1969, McGraw-Hill Book Co., pp. 362-374.
7. Havelock, Ronald G.: The change agent's guide to innovation in education, Englewood Cliffs, N.J., 1973, Educational Technology Publications.
8. Mager, Robert F., and Pipe, Peter: Analyzing performance problems or "You really oughta wanna," Belmont, Calif., 1970, Fearon Publishers.
9. Miller, George E., M.D.: Continuing education for what? J. Med. Educ. 42:320-326, Apr. 1967.
10. Quality assurance of medical care, monograph, Regional Medical Programs Service, Health Services and Mental Health Administration, Washington, D.C., Feb. 1973, U.S. Department of Health, Education, and Welfare.
11. Williamson, John W., Alexander, Marshal, and Miller, George E.: Priorities in patient-care research and continuing medical education, J.A.M.A. 204(4):93-98, Apr. 22, 1968.

Model concurrent and retrospective criteria

Abdomen, surgical conditions, group

Abdominal pain, etiology unknown, with exploratory celiotomy (Code: 780)
Abdominal trauma, with surgical intervention (Code: 863)
Appendectomy (Codes: 540, 540.1, 542, 543)
Cholecystitis resulting in cholecystectomy (Codes: 475, 574, 575, 575.1, 576-576.5, 576.9)

CONCURRENT REVIEW CRITERIA
Identification of patient's physical and psychosocial needs and/or concerns

Relief of symptoms and control of pain

Understanding of surgical procedure and the expected preoperative and postoperative course, emotional support for surgical invasion of body, and alleviation of fear about pain of unknown origin (for abdominal pain, etiology unknown with exploratory celiotomy)

Maintenance of physiological responses including blood pressure, respiration, temperature, adequate intake and output, and electrolyte balance

Prevention of postoperative complications, including respiratory, wound, urinary, and intestinal

Acceptance of low-fat diet restriction (for cholecystectomy)

Recommended nursing action consistent with diagnosis
Nursing services

Provide preoperative and postoperative information and reassurance

Relieve pain through medication, positioning, and other measures

Monitor and assess physiological responses; report to the physician any deviations from normal physiological response parameters and initiate treatment

Assist with turning, coughing, and deep breathing every 2 to 4 hours for 48 hours and as needed

Inspect the wound and dressing for signs of hemorrhage, infection, drainage, and dehiscence and change dressing as needed to promote wound healing

Health education

Instruct patient on technique of coughing and deep breathing and impress on patient the rationale for this; reinforce postoperatively

Instruct patient in the need for early self-care, ambulation, and regaining of independence

Discuss condition, course, prognosis, and limitations (if any)

Teach patient the importance of avoiding constipation through diet, laxatives, stool softeners

Indicators for discharge
Adaptation to health status

Independence reestablished in activities of daily living

Normal physiological responses reestablished including tolerating discharge diet for 2 to 3 days

Wound healed

Examples of community resources

Referral usually not indicated

RETROSPECTIVE CRITERIA
Health

Normal physiological responses reestablished

Wound healed

Pain controlled

Activity

Independence exhibited in ambulation and in activities of daily living

Knowledge

Understands wound care

Understands activity and/or diet restrictions

Understands importance of avoiding constipation

COMPLICATIONS

Acute peritonitis
Adhesions
Intestinal obstruction

Intra-abdominal sepsis
Pancreatitis
Postoperative intestinal obstruction
Respiratory infection (pneumonia)
Thrombophlebitis
Wound infection

Abscess of anal and rectal regions (Codes: 566, 590.2)

CONCURRENT CRITERIA
**Identification of patient's physical and
psychosocial needs and/or concerns**

Relief of acute pain during and after
defecation, spotting of bright red blood
at stool, constipation, spasm of anal
canal, and infection
Understanding of surgical procedure,
expected preoperative and postoperative course, medical and nursing management, and duration of hospitalization
Fear of surgical invasion of body and,
possibly, of inflammatory bowel disease
Prevention of constipation and/or diffi-
cult bowel movements

**Recommended nursing action consistent
with diagnosis**
Nursing services

Control pain and relieve fears
Initiate preoperative nursing care, including nutrition, elimination, and hydration, and preparation of patient for
surgery
Explain surgical procedure, recovery
room, postoperative chest physiology,
and sitz bath procedures
Implement postoperative nursing care,
including assessment of physiological
response parameters and vital signs,
prevention of complications, hot sitz
baths to hasten process of localization,
and stool softeners; give adjustment to
surgical invasion of body; teach and
wound care

Health education

Instruct about treatment and medications,
including frequency, duration, and
effects to report to physician
Instruct about nutrition and fluid to
prevent constipation
Explain disease process, course, treatment, medical and nursing management, and expected outcome

Indicators for discharge
Adaptation to health status

Soft bowel movements reestablished
Wound healing
Acute pain during and after defecation
relieved or controlled
Complications not evident
Health education completed

Examples of community resources

Referral usually not indicated

RETROSPECTIVE CRITERIA
Health

Abscess surgically removed
Normal physiological responses reestab-
lished, including bowel movements
Complications not evident
Wound healing
Acute pain during and after defecation
reduced or controlled

Activity

Ambulatory
Independent in activities of daily living
Performing own sitz baths and dressing
changes, if indicated

34

Knowledge

Understands and can verbalize disease process, treatment, medication instructions, nutrition and fluid instructions, and symptoms to report to physician

COMPLICATIONS

Fecal impaction
Persistent fistula
Postoperative hemorrhage
Sepsis
Urinary retention and/or infection

Abscess, brain (Code: 322)

CONCURRENT CRITERIA
Identification of patient's physical and psychosocial needs and/or concerns

Relief from symptoms, including visual field defects, motor and sensory changes, aphasia, headache, rigidity of neck, or increased intracranial pressure

Explanation of infectious process, including cause as related to primary infections such as otitis media, mastoiditis, sinusitis, or infected head injuries; course; prognosis; and outcome in terms of possible hemiparesis, seizures, visual defects, or learning problems (in a child)

Patient/family understanding of the diagnostic and therapeutic medical and surgical procedures, including purpose, preparation, outcome, special care units (if indicated), special aftercare, isolation, bed rest, and antibiotic therapy

Patient/family understanding of medical management, including isolation, bed rest, and antibiotic therapy

Patient/family awareness of community agencies available to assist in case of residual neurological deficits

Fear of death, contagion, increased dependency, change in body image

Recommended nursing action consistent with diagnosis
Nursing services

Closely observe for signs and symptoms of increased intracranial pressure and desired and side effects of drug therapy; administer prompt nursing intervention should side effects or increased intracranial pressure occur

Establish safety measures to prevent injury resulting from restlessness, disorientation, impaired judgment, visual defects, or seizures

Maintain vital body functions, including adequate hydration, nutrition, elimination, respiration, and cardiovascular function

Implement measures to prevent complications, such as contractures, pneumonia, circulatory stasis, impactions, or decubitus ulcers, caused by immobility or bed rest

Isolate patient and provide comfort measures to reduce severity of anxiety, pain, or visual impairment

Health education

Educate patient/family about prompt medical attention of primary infections and avoidance of infections

Educate patient/family concerning isolation techniques, purpose, duration, and methods of maintenance

Provide patient/family preoperative and postoperative teaching, including explanation of procedure, special care units (if any), dressings, intravenous equipment, turning, coughing, positioning, comfort measures, and the like

Provide patient/family teaching concerning rehabilitation measures should residual neurological deficits occur, including bladder and bowel control, measures, techniques for minimizing speech difficulties, range of motion exercises, transfer techniques, good nutrition and hydration principles and methods, skin care procedures, positioning, alignment, use of supportive devices and equipment, epileptic care, and medications

Teach patient/family concerning community agencies available for assisting with care after discharge

Indicators for discharge
Adaptation to health status

Afebrile

Maximal improvement after medical and/or surgical therapy

Understanding by patient/family of care necessary for home care of convalescence

Referral agencies contacted for follow-up care

Examples of community resources

Visiting Nurse Association or public health nurse

Social services for financial assistance or other appropriate referrals

Speech, physical, or vocational rehabilitation centers

Public school (school nurse to survey health status of child, teacher for guidance when learning disability may be present, or referral to an exceptional child center)

Medical, surgical, or epileptic clinics

Vocational rehabilitation center

RETROSPECTIVE CRITERIA
Health

Afebrile

Neurological deficits diminishing

Abscess resolving, wound healing, coping with fears

Activity

Able to carry out activities of daily living with little or no assistance

Knowledge

Family understands importance of prompt medical attention to eye, ear, nose, and throat infections

Family understands rehabilitiative care necessary for home management of patient with residual neurological deficits

Patient/family understands care as related to the epileptic individual, including medications, safety precautions, measures of decreasing occurrence, and legal implications

Patient/family are aware and understand function of community agencies that can appropriately help after discharge

COMPLICATIONS

Chemotherapy complications
Contractures
Decubitus ulcers
Drug reaction
Intracranial pressure increased
Neurological deficits
Persistent fever
Pneumonia
Wound infection

Alcoholism (Codes: 303, 303.1, 303.2)

CONCURRENT CRITERIA
Identification of patient's physical and psychosocial needs and/or concerns

Total and permanent abstinence from alcohol intake

Relief from repetitive or chronic use of alcohol in any form to solve personal problems; emotional difficulties such as depression, insecurity, feelings of inadequacy, or the need for control over others

Identification of continuing problems

related to use of alcohol, such as economic, social, family relationships, physical well-being, or self-deprecation

Determination of physical health status, such as personal hygiene, nutritional status, and mental status

Expression of attitude regarding hospitalization and concern regarding family, job, and others

Counseling or psychotherapy for patient and spouse

Recommended nursing action consistent with diagnosis
Nursing services

Observe closely for symptoms of withdrawal; use medications, as required, to manage symptoms

Provide for improvement/maintenance of health status, including hygiene, nutrition, and fluids

Observe patient for continued alcohol intake or drug abuse

Give emotional support; motivate continued abstinence

Make recommendations for treatment plan

Health education

Inform patient and significant others of treatment plan and realistic expectations of that plan

Teach patient and significant others of the physical effects of alcoholism

Indicators for discharge
Adaptation to health status

Achievement of inpatient treatment goals

Establishment of follow-up treatment

plan that is understood by patient and significant others

Examples of community resources

Alcoholics Anonymous
Alanon
Alateen
Community half-way house

RETROSPECTIVE CRITERIA
Health

Withdrawal from alcohol dependency
Nutritional state improved
Mentally accepting necessity of abstaining from alcohol ingestion
Complications not evident

Activity

Ambulatory
Abstaining from alcohol intake

Knowledge

Patient verbalizes understanding of instructions for taking of medications, signs and symptoms of untoward reactions, and the need to report these to the physician

Patient verbalizes a positive attitude toward abstinence

COMPLICATIONS

Acute alcohol hallucinations
Anxiety and guilt feelings
Cirrhosis of liver
Continued drinking during hospitalization
Convulsive state
Delirium tremens or withdrawal seizures
Drug reaction
Malnutrition
Trauma

Amputation of foot and ankle, acquired (Code: Y56.6)

CONCURRENT CRITERIA
Identification of patient's physical and psychosocial needs and/or concerns

Relief from symptoms such as pain, infection, circulatory impairment, or deformity

Understanding of surgical treatment as well as nursing management, so that realistic plans for health maintenance can be made for after discharge

Preventive measures as related to problems caused by immobility

Rehabilitative measures to regain ambulatory status

Concern or grief over change in body image

Recommended nursing action consistent with diagnosis
Nursing services

Implement preoperative care and teaching, including pain-reducing measures, such as measures to provide adequate hydration, nutrition, and elimination; explain operative procedure, possibility of phantom limb discomfort, possibility of using a prosthesis, recovery room, expected duration of hospitalization, and expected graduated steps to ambulation; teach through demonstration, explanation, and return demonstration by the patient of muscle-strengthening exercises of arms in preparation for crutch walking, such as push-ups from prone position, weight flexion and extension exercises of arms, sit-ups, and crutch walking, as well as quadriceps and gluteal setting, and leg lift exercises when not contraindicated; instruct in deep-breathing and coughing exercise and the need for frequent turning; explain the possible use of traction or a rigid plaster dressing with IPSF; assist the patient in coping with changes in body image; prepare patient physically for surgery

Implement postoperative nursing care, including observation for signs and symptoms of complications with prompt nursing intervention should any occur; maintain traction properly, if used; prevent contracture by use of proper positioning and alignment as well as by the use of supportive devices; control bleeding; prevent wound infection and problems resulting from immobility

Implement rehabilitation measures, including bed exercises consisting of push-ups from the prone position, active range of motion exercises, partial sit-ups and standing exercises consisting of stationary hopping, hopping with advancement with and without a walker, balancing, standing, with knee flexion exercises, and crutch walking; facilitate stump healing conducive to the use of a prosthetic device; assist the patient in the proper use of crutches or prosthesis

Initiate health teaching and appropriate referrals

Health education

Instruct patient as to name, purpose, frequency, dosage, side effects, action to take if side effects occur, and precautions regarding all discharge medications

Instruct patient on stump care, as to daily hygiene of stump, including massage of suture line, application of Ace bandages, signs and symptoms of infection, and actions to take should such signs appear

Instruct patient on proper care and use of prosthesis

Instruct patient on therapeutic and restricted activities

Instruct patient when and why it is necessary to return to the physicians' office or clinic for follow-up medical care

Indicators for discharge
Adaptation to health status

Wound healing
Pain controlled
Complications not evident
Health teaching completed
Referrals made

Examples of community resources

Visiting Nurse Association or public
health nurse
Orthopedic clinic
Physical and vocational rehabilitation
Social services

RETROSPECTIVE CRITERIA
Health

Symptoms relieved or controlled
Wound healing
Mentally accepting loss of body part and
change in body image
Complications not evident

Activity

Ambulatory
Able to apply and use prosthesis prop-
erly
Able to use crutches correctly and safely
Able to implement exercise program and
stump care

Knowledge

Knows the name of each discharge medication and understands the purpose,
dosage, frequency, side effects, action
to take if side effects occur, and precautions for each drug
Understands therapeutic and restricted
activities and can implement therapeutic ones
Understands and can implement stump
care
Understands and can implement proper
use and care of prosthesis
Understands when and why it is necessary to return to physician's office or
clinic for follow-up medical care

COMPLICATIONS

Circulatory impairment
Contracture of joint
Difficulty in breathing
Drug reaction
Hemorrhage
Malpositioning, drainage, infection, or
circulatory impairment from rigid plas-
ter dressing and IPSF
Mental depression
Phantom pain sensation
Pneumonia
Pulmonary embolism
Shock
Tissue necrosis
Wound infection

Amputation of foot and ankle, traumatic (Codes: 896, 896.1, 896.9)

CONCURRENT CRITERIA
Identification of patient's physical and
psychosocial needs and/or concerns

Relief from hemorrhage, shock, infection,
and pain
Maintenance of vital body functions
Understanding of surgical treatment as
well as nursing management, so that
realistic plans for health maintenance
can be made for after discharge
Concern over change in body image
Preventive measures concerning problems due to immobility

Recommended nursing action consistent
with diagnosis
Nursing services

Implement measures to interrupt life-
threatening, traumatic process, including pain-reducing measures; maintain
adequate ventilation and adequate cardiovascular functioning, such as control of bleeding, maintenance of arterial
pressure, replacement of lost fluid, and
administration of appropriate cardiotonics and vasopressors as ordered;
implement measures to reduce the

effects of fluid loss, such as conservation of body heat and proper positioning; observe closely for the effects of measures taken as well as for signs of physical deterioration by frequent monitoring of sensorium, pupils, pulse rate and character, blood pressure (including pulse pressure), hourly urinary output, and the presence and quality of the peripheral pulse; administer appropriate antibiotics as ordered; physically prepare patient for surgery

Implement postoperative nursing care, including observation for signs and symptoms of complications with prompt nursing intervention should any signs occur; maintain traction properly, if used, and prevent contractures by use of proper positioning and alignment as well as the use of supportive devices; control bleeding; prevent infection of the wound; implement pain-reducing measures; provide adequate hydration, nutrition, and elimination; assist the patient through the grief process of change in body image; prevent problems resulting from immobility

Implement rehabilitative measures, including bed exercises consisting of push-ups from the prone position, active range of motion exercises, partial sit-ups, standing and stationary hopping, hopping with advancement with or without a walker, and standing, flexing the knees and balancing on one leg, and crutchwalking; facilitate stump healing conducive to the use of a prosthesis by application of Ace bandages to promote shrinkage, stump exercises, and stump massage; assist the patient in proper use of crutches or prosthesis

Initiate appropriate referrals

Health education

Instruct as to name, purpose, dosage, frequency, side effects, action to take if side effects occur, and precautions relating to all discharge medications

Instruct on stump care, as to daily hygiene of stump, daily massage of suture line, application of Ace bandages, signs and symptoms of infection, and action to take should any signs of infection or other problems, such as shrinkage, occur

Instruct on proper use and care of prosthesis

Instruct as to therapeutic and restricted activities

Instruct as to when and why it is necessary for the patient to return to the physician's office or clinic for follow-up medical care

Indicators for discharge
Adaptation to health status

Condition stable
Wound healing
Complications not evident
Health teaching completed
Referrals made

Examples of community resources

Visiting Nurse Association or public health nurse
Orthopedic clinic
Physical and vocational rehabilitation center
Social services

RETROSPECTIVE CRITERIA
Health

Wound healing
Mentally accepting changes in body image
Complications not evident

Activity

Ambulatory
Able to apply and use prosthesis properly
Able to use crutches properly
Implements stump care and exercise program

Knowledge

Knows the name of each discharge medication and understands the purpose, dosage, frequency, side effects, action to take if side effects occur, and precautions for each drug

Understands and can implement stump care

Understands therapeutic and restricted activities and can implement therapeutic ones

Understands and can implement proper use and care of prosthesis

Understands when and why it is necessary to return to physician's office or clinic for follow-up medical care

COMPLICATIONS
Circulatory impairment
Contractures of joint

Difficulty in breathing
Drug reaction
Hemorrhage
Malpositioning, drainage, infection, or circulatory impairment from rigid plaster dressing and IPSF
Mental depression
Phantom pain sensation
Pneumonia
Pulmonary embolism
Shock
Tissue necrosis
Wound infection

Amputation of leg above knee, traumatic (Code: 897.1)

CONCURRENT CRITERIA
Identification of patient's physical and psychosocial needs and/or concerns

Relief from hemorrhage, shock, pain, or infection

Maintenance of vital body functions

Understanding of surgical treatment as well as nursing management, so that realistic plans for health maintenance can be made

Concern or grief over change in body image and life-style

Preventive measures relating to problems resulting from immobility

Recommended nursing action consistent with diagnosis
Nursing services

Implement measures to interrupt life-threatening situations, including pain-reducing measures; maintain adequate ventilation; maintain adequate cardiovascular functioning, such as control of bleeding, maintenance of arterial pressure, replacement of fluid loss, administration of appropriate cardiotonics and vasopressors as ordered; implement measures to reduce effects of fluid loss, such as conservation of body heat and proper positioning; observe closely for effects of measures taken as well as for signs of physical deterioration through frequent monitoring of sensorium, pupils, pulse rate and character, blood pressure (including pulse pressure), hourly urinary output, and the presence and quality of peripheral pulse; administer appropriate antibiotics as ordered; and prepare patient physically for surgical treatment

Implement postoperative nursing care, including observation for signs and symptoms of complications, with prompt nursing intervention should any occur; maintain traction properly, if used, and prevent contractures by use of proper positioning and alignment as well as the use of supportive devices, such as a trochanter roll; control bleeding; prevent infection of wound; reduce pain; provide adequate hydration, nutrition, and elimination; assist the patient through grief process of change in body image; prevent problems of immobility

Implement rehabilitative measures, including bed exercises consisting of push-ups from the prone position, active range of motion exercises, and partial sit-ups, and standing exercises consisting of hopping in stationary position, hopping with advancement with and without a walker, standing and flexing knee, balancing on one leg, and crutchwalking; implement measures to facilitate stump healing conducive to comfort, use of a prosthesis, and properly healed incision with such measures as application of Ace bandages to promote shrinkage, stump exercises to toughen the skin and muscles, and stump massage to promote circulation and healing; assist the patient in proper usage of crutches or prosthesis

Initiate appropriate referrals

Health education

Instruct on discharge medications, as to name, purpose, dosage, frequency, side effects, action to take if side effects occur, and precautions

Instruct on stump care, as to daily hygiene of stump, daily massage of suture line, application of Ace bandages, signs and symptoms of infection, and actions to take should any signs of infection or other problems, such as shrinkage, occur

Instruct on proper care and use of prosthesis

Instruct as to therapeutic and restricted activities

Instruct patient when and why it is necessary to return to the physician's office or clinic for follow-up medical care

Indicators for discharge
Adaptation to health status

Condition stable
Wound healing
Complications not evident
Health teaching completed
Referrals made

Examples of community resources

Visiting Nurse Association or public health nurse
Orthopedic clinic
Physical and possibly vocational rehabilitation centers
Social services

RETROSPECTIVE CRITERIA
Health

Relief of symptoms
Wound healing
Mentally accepting change in body image
Complications not evident

Activity

Ambulatory
Able to use crutches or walker properly and safely
Able to apply and use prosthesis correctly
Implements stump care and exercise program

Knowledge

Knows the name of each discharge medication and understands the purpose, dosage, frequency, precautions, side effects, and actions to take if side effects occur for each drug
Understands and can implement stump care
Understands and can implement proper care and use of prosthesis
Understands therapeutic and restricted activities and can implement therapeutic ones
Knows when and why it is necessary to return to the clinic for follow-up medical care

COMPLICATIONS

Abduction deformity
Circulatory impairment
Contractures of joint
Difficulty in breathing
Drug reaction
Hemorrhage
Malpositioning, drainage, infection, and

circulatory impairment from rigid plaster dressing and IPSF
Mental depression
Phantom pain
Pneumonia

Pulmonary embolism
Shock
Tissue necrosis
Wound infection

Amputation of leg, acquired (Code: Y56.8)

CONCURRENT CRITERIA
Identification of patient's physical and psychosocial needs and/or concerns

Relief from symptoms and disability, such as circulatory impairment, pain, and gangrene

Concern over change in body image and possibly life-style

Understanding of surgical treatment and nursing management, so that realistic plans for health maintenance can be made for after discharge

Preventive measures in regard to problems caused by immobility

Rehabilitative measures to regain ambulatory status

Recommended nursing action consistent with diagnosis
Nursing services

Implement preoperative care and teaching, including pain-reducing measures and adequate hydration, nutrition, and elimination; explain operative procedure, possibility of phantom limb discomfort, and the possibilities of using a prosthesis, recovery room, expected duration of hospitalization, and expected graduated steps to ambulation; teach through demonstration, explanation, and return demonstration by the patient of muscle-strengthening exercises of arms in preparation for crutch walking, such as push-ups from prone position, weight flexion and extension exercises of the arms, sit-ups, and crutch walking, as well as quadriceps and gluteal setting, and leg lift exercises when not contraindicated; instruct in deep-breathing and coughing exercises and the need for frequent turning; explain possible use of traction or plaster dressing with IPSF; assist the patient in coping with changes of body image; maintain proper traction, if traction is used; and physically prepare patient for surgery

Implement postoperative nursing care, including observation for signs and symptoms of complications with prompt nursing intervention should any signs occur; properly maintain traction, if used; prevent contractures by use of proper positioning and alignment as well as by the use of supportive devices such as a trochanter roll; implement measures to control bleeding, prevent excessive bleeding or wound infection; prevent problems resulting from immobility

Implement rehabilitation measures, including bed exercises consisting of push-ups from the prone position, active range of motion exercises, partial sit-ups and standing exercises consisting of stationary hopping, hopping with advancement with and without a walker, balancing, standing, with knee flexion exercises, and crutch walking; facilitate stump healing conducive to the use of a prosthetic device; assist the patient in the proper use of crutches or prosthesis

Initiate appropriate referrals

Health education

Instruct as to name, purpose, dosage, frequency, side effects, action to take if side effects occur, and precautions relating to all discharge medications

Instruct on stump care, as to daily hygiene of stump, daily massage of suture line, application of Ace bandages, signs and symptoms of infection, and action to take should any signs of infection or other problems, such as shrinkage, occur

Instruct on proper use and care of prosthesis

Instruct as to therapeutic and restricted activities

Instruct as to when and why it is necessary for the patient return to the physician's office or clinic for follow-up medical care

Indicators for discharge
Adaptation to health status

Condition stable
Wound healing
Complications not evident
Health teaching completed
Referrals made

Examples of community resources

Visiting Nurse Association or public health nurse
Orthopedic clinic
Physical and vocational rehabilitation centers
Social services

RETROSPECTIVE CRITERIA
Health

Relief from symptoms and disability
Wound healing
Mentally accepting change in body image
Complications not evident

Activity

Ambulatory
Able to apply and use prosthesis properly
Able to use crutches properly
Implements stump care and exercise program

Knowledge

Knows the name of discharge medications and understands the purpose, dosage, frequency, side effects, action to take if side effects occur, and precautions for each drug

Understands and can implement stump care

Understands therapeutic and restricted activities and can implement therapeutic ones

Understands and can implement proper use and care of prosthesis

Understands when and why it is necessary to return to physician's office or clinic for follow-up medical care

COMPLICATIONS

Circulatory impairment
Contractures of joint
Difficulty in breathing
Drug reaction
Hemorrhage
Malpositioning, drainage, infection, or circulatory impairment from rigid plastic dressing and IPSF
Mental depression
Phantom pain sensation
Pneumonia
Pulmonary embolism
Shock
Tissue necrosis
Wound infection

Amputation of leg below knee, acquired (Code: Y56.7)

CONCURRENT CRITERIA
Identification of patient's physical and psychosocial needs and/or concerns

Relief from symptoms such as pain, infection, circulatory impairment, or deformity

Concern over change in body image

Understanding of surgical treatment as well as nursing management, so that realistic plans for health maintenance can be made for after discharge

Preventive measures as related to problems caused by immobility

Rehabilitative measures to regain ambulatory status

Recommended nursing action consistent with diagnosis
Nursing services

Implement preoperative care and teaching, including pain-reducing measures and measures to provide adequate hydration, nutrition, and elimination; assist patient in coping with changes in body image; explain operative procedure, possibility of phantom limb discomfort, possibility of using a prosthesis, recovery room, expected duration of hospitalization, and expected graduated steps to ambulation; teach by demonstration, explanation, and return demonstration by the patient of muscle-strengthening exercises of the arms in preparation for crutch walking, such as push-up exercises from a prone position, weight flexion and extension exercises of the arms, sit-ups, and crutch walking, as well as quadriceps and gluteal setting and leg lift exercises when not contraindicated; instruct in deep-breathing and coughing exercises and the need for frequent turning; explain possible use of traction or a plaster dressing with IPSF; physically prepare patient for surgery

Implement postoperative nursing care to include observation for signs and symptoms of complications with prompt nursing intervention should any occur; implement measures to properly maintain traction, if used, and to prevent contractures by use of proper positioning and alignment as well as by the use of supportive devices; control bleeding; prevent wound infection; implement measures to prevent problems resulting from immobility

Implement rehabilitation measures including bed exercises consisting of push-ups from prone position, active range of motion exercises, partial sit-ups and standing exercises consisting of stationary hopping, hopping with advancement with and without a walker, and standing, flexing knees or balancing on one leg, and crutch walking; implement measures to facilitate stump healing conducive to comfort, use of prosthetic device, and properly healed incision, by application of Ace bandages to promote shrinkage; stump exercise to toughen the skin, and stump massage; implement measures to assist the patient in proper use of crutches or prosthesis

Initiate appropriate referrals

Health education

Instruct as to name, purpose, dosage, frequency, side effects, action to take if side effects occur, and precautions regarding all discharge medications

Instruct on stump care, as to daily hygiene of stump, including daily massage of suture line, application of Ace bandages, signs of infection, and actions to take should any signs of infection or other problems, such as shrinkage, occur

Instruct on proper care and use of prosthesis

Instruct on therapeutic and restricted activities

Instruct as to when and why it is necessary to return to the physician's office or clinic for follow-up medical care

Indicators for discharge
Adaptation to health status

Condition stable
Wound healing
Complications not evident
Health teaching completed
Referrals made

Examples of community resources

Visiting Nurse Association or public health nurse
Orthopedic clinics
Physical and vocational rehabilitation centers
Social services

RETROSPECTIVE CRITERIA
Health

Relief from symptoms
Wound healing
Mentally accepting change in body image
Complications not evident

Activity

Ambulatory
Able to use crutches or prosthesis correctly, if prescribed
Implements stump care and exercise program

Knowledge

Knows name of each discharge medication and understands purpose, dosage, frequency, side effects, action to take should side effects occur, and precautions for each drug
Understands and can implement stump care properly
Understands and can implement proper care and use of prosthesis
Understands both therapeutic and restricted activities and can implement therapeutic ones
Understands when and why it is necessary to return to the physician's office or clinic for follow-up care

COMPLICATIONS

Circulatory impairment
Contractures of joint
Difficulty in breathing
Drug reaction
Hemorrhage
Malpositioning, drainage, infection, or circulatory impairment from rigid plaster dressing and IPSF
Mental depression
Phantom pain sensation
Pneumonia
Pulmonary embolism
Shock
Tissue necrosis
Wound infection

Amputation of leg below knee, traumatic (Code 897)

CONCURRENT CRITERIA
Identification of patient's physical and psychosocial needs and/or concerns

Relief from hemorrhage, shock, pain, or infection
Maintenance of vital body functions
Understanding of the surgical treatment as well as nursing management, so that realistic plans for health maintenance can be made for after discharge
Concern or grief over change in body image
Preventive measures concerning problems resulting from immobility

Recommended nursing action consistent with diagnosis

Nursing services

Implement measures to interrupt life-threatening, traumatic process, including pain-reducing measures, adequate ventilation and adequate cardiovascular functioning, such as control of bleeding, maintenance of arterial pressure, replacement of fluid loss, and administration of appropriate cardiotonics and vasopressors as ordered; implement measures to reduce the effects of fluid loss, such as conservation of body heat and proper positioning; observe closely for effects of measures taken as well as for signs of physical deterioration by frequent monitoring of the sensorium, pupils, pulse rate and character, blood pressure (including pulse pressure), hourly urinary output, and the presence and quality of the peripheral pulse; administer appropriate antibiotics as ordered; physically prepare patient for surgery

Implement postoperative nursing care, including observation for signs and symptoms of complications with prompt nursing intervention should any occur; implement measures to maintain traction properly, if used, and to prevent contractures by use of proper positioning and alignment as well as the use of supportive devices; provide adequate hydration, nutrition, and elimination; control bleeding; prevent infection of wound; implement measures to reduce pain; assist patient through the grief process of change in body image; implement measures to prevent problems caused by immobility

Implement rehabilitative measures, including bed exercises consisting of push-ups from the prone position, active range of motion exercises, partial sit-ups; standing exercises consisting of hopping in a stationary position, hopping with advancement with and without a walker, and standing, flexing knees and balancing on one leg, and crutch walking; facilitate stump healing conducive to the use of a prosthesis by application of Ace bandages to promote shrinkage, stump exercises, and stump massage; assist patient in proper use of crutches or prosthesis

Initiate appropriate referrals

Health education

Instruct as to name, purpose, dosage, frequency, side effects, action to take if side effects occur, and precautions for all discharge medications

Instruct about stump care, as to daily hygiene of stump, daily massage of suture line, application of Ace bandages, signs and symptoms of infection, and actions to take should any signs of infection or other problems, such as shrinkage, occur

Instruct on proper use and care of prosthesis

Instruct as to therapeutic and restricted activities

Instruct as to when and why it is necessary for return to the physician's office or clinic for follow-up medical care

Indicators for discharge
Adaptation to health status

Condition stable
Wound healing
Complications not evident
Health teaching completed
Referrals made

Examples of community resources

Visiting Nurse Association or public health nurse
Orthopedic clinic
Physical and vocational rehabilitation centers
Social services

RETROSPECTIVE CRITERIA
Health

Relief of symptoms
Wound healing

Mentally accepting change in body image

Complications not evident

Activity

Ambulatory

Able to use crutches or prosthesis (if prescribed) correctly

Implements stump care and exercise program

Knowledge

Knows the name of each discharge medication and understands the purpose, dosage, frequency, side effects, action to take if side effects occur, and precautions for each drug

Understands and can implement stump care properly

Understands both therapeutic and restricted activities and can implement therapeutic ones

Understands when and why it is necessary to return to the physician's office or clinic for follow-up care

COMPLICATIONS

Circulatory impairment

Contractures of joint

Difficulty in breathing

Drug reaction

Hemorrhage

Malpositioning, drainage, infection, or circulatory impairment from rigid plaster dressing and IPSF

Mental depression

Phantom pain sensation

Pneumonia

Pulmonary embolism

Shock

Tissue necrosis

Wound infection

Amputation of leg, congenital (Code: 755.2)

CONCURRENT CRITERIA
Identification of patient's physical and psychosocial needs and/or concerns

Relief of physical impairment and deformity

Understanding of surgical treatment as well as nursing management, so that realistic plans for health maintenance after discharge can be made

Rehabilitative measures to regain ambulatory status

Preventive measures for problems resulting from immobility

Concern over changes in body image

Recommended nursing action consistent with diagnosis
Nursing services

Implement preoperative care and teaching, including pain-reducing measures and provision of adequate nutrition, hydration, and elimination; aid patient in coping with changes in body image; explain surgical procedure, recovery room, estimated period of hospitalization, graduated steps to ambulation, postoperative pain-reducing measures, the possibility of phantom pain, the possibility of traction, rigid plaster dressings and IPSF, the importance of deep breathing, coughing, and frequent turning, and muscle strengthening exercises such as push-ups, partial sit-ups, arm flexion, and extension exercises with weights; physically prepare patient for surgery

Implement postoperative nursing care, including close observation for signs of complications, with prompt nursing intervention if any signs occur; maintain proper alignment and traction, if used; control bleeding; prevent wound infection and problems caused by immobility

Implement rehabilitation measures, including bed exercises such as push-ups from the prone position, active range of motion exercises, and partial sit-ups, standing exercises, stationary hopping, hopping with advancement, and knee flexing and balancing exercises; facilitate stump healing conducive to the use of prosthetic device; aid the patient in proper use of crutches and/or prosthesis

Initiate appropriate referrals

Health education

Instruct as to name, purpose, dosage, frequency, side effects, action to take if side effects occur, and precautions relating to all discharge medications

Instruct on daily stump care

Instruct on proper care and use of prosthetic device

Instruct on therapeutic and restricted activities

Instruct on when and why it is necessary for the patient to return to the clinic or physician's office for follow-up medical care

Indicators for discharge
Adaptation to health status

Condition stable
Wound healing
Complications not evident
Health teaching completed
Referrals made

Examples of community resources

Visiting Nurse Association or public health nurse
Orthopedic clinic
Vocational and physical rehabilitation centers
Social services

RETROSPECTIVE CRITERIA
Health

Relief from impairment or deformity of leg

Wound healing
Mentally accepting change in body image
Complications not evident

Activity

Ambulatory
Able to use crutches or prosthesis properly
Implements stump care and exercise program

Knowledge

Knows the name of each discharge medication and understands purpose, dosage, frequency, side effects, action to take if side effects occur, and precautions

Understands therapeutic and restricted activities, and can implement therapeutic ones

Understands and can implement proper care and use of prosthesis

Understands when and why it is necessary to return for follow-up medical care

COMPLICATIONS

Circulatory impairment
Contractures of joint
Difficulty in breathing
Drug reaction
Hemorrhage
Malpositioning, drainage, infection, or circulatory impairment from rigid plaster dressing and IPSF
Mental depression
Phantom pain sensation
Pneumonia
Pulmonary embolism
Shock
Tissue necrosis
Wound infection

Amputation of legs, acquired (Code: 896.9)

CONCURRENT CRITERIA
Identification of patient's physical and psychosocial needs and/or concerns

Relief from pain, infection, circulatory impairment, or deformity

Understanding of surgical treatment as well as nursing management, so that realistic plans for health maintenance can be made for after discharge

Rehabilitative measures to regain ambulatory status

Concern over change in body image

Preventive measures in relation to problems resulting from immobility

Recommended nursing action consistent with diagnosis
Nursing services

Implement preoperative care and teaching, including pain-reducing measures; provide adequate hydration, nutrition, and elimination; implement measures to aid the patient in coping with changes in body image; explain surgical procedure, recovery room, estimated period of hospitalization, postoperative pain-reducing measures, the importance of deep breathing, coughing, and turning (if turning is not contraindicated), the possibility of phantom limb sensation, muscle-strengthening exercises in preparation to use crutches and prostheses, and possible traction or rigid plaster dressings with IPSF; prepare patient physically for surgery

Implement postoperative nursing care including observation for signs and symptoms of complications with prompt nursing intervention if any occur; implement measures to maintain proper positioning and alignment; control bleeding; prevent wound infection and problems caused by immobility

Implement rehabilitation measures, including bed exercises, such as push-ups

from the prone position, active range of motion exercises, and partial sit-ups; implement measures to facilitate stump healing conducive to the use of prosthetic devices; assist patient in proper usage of crutches and prosthetic devices; initiate appropriate referrals

Health education

Instruct as to the name, purpose, frequency, side effects, action to take if side effects occur, and precautions regarding all discharge medications

Instruct as to daily stump care

Instruct as to proper care and use of prosthetic devices

Instruct as to therapeutic and restricted activities

Instruct as to when and why it is necessary for the patient to return to the physician's office or clinic for follow-up medical care

Indicators for discharge
Adaptation to health status

Condition stable

Wound healing

Complications not evident

Health teaching completed

Referrals made

Examples of community resources

Visiting Nurse Association or public health nurse

Orthopedic clinic

Vocational and physical rehabilitation centers

Social services

RETROSPECTIVE CRITERIA
Health

Relief of pain, infection, circulatory impairment, or deformity

Wound healing

Mentally accepting change in body image

Complications not evident

Activity

Ambulatory

Able to use crutches correctly and safely

Able to apply and use prostheses correctly

Implements stump care and exercise program

Knowledge

Knows the name of each discharge medication and understands the purpose, dosage, frequency, side effects, action to take should side effects occur, and precautions for each drug

Understands and can implement stump care

Understands therapeutic and restricted activities and can implement therapeutic ones

Understands and can implement proper care and use of prostheses

Understands when and why it is necessary to return to physician's office or clinic for follow-up care

COMPLICATIONS

Circulatory impairment

Contractures of joints

Difficulty in breathing

Drug reaction

Hemorrhage

Malpositioning, drainage, infection, and circulatory infection from rigid plaster dressing and IPSF

Mental depression

Phantom pain sensation

Pneumonia

Pulmonary embolism

Shock

Tissue necrosis

Wound infection

Amputation of legs, traumatic (Codes: 897, 897.1, 897.9)

CONCURRENT CRITERIA
Identification of patient's physical and psychosocial needs and/or concerns

Relief from hemorrhage, shock, pain, or infection

Maintenance of vital body functions

Understanding of surgical treatment as well as nursing management, so that realistic plans for health maintenance can be made for after discharge

Concern or grief over change in body image

Preventive measures concerning problems caused by immobility

Recommended nursing action consistent with diagnosis
Nursing services

Implement measures to interrupt life-threatening, traumatic process, including pain-reducing measures; maintain adequate ventilation, adequate cardiovascular functioning, such as control of bleeding, maintenance of arterial pressure, replacement of fluid loss, and administration of appropriate cardiotonics and vasopressors as ordered; implement measures to reduce effects of fluid loss, such as conservation of body heat and proper positioning; observe closely for effects of measures taken as well as for signs of physical deterioration by frequent monitoring of sensorium, pupils, pulse rate and character, blood pressure (including pulse pressure), hourly urinary output, and the presence and quality of the peripheral pulse; administer appropriate antibiotics as ordered; prepare patient physically for surgery

Implement postoperative nursing care, including observation for signs and symptoms of complications with prompt nursing intervention should any occur; implement measures to maintain traction properly, if used, and to prevent contractures by use of proper positioning and alignment as well as

51

the use of supportive devices; implement measures to provide adequate hydration, nutrition, and elimination; control bleeding; prevent infection of wound; reduce pain; assist patient through the grief process of change in body image; implement measures to prevent problems from immobility

Implement rehabilitative measures, including bed exercises consisting of push-ups from the prone position, active range of motion exercises, and partial sit-ups; facilitate stump healing conducive to the use of a prosthesis, by such measures as application of Ace bandages to promote shrinkage, stump exercises, and stump massage; assist patient in proper use of crutches or prostheses

Initiate appropriate referrals

Health education

Instruct as to name, purpose, dosage, frequency, side effects, action to take if side effects occur, and precautions for each discharge medication

Instruct as to daily stump care

Instruct on proper use and care of prostheses

Instruct as to therapeutic and restricted activities

Instruct as to when and why it is necessary for the patient to return to the physician's office or clinic for follow-up medical care

Indicators for discharge
Adaptation to health status

Condition stable
Wound healing
Complications not evident
Health teaching completed
Referrals made

Examples of community resources

Visiting Nurse Association or public health nurse
Orthopedic clinic
Physical and vocational rehabilitation centers
Social services

RETROSPECTIVE CRITERIA
Health

Absence of pain or infection
Wound healing
Mentally accepting change in body image
Complications not evident

Activity

Ambulatory
Able to use crutches correctly and safely
Able to apply and use prostheses correctly
Implements stump care and exercise program

Knowledge

Knows the name of each discharge medication and understands the purpose, dosage, frequency, side effects, action to take should side effects occur, and precautions for each drug

Understands and can implement stump care

Understands therapeutic and restricted activities and can implement therapeutic ones

Understands proper care and use of prostheses

Understands when and why it is necessary to return to physician's office or clinic for follow-up care

COMPLICATIONS

Circulatory impairment
Contractures of joints
Difficulty in breathing
Drug reaction
Hemorrhage
Malpositioning, drainage, infection, and circulatory infection from rigid plaster dressing and IPSF
Mental depression
Phantom pain sensation
Pneumonia
Pulmonary embolism
Shock
Tissue necrosis
Wound infection

Amputation of thumb, fingers, or hand, traumatic
(Codes: 885-887)

CONCURRENT REVIEW CRITERIA
Identification of patient's physical and psychosocial needs and/or concerns

Relief of pain, control of hemorrhage, and prevention of infection

Adaptation of activities of daily living, may include adaptive functions of upper extremity

Grief over loss of body part and fear related to change in body image

Understanding of condition, cause, treatment, medical and nursing management, and rehabilitation potential

Recommended nursing action consistent with diagnosis
Nursing services

Provide sterile stump care with observation for symptoms of infection, such as fever, purulent drainage, or odor

Give emotional support and counseling for body image alteration and alteration in life-style

Instigate activity of daily living assessment and program to promote independence

Initiate discharge planning and referrals

Health education

Instruct on care of stump or operative site

Instigate activities of daily living program, including use of assistive device or prosthesis

Explain condition, cause, prognosis, surgical treatment, medical and nursing management, and discharge care

Indicators for discharge
Adaptation to health status

Successful adaptation to activities of daily living

Stump or operative site healed

Complications not evident

Adjustment to loss of body part evident

Examples of community resources

Vocational and occupational rehabilitation centers

Visiting Nurse Association or public health nurse

RETROSPECTIVE REVIEW CRITERIA
Health

Stump or operative site healed

Loss of body part accepted

Activity

Activities of daily living adapted or transferred to inpatient rehabilitation center

Implements stump care

Knowledge

Understands and can verbalize stump care, adaptive activities of daily living, and condition process and symptoms to report to physician

COMPLICATIONS

Contractures of joint
Drainage
Drug reaction
Hemorrhage
Mental depression
Phantom pain sensations
Shock
Tissue necrosis
Wound infection

Amputation of toes, acquired (Code: 856.5)

CONCURRENT CRITERIA
Identification of patient's physical and psychosocial needs and/or concerns

Relief from pain, infection, circulatory impairment, or deformity

Understanding of surgical treatment as well as nursing management, so that realistic plans for health maintenance can be made for after discharge

Preventive measures as related to problems resulting from immobility

Rehabilitative measures to regain ambulatory status

Concern or grief over change in body image

Recommended nursing action consistent with diagnosis
Nursing services

Implement preoperative care and teaching, including pain-reducing measures and measures to provide adequate hydration, nutrition, and elimination; assist patient in coping with changes in body image; initiate preoperative teaching, such as explanation of operative procedure, recovery room, possibility of phantom limb discomfort, estimated duration of hospitalization, and expected steps to ambulation, including demonstration and instruction related to use of crutches and to postoperative pain-reducing measures, and the importance of frequent turning, coughing, and deep breathing

Implement postoperative nursing care, including observation for signs and symptoms of complications with prompt nursing intervention should they occur; maintain proper positioning and alignment; prevent problems caused by immobility

Implement rehabilitative measures, including bed exercises to strengthen arms for crutch walking, standing exercises, hopping and balancing exercises;

facilitate proper stump healing; assist patient in proper use of crutches

Initiate appropriate referrals

Health education

Instruct as to name, purpose, frequency, side effects, action to take should side effects occur, and precautions regarding all discharge medications

Instruct in stump care, such as instruction as to daily hygiene of stump, including massage of suture line, application of special dressings, signs and symptoms of infection, and actions to take should such signs appear

Instruct patient on therapeutic and restricted activities

Instruct patient on proper, safe use of crutches, walker, or cane

Instruct patient when and why it is necessary to return to the physician's office or clinic for follow-up medical care

Indicators for discharge
Adaptation to health status

Condition stable
Complications not evident
Health teaching completed
Referrals made

Examples of community resources

Visiting Nurse Association or public health nurse
Orthopedic clinic
Physical and vocational rehabilitation centers
Social services

RETROSPECTIVE CRITERIA
Health

Condition stable
Stump circulation within normal limits
Complications not evident

Activity

Ambulatory

Able to use crutches, cane, or walker properly

Knowledge

Knows the name of each discharge medication and understands the purpose, dosage, frequency, side effects, action to take should side effects occur, and precautions for each drug

Understands and can implement stump care

Understands therapeutic and restricted activities and can implment therapeutic ones

Understands when and why it is necessary to return to physician's office or clinic for follow-up care

COMPLICATIONS

Circulatory impairment
Contractures of joint
Drug reaction
Hemorrhage
Mental depression
Phantom pain sensation
Shock
Tissue necrosis
Wound infection

Amputation of toes, traumatic (Codes: 895, 895.1, 895.9)

CONCURRENT CRITERIA
Identification of patient's physical and psychosocial needs and/or concerns

Relief from hemorrhage, shock, infection, or pain

Maintenance of vital body functions

Understanding of surgical treatment as well as nursing management, so that realistic plans for health maintenance can be made for after discharge

Grief over change in body image

Preventive measures concerning problems resulting from immobility

Recommended nursing action consistent with diagnosis
Nursing services

Implement measures to interrupt life-threatening traumatic process, including pain-reducing measures, adequate ventilation, and adequate cardiovascular functioning; maintain measures to reduce the effects of fluid loss, such as conservation of body heat and proper positioning; observe closely for the effects of measures taken as well as for signs of physical deterioration by frequent monitoring of the sensorium, pupils, pulse rate and character, blood pressure (including pulse pressure), hourly urinary output, and the presence and quality of peripheral pulse; administer appropriate antibiotics as ordered; physically prepare patient for surgery

Implement postoperative nursing care, including observation for signs and symptoms of complications with prompt nursing intervention should any signs occur; implement measures to prevent contractures, control bleeding, prevent wound infection, and reduce pain; assist patient through the grief process of change in body image; ensure proper hydration, nutrition, and elimination; initiate measures to prevent problems caused by immobility

Implement rehabilitative measures, including exercises for balancing and use of crutches, walker, or cane; facilitate stump healing; assist patient in safe and proper use of crutches, cane, or walker

Initiate appropriate referrals

Health education

Instruct as to the name, purpose, dosage, frequency, side effects, action to take should side effects occur, and precautions related to each discharge medication

Instruct about stump care, as to daily hygiene, daily massage of suture line, application of special dressings, signs and symptoms of infection, and the appropriate actions to take should infection appear

Instruct as to therapeutic and restricted activities

Instruct as to proper and safe use of crutches, walker, and cane

Instruct as to when and why it is necessary to return to the physicians' office or clinic for follow-up medical care

Indicators for discharge
Adaptation to health status

Condition stable
Complications not evident
Health teaching completed
Referrals made

Examples of community resources

Visiting Nurse Association or public health nurse
Orthopedic clinic
Physical and vocational rehabilitation centers
Social services

RETROSPECTIVE CRITERIA
Health

Condition stable
Stump circulation within normal limits
Complications not evident

Activity

Ambulatory
Able to use crutches, cane, or walker properly

Knowledge

Knows the name of each dishcarge medication and understands the purpose, dosage, frequency, side effects, action to take if side effects occur, and precautions for each drug

Understands and can implement stump care

Understands therapeutic and restricted activities and can implement therapeutic ones

Understands when and why it is necessary to return to physician's office or clinic for follow-up medical care

COMPLICATIONS

Circulatory impairment
Contractures of joint
Drug reaction
Hemorrhage
Mental depression
Phantom pain sensation
Shock
Tissue necrosis
Wound infection

Amyotrophic lateral sclerosis (Code: 348)

CONCURRENT CRITERIA
Identification of patient's physical and psychosocial needs and/or concerns

Relief of symptoms, as much as possible, such as progressive weakness, atrophy, spasticity, fibrillation of the affected muscles, and difficulty in chewing and swallowing in advanced cases

Fear of possible death, which usually occurs from 3 to 5 years after the patient has been diagnosed, and anxiety about increased dependence and changes in body image and in role

Understanding of disease disorder as related to cause (trauma, hereditary, syphilis, lead poisoning), prognosis, course, and management, so that realistic plans can be made for care after discharge and for any necessary screening of family members, such as genetic counseling

Assistance in coping with increased dependence, changes in body image, and role, and eventual death

Awareness of community agencies that can most appropriately assist with care after discharge

Recommended nursing action consistent with diagnosis
Nursing services

Assist the patient and family with coping with increased dependence, changes in body image and role, and eventual death

Maintain adequate nutrition, hydration, and elimination

Prevent complications resulting from immobility or decreased activity

Implement measures designed for maintaining maximum functional ability for as long as possible, such as active and passive exercises and use of adaptive devices, braces, walker, and canes

Initiate appropriate referrals

Health education

Family/patient education regarding measures to avoid fatigue, such as pacing techniques, scheduled rest periods, therapeutic and restricted activities

Family/patient education regarding diet and hydration, such as soft or regular (depending on stage of disease), small frequent 2-hour feedings, method of tube feedings, if necessary, daily fluid intake required to maintain adequate hydration and urinary output to reduce the occurrence of urinary infections and renal calculi (should be at least 2,500 to 3,000 ml) and foods to aid in preventing constipation

Family/patient instruction in the use of adaptive devices, range of motion, active and passive, flexor and extensor, and resistive exercises, the need and method of good skin hygiene, the need for frequent turning (if bedridden), Foley catheter care (if applicable), transfer techniques, and the use of safety devices and measures

Family/patient education concerning names of each discharge medication and the dosage, frequency, side effects, measures to reduce side effects, and precautions for each drug

Family/patient education concerning community agencies available for assistance

Indicators for discharge
Adaptation to health status

Condition stable
Vital signs stable
Complications not evident
Referrals made

Examples of community resources

Multiple Sclerosis Association
Visiting Nurse Association and Home Health Aide Program

Meals on Wheels
Social services
Physiotherapy or vocational rehabilitation centers (for patient or family members)

Health

Condition stable
Complications not evident
Coping with aspects of terminal disease
Intake and output between 2,500 and 3,000 ml daily
Weight maintained

Activity

Ambulatory
Able to carry out activities of daily living

Knowledge

Understands and is able to implement measures to maintain adequate hydration and nutrition
Understands and is able to use adaptive devices
Understands the need for and can imple-
ment range of motion, flexor and extensor, and active and passive exercises
Understands the need for proper rest and avoidance of fatigue and has developed pacing techniques
Understands the need for good skin hygiene and can implement methods to obtain it
Understands the need for maintaining proper Foley catheter care, alignment, frequent change of position and can implement methods of maintenance
Understands transfer techniques and safety measures
Understands and knows the name of each discharge medication and understands the purpose, dosage, frequency, side effects, action to take should side effects occur, and precautions for each drug
Understands the possible genetic relationship of disease

COMPLICATIONS

Contractures
Decubitus ulcers
Pneumonia
Urinary tract infection

Anemia, aplastic (Code: 284)

CONCURRENT CRITERIA
Identification of patient's physical and psychosocial needs and/or concerns

Relief of symptoms, including lassitude, pallor, purpura, bleeding, fatigue, tachycardia, thrombocytopenia, or infection with high fever
Identification of possible toxic agents in patient's personal or work environment, including medications or agents for infection, arthritis, or convulsions, exposure to radiation, hair dyes, plant sprays, insecticides, volatile solvents, or large doses of antileukemic drugs
Meticulous attention to personal hygiene and avoidance of exposure to infections
Understanding of disease process, course, medical and nursing management, treatment with androgenic steroids, transfusions, or splenectomy
Fear of death, prolonged illness, possible need to be maintained on transfusions, change in life-style, change in role, and loss of time from normal activities

Recommended nursing action consistent with diagnosis
Nursing services

Place in reverse isolation, with explanation of procedure, duration, and need for noninfectious environment
Organize nursing care to conserve pa-

tient's energy, avoid fatigue, and maintain activity as tolerated

Maintain body functions, including monitoring vital signs and positioning patient to maximize chest expansion; turn patient; assist patient in coughing and deep breathing; check stools for blood; monitor intake and output and diet of preference for nutrition

Administer treatments; observe for side effects, including virilism, sodium and water retention, hepatic changes, and muscle cramps, side effects of androgenic steroids and leukoagglutinins manifested by chills and fever following transfusion

Give emotional support to patient/family about disease process and fear of death

Health education

Teach conservation of energy and how to plan life-style to permit rest periods or avoid fatigue

Teach prevention of infections through personal hygiene and avoiding exposure to persons with infections, especially upper respiratory infections

Teach avoidance of constriction of blood vessels by not wearing tight clothing, elastic garters, or tight belts and by not sitting in the same position for long periods of time

Explain disease process and observation of symptoms requiring immediate reporting to physician

Teach techniques of oral hygiene, including gentle brushing with soft toothbrush and frequently using diluted mouthwash; observing for hemorrhage of gums

Indicators for discharge
Adaptation to health status

Symptoms subsided or controlled
Complications not evident
Health teaching completed
Red cell count increased

Examples of community resources

Visiting Nurse Association or public health nurse

RETROSPECTIVE CRITERIA
Health

Afebrile
Symptoms resolved or controlled
Complications not evident
Red cell count increased

Activity

Minimal assistance needed in activities of daily living
Ambulatory without undue fatigue
Oral hygiene before and after meals

Knowledge

Patient and/or family can verbalize essential life-style to conserve energy, preventive measures for infection or bleeding, medication information, and symptoms to report to physician

COMPLICATIONS

Hemorrhage
Infection, severe
Leukoagglutinins after transfusion
Side effects of androgenic steroids

Anemia group in children

Sickle cell (Code: 282.6)
Undetermined origin (Code: 280)

CONCURRENT CRITERIA
Identification of patient's physical and psychosocial needs and/or concerns

Freedom from anxiety and cardiorespiratory distress
Relief of abdominal distention and pain
Relief of pain and spasms of muscles
Freedom from fatigue and weakness in daily activites
Patient/parental understanding of diagnostic and treatment procedures and long-term implications of condition

Recommended nursing action consistent with diagnosis
Nursing services

Provide comfort measures to relieve cardiorespiratory distress, pain, and functional limitations, by positioning; carry out medical orders, such as providing oxygen, intravenous therapy with electrolytes, blood transfusion, and pain-relieving measures of packs, analgesics, administration of stimulants, antipyretics, analgesics, and iron; time of laboratory procedures; provide play therapy or physical comfort through cuddling or rocking
Consistently monitor vital signs (particularly during transfusions), fluid intake and output, activity, rest, and mental affect
Instruct and explain appropriately for age for all diagnostic and follow-up procedures
Provide adequate nutrition and hydration, including slow and timely feeding, especially during periods of least respiratory distress; individualize therapeutic diet high in iron and vitamin C
Prevent infection, by bed placement and administration of antibiotics as ordered

Health education

Educate parents about disease condition, genetic counseling, where appropriate, and implication for priorities in care of child, including immediate in-house diagnostic and treatment procedures
Provide specific instruction and, when possible, written information for parents about dietary, hygiene, activity, program and instructions for child based on assessment of home environment and ability to comply
Instruct parents regarding danger signs, including respiratory and pulse rate, pain, color, loss of consciousness, and fatigue, and modes of intervention
Explain services offered by referral agencies
Provide child with information, appropriate for age and developmental level, about diet, activity, signs and symptoms, and potential for normal lifestyle

Indicators for discharge
Adaptation to health status

Afebrile; vital signs within normal limits
Corrections of anemic crisis and potential for home care indicated by laboratory blood reports
Cardiorespiratory distress, pain, or severe functional limitations relieved
Normal eating, sleeping, and activity patterns reestablished

Examples of community resources

Public health nurse or Visiting Nurse Association

RETROSPECTIVE CRITERIA
Health

Afebrile
Vital signs stable, within normal limits

Infection not evident
Anemic crisis corrected

Activity

Resumption of normal patterns, including diet, sleep, and physical activity, consistent with age and developmental level

Knowledge

Child/parents understand permitted and restricted activities
Child/parents aware of danger signs and response required
Parents able to implement medications, diet, hygiene, and activity schedule as ordered
Parents understand genetic implications of sickle cell anemia

COMPLICATIONS

Aplastic crises
Aseptic necrosis of femoral head
Bone infarction
Cardiac enlargement
Cholelithiasis
Infections
Leg ulcers
Osteomyelitis
Recurrent gross hematuria

Anemia, hemolytic, acquired (Code: 283)

CONCURRENT CRITERIA
Identification of patient's physical and psychosocial needs and/or concerns

Relief from chills, fever, headaches, precordial spasm and pain, nausea and vomiting
Reduction of irritability
Increased urinary output

Recommended nursing action consistent with diagnosis
Nursing services

Carefully observe for pale conjunctiva, mucous membranes, nail beds, and palms
Maintain electrolyte balance
Measure intake and output
Administer oxygen as ordered
Maintain communication with patient; explain procedures; provide opportunity for discussion

Health education

Help patient determine realistic goals
Continue medical care and treatment
Contribute to life-style planning, so that patient can remain productive and contributory member of society

Indicators for discharge
Adaptation to health status

Afebrile
No chest pain
No gastrointestinal symptoms
Ambulatory
Patient/family can verbalize essentials of medical care requirements

Examples of community resources

Referral usually not indicated

RETROSPECTIVE CRITERIA
Health

Afebrile
No chest pain
No nausea or vomiting
Urinary output improved

Activity

Ambulatory without undue fatigue

Knowledge

Patient/family verbalizes understanding of maintaining a realistic health program, the importance of intake and output, and the dosage, frequency, purpose, and toxicity of medications

Understands importance of continued medical supervision

COMPLICATIONS

Aplastic crisis
Cholelithiasis

Myocardial infarction
Prostration
Shock
Thrombocytopenic purpura
Upper abdominal pain

Anemia, iron deficiency (Code: 280)

CONCURRENT CRITERIA
Identification of patient's physical and psychosocial needs and/or concerns

Relief of symptoms including pallor, lassitude, fatigue, dyspnea, palpitation, angina, brittle hair and/or nails, smooth tongue, excessive bleeding frequently in stool
Understanding of disease, course, prognosis, medical and nursing management

Recommended nursing action consistent with diagnosis
Nursing services

Plan organization of nursing care to prevent fatigue, dyspnea, palpitation, or angina through use of rest periods
Administer oral or parenteral iron therapy; monitor laboratory reports for presence of hypochromia, microcythemia, or red blood count less reduced than hemoglobin
Encourage adequate nutrition, hydration, and elimination by providing foods and fluids reflecting basic nutrition and individual preferences
Assist with oral hygiene every 2 hours

Health education

Instruct about medication, including name, purpose, frequency, dosage, side effects, and actions to initiate if side effects occur
Explain symptoms and results of observations to be reported to physician
Instruct about diet
Explain importance of continued medical supervision

Help design life-style that allows for rest periods and avoidance of fatigue

Indicators for discharge
Adaptation to health status

Cessation of symptoms including fatigue or dyspnea
Rise in hemoglobin
Provision of own oral hygiene
No evidence of excessive bleeding

Examples of community resources

Referral usually not indicated

RETROSPECTIVE CRITERIA
Health

Dyspnea not evident
Fatigue subsided
Hemoglobin rising

Activity

Ambulatory
Independent in activities of daily living

Knowledge

Patient/family can verbalize design of life-style that permits rest and prevents fatigue; understands diet, medication instructions, and symptoms of disease process to report to physician

COMPLICATIONS

Angina pectoris
Congestive heart failure
Hypochromia
Microcythemia
Severe dysphagia

Anemia, pernicious (Code: 281.0)

CONCURRENT CRITERIA
Identification of patient's physical and psychosocial needs and/or concerns

Relief of symptoms including anorexia; dyspepsia; smooth, sore tongue; constant, symmetrical numbness and tingling of the feet; pallor or trace of jaundice; fatigue; dyspnea; palpitation; angina; mental disturbances; and/or loss of vibration sense and deep reflexes

Understanding of disease, course, prognosis, and medical and nursing management

Encouragement to continue treatment, since untreated pernicious anemia is fatal and early treatment will reverse central nervous system symptoms if they have been present for less than 6 months

Understanding that vitamin B_{12} injections will continue for the rest of patient's life

Adjustment to regular intramuscular injections of medications

Recommended nursing action consistent with diagnosis
Nursing services

Plan organization of nursing care to prevent fatigue, dyspnea, palpitation, or angina through use of rest periods

Provide special oral hygiene every 2 hours and document complaints of sore or burning tongue

Encourage adequate nutrition, hydration, and elimination by providing foods and fluids reflecting basic nutrition and individual preferences

Administer medications, especially vitamin B_{12}; monitor laboratory reports for presence of oval macrocytes, pancytopenia, hypersegmented neutrophils, or megaloblastic bone marrow

Encourage communication for expression of feelings and adjustment to treatment regime

Health education

Instruct about essentials for a balanced diet

Teach patient/family, with return demonstrations, to administer injections; teach the name, purpose, duration, frequency, and side effects of medications, actions to take if side effects occur

Teach methods of progressive ambulation for patients with a neurological residual deficit

Advise patient in planning life-style to provide appropriate activities and independence

Indicators for discharge
Adaptation to health status

Hemoglobin values nearing normal or rising since admission

Nutritional status improved

Ambulation without numbness and/or tingling of feet

Central nervous system symptoms improved or controlled

Examples of community resources

Visiting Nurse Association or public health nurse

RETROSPECTIVE CRITERIA
Health

Pesenting signs and symptoms, especially fatigue, reduced

Nutritional status improved

Numbness and/or tingling of feet relieved

Hemoglobin values rising

Activity

Ambulatory with minimal assistance

Independent in activities of daily living

Medication injections administered by self or family member

Knowledge

Patient/family understands disease process and necessity for continued treatment, method of medication administration and injections, importance of blood test to monitor disease process, and that central nervous system symptoms are usually reversible

Patient/family knows name, purpose, duration, frequency, side effects, and action to initiate if side effects occur of each medication

Understands importance of continuing vitamin B_{12} injections; patient/family member can administer injections

COMPLICATIONS

Acute gout attack
Congestive heart failure
Infection of intramuscular injection sites
Neurological residual deficit
Peripheral neuropathy
Pulmonary edema

Aortic aneurysm, abdominal (Codes: 441.3, 441.4)

CONCURRENT CRITERIA
Identification of patient's physical and psychosocial needs and/or concerns

Relief from pain, hoarseness, "fox-like bark" when coughing, dysphagia, dyspnea, left-sided lumbar back pain, and indigestion
Bed rest
Fear of surgery; fear of death
Sudden dependency on others and restriction of activities
Physiological deficits associated with hypotension

Recommended nursing action consistent with diagnosis
Nursing services

Give nothing by mouth, pending surgery
Restrict any exertion; require bed rest
Give immediate, calm response to patient's requests and queries
Monitor vital signs every 15 minutes
Keep patient/family informed of progress of diagnostic tests and preparations for surgery

Health education

Defer complex teaching during acute phase, remaining open to questions from patient
Explain relationship of restrained movement to comfort and vessel integrity

Describe to family anticipated surgery, with probable time of return to room
Explain presence of and need for tubes and devices used postoperatively

Indicators for discharge
Adaptation to health status

Patient plans for own future
Patient demonstrates knowledge of the nature of the surgery
Patient understands any physical limitations incurred
Family ready to receive patient and has made appropriate positive plans for patient's discharge

Examples of community resources

Visiting Nurse Association

RETROSPECTIVE CRITERIA
Health

Wound closed
Abdominal pain absent

Activity

At preacute levels

Knowledge

Limitations, if any
Medication regime
Nature of surgery

COMPLICATIONS

Aneurysmal rupture (preoperative)
Bone marrow depression
Hemoptysis

Intestinal obstruction
Pneumonia
Sepsis
Wound infection

Appendicitis in children (Codes: 540, 542, 543)

CONCURRENT REVIEW CRITERIA
Identification of patient's physical and psychosocial needs and/or concerns

Reassurance and relief from pain

Understanding of diagnostic and treatment procedures

Knowledge of level of activity permitted and plan for return to normal schedule and life-style

Assistance in adapting to hospitalization, consistent with age and developmental level

Recommended nursing action consistent with diagnosis
Nursing services

Reassure by explanation to child and parents; relieve pain, by positioning and administering medication as ordered

Prepare patient for surgery, including laboratory procedures, medications, and intravenous and postoperative equipment; physically prepare patient for surgery, with instruction and practice in deep breathing; explain postoperative turning and administration of preoperative medications

Monitor and record vital signs; locations, intensity, frequency, aggravating factors, such as pain or color affect, and symptoms of digestive disorder, such as nausea, vomiting, or mass pressure distention, and promptly intervene if necessary

Maintain and monitor adequate fluid intake and output

Implement postoperative nursing care and/or intervention regarding vital signs, skin color, temperature, sensory-motor fuction and affect, incision and dressing, condition of dryness or oozing, nasogastric tube (if present) for patency and irrigation; position in semi-Fowler's position or as ordered; maintain adequate ventilation by aiding patient in turning, coughing, deep breathing and being supported every 2 hours

Maintain adequate fluids, nutritional intake, and output via individual diet planned to meet physician's order and patient preference; monitor intake and output plus voluntary urination within 8 hours postoperatively

Relieve pain via positioning and analgesics, as ordered

Prevent infection via sterile technique in dressing change, frequent turning, deep breathing, hygienic measures, and separation from potentially infectious persons

Health education

Explain to parent diagnostic, surgical, and follow-up procedures; care of incision; dressing change; permissible and restricted activities; administration, purpose, dosage, mode, frequency of medications

Give ongoing explanation to child, commensurate with age and developmental level, of diagnostic and treatment procedures

Indicators for discharge
Adaptation to health status

Afebrile

Vital signs stable and within normal limits

Food and fluids tolerated
Wound healing satisfactorily
Normal activity for age and developmental level resumed

Examples of community resources

Referral not usually indicated

RETROSPECTIVE REVIEW CRITERIA
Health

Afebrile
Resolution of symptoms
Satisfactory wound healing
Tolerating food and fluids

Activity

Alert
No limitation in movement

Resumption of normal activity for age and developmental level

Knowledge

Completion of education regarding postoperative care

COMPLICATIONS

Appendiceal abscess
Generalized peritonitis
Hemorrhage
Intestinal obstruction
Intra-abdominal sepsis
Perforation
Pneumonia
Pylephlebitis
Subphrenic abscess
Wound infection

Arterial occlusive disease, aortoiliac, chronic (Codes: 444, 444.4, 445)

CONCURRENT CRITERIA
Identification of patient's physical and psychosocial needs and/or concerns

Relief from pain of intermittent claudications, ischemic neuritis, or paresthesias
Decrease in capacity for protection against and healing of infections of extremities
Relief from fear of chronic pain and limited mobility in order *not* to further increase peripheral vascular resistance, as the result of stress

Recommended nursing action consistent with diagnosis
Nursing services

Take bilateral pedal pulses twice a day; use oscillometer if available
Install foot cradle
Maintain room temperature at a constant 78° to 80° F
Place head of bed on 12 to 15-inch blocks (do not use Gatch bed)
Provide unhurried time for exploring uncertainties at least once every evening

Health education

Demonstrate foot care, with return demonstration
Explain relationship between fear and stress and vasoconstriction
Interpret physician's activity limitation directives in individualized, specific terms

Indicators for discharge
Adaptation to health status

Satisfactory return demonstration of foot care
Willingness to initiate questions about own care
No apparent potential for change in physical or psychosocial status
Demonstration of desire for discharge

Examples of community resources

Local Loan Closet for wheel chair and bed blocks, as needed
Visiting Nurse Association for adaptation assistance in home

RETROSPECTIVE CRITERIA
Health

No open wounds
Free of extremity pain during activities of
daily living
Afebrile

Activity

At or above admission level

Knowledge

Understands dosage and purpose of
drugs
Understands and can implement foot
care

COMPLICATIONS

Arterial aneurysm
Arterial thrombosis
Cardiac failure
Death of limb
Gangrene
Hemorrhage
Impotence, in men
Infection
Ischemia
Leriche's syndrome
Pneumonia
Postoperative complication
Pulmonary edema
Pulmonary embolism
Renal failure
Respiratory insufficiency
Retrograde ejaculation
Urinary retention

Arterial occlusive disease, extracranial (Codes: 432, 432.1, 435, 435.1, 446.6, 447.2, 447.9)

CONCURRENT CRITERIA
Identification of patient's physical and psychosocial needs and/or concerns

Control of alterations in consciousness or
orientation
Control of alterations in behavior
Improvements in deficits in motor and
verbal skills
Acceptance of changed relations with
family members because of greater
dependency

Recommended nursing action consistent with diagnosis
Nursing services

Explain procedures slowly, being responsive to verbal and nonverbal clues to
understanding
Report blood pressure changes, bruits, or
changes in consciousness immediately
Position patient so that affected side is
not the determinant of balance
Provide sensory and motor stimulation

Control oral intake to maintain positive
nitrogen balance

Health education

Explain patient's limitations to family,
emphasizing strengths remaining and
how to capitalize on them
Teach crutchwalking or use of walker
Explain diagnostic and/or surgical procedures and the sensations usually
accompanying them
Explain need for avoiding immobilization except in immediate postoperative
phase

Indicators for discharge
Adaptation to health status

Patient able to control frustration regarding any remaining motor or speech
deficits
Patient expresses readiness to be discharged

Family understands patient's limitations and shows willingness to accept patient

Patient/family member demonstrates understanding of medication, purpose, and dosage

Patient/family recognizes patient's ability to remain unattended for half-day periods

Examples of community resources

Visiting Nurse Association
Meals on Wheels

RETROSPECTIVE CRITERIA
Health

Acceptance of condition
Absence of inappropriate dependence

Activity

Ability to carry out activities of daily living

Knowledge

Knows physical limits
Understands probable prognosis
Knows purpose, dosage, and effects of medication
Understands new coping methods as alternatives to lost functions

COMPLICATIONS

Neurological deficit
Peripheral nerve deficit
Pneumonia
Postoperative stroke
Unrealistic hopelessness
Wound infection

Arterial occlusive disease, peripheral, of lower extremity, chronic
(Codes: 444, 445)

CONCURRENT CRITERIA
Identification of patient's physical and psychosocial needs and/or concerns

Relief of pain, blanching, rubor, cyanosis, coldness, ulcerations of extremities
Adjustment to limited mobility
Understanding of diminished capacity for protection against and healing of infections of extremities
Fear of meaning of chronic pain and limited mobility (prognosis and treatment)
Relief from further increase in peripheral vascular resistance, resulting from stress or fear

Recommended nursing action consistent with diagnosis
Nursing services

Take bilateral pedal pulses twice daily (use oscillometer where available)
Use foot cradle and other measures to increase circulation and avoid further occlusion

Keep room temperature constant at 78° to 80° F
Put head of bed on 12- to 15-inch blocks (do not use Gatch bed)
Provide unhurried time for exploring uncertainties at least every night

Health education

Demonstrate foot care
Explain relationship between fears and stress and vasoconstriction
Explain relationship between smoking and vasoconstriction
Interpret physician's activity limitations directives in individualized, specific terms
Teach measures that increase and decrease blood flow to lower extremities

Indicators for discharge
Adaptation to health status

Satisfactory return demonstration of foot care

Demonstration of willingness to initiate questions about own care and medical regime

No apparent potential for change in physical or psychosocial status

Demonstration of desire for discharge

Understanding of vasoconstricting and vasodilating adjuncts

Examples of community resources

Local Loan Closet for wheelchair and bed blocks, as necessary

Visiting Nurse Association or public health nurse for adaptation assistance in home

RETROSPECTIVE CRITERIA
Health

No open wounds

Free of extremity pain during activities of daily living

Afebrile

Activity

At or above admission level

Knowledge

Understands and can implement foot care

Knows discharge medication, including name, dosage, and purpose

COMPLICATIONS

Intraperitoneal abscess
Pulmonary embolism
Wound infection

Arthritis of knee, degenerative (Code: 713)

CONCURRENT CRITERIA
Identification of the patient's physical and psychosocial needs and/or concerns

Relief from pain or impaired function of knee

Concern over increased dependence and change in role, life-style, or body image

Understanding of medical, surgical, and nursing management of disease, so that realistic plans for health maintenance, after discharge can be made

Rehabilitative measures to regain or promote fullest degree of functioning within restriction of disease

Preventive measures regarding problems caused by immobility

Recommended nursing action consistent with diagnosis
Nursing services

Implement pain-reducing measures, including use of braces and splints

Implement measures to maintain safety

Implement measures to ensure adequate hydration, nutrition, and elimination

Implement measures to prevent problems caused by immobility

Implement preoperative and postoperative nursing care, including explanation of surgical procedure, recovery room, deep-breathing and coughing exercises, preliminary steps to ambulation (crutchwalking and muscle-strengthening exercises), estimated period of hospitalization, and measures used postoperatively to reduce discomfort; physically prepare patient for surgery; closely observe for signs of complications, with prompt nursing intervention should any occur; if cast is used, implement cast care and proper positioning and alignment appropriate for particular surgical procedure used to promote maximum functioning of joint and to support surgical treatment; implement prescribed postoperative exercises and measures to teach proper use of crutches, canes, and walker

Health education

Instruct on name of each discharge medication and the purpose, dosage, frequency, side effects, action to take should side effects occur, and precautions for each drug

Instruct on measures to prevent problems caused by decreased activity during convalescence

Instruct on therapeutic and restricted activities and safety measures related to convalescence and prevention of future damage to joint by improper body mechanics

Instruct on proper use of crutches, walker, or canes

Instruct on measures to reduce discomfort

Indicators for discharge
Adaptation to health status

Condition stable
Complications not evident
Health teaching completed
Referrals made

Examples of community resources

Visiting Nurse Association or public health nurse
Orthopedic clinic
Social worker
Physical therapy clinic
Vocational rehabilitation services

RETROSPECTIVE CRITERIA
Health

Condition stable
Complications not evident

Activity

Ambulatory
Able to use crutches, canes, or walker properly

Knowledge

Knows the name and purpose of each discharge medication and understands dosage, frequency, side effects, action to take should side effects occur, and precautions for each drug

Understands therapeutic and restricted activities and can implement therapeutic ones

Understands and can implement safety measures

Understands and can implement measures to reduce problems related to decreased activity

Understands the importance of keeping appointments with physician or clinic for follow-up care and knows when appointments are scheduled

COMPLICATIONS

Circulatory impairment
Dehydration
Drug reaction
Hemorrhage
Infection
Shock
Thromboembolism

Arthritis, rheumatoid (Code: 712.9)

CONCURRENT CRITERIA
Identification of patient's physical and psychosocial needs and/or concerns

Relief from malaise, fatigue, fever, weight loss, weakness, anemia, joint pain, joint swelling, or enlarged lymph nodes

Understanding of course of disease, prognosis, medical, surgical, and nursing management in order to make realistic plans for health maintenance after discharge

Nursing measures to prevent problems of immobility

Concern over increased dependence and change in body image or life-style

Rehabilitative measures to maintain function to optimal level within restrictions of disease

Recommended nursing action consistent with diagnosis
Nursing services

Implement pain-reducing measures and measures to prevent problems resulting from immobility or decreased activity; maintain hydration, nutrition, and elimination; implement measures to assist patient/family in coping with increasing dependency of patient, change in body image, change in life-style, and role changes

Implement measures consistent with medical treatment, including measures to maintain function of all joints and strengthen muscles that support joints, such as by isometric, range of motion, and progressive resistive exercises after inflammatory process is under control; implement use of adaptive devices for ambulation and activities of daily living, such as adapted eating utensils, raised seats on chairs and toilets, fastening equipment for clothing, and crutches, canes, or walkers; implement measures to provide rest for joints during acute inflammatory process and reduce deformities, such as regular rest periods, maintenance of correct positioning and alignment, use of supportive devices to prevent contractures and deformities, application of splints to maintain correct positioning of joints, placement of patient in prone position at least twice daily to prevent hip flexion and knee contractures

Observe for therapeutic effects of antiarthritic drugs; initiate nursing action to intervene should side effects occur

Implement diversional therapy

Implement nursing measures consistent with surgical treatment, including preoperative nursing care and teaching, such as through explanation of deep-breathing exercises, turning procedures, estimated period of hospitalization, specific exercises for restoring function or preventing deterioration in function of joints, and actual physical preparation of patient for surgery; implement postoperative pain-reducing measures and measures to maintain correct positioning and alignment, to prevent problems caused by immobility, to maintain adequate hydration, nutrition, and elimination, and to prevent wound infection; implement therapeutic exercises for regaining use of joints and adaptive devices as prescribed

Health education

Instruct on the name of each discharge medication and the purpose, dosage, frequency, side effects, action to take should side effects occur, and precautions for each drug

Instruct in use of adaptive devices, particularly crutches, walker, and canes

Instruct on therapeutic and restricted activities and on the importance of adequate daily rest periods

Instruct on specific treatments to be done at home, such as the paraffin treatment and on measures to reduce the occurrence of problems caused by decreased activity

Instruct on any necessary wound care and on use of adaptive devices

Indicators for discharge
Adaptation to health status

Condition stable
Complications not evident
Health teaching completed
Referrals made

Examples of community resources

Physiotherapy clinic
Orthopedic clinic
Social worker
Visiting Nurse Association or public health nurse
Meals on Wheels

RETROSPECTIVE CRITERIA
Health

Condition stable
Complications not evident

Activity

Ambulatory
Able to carry out activities of daily living

Able to use adaptive devices properly

Knowledge

Understands purpose and name of each discharge medication, as well as dosage, frequency, side effects, action to take if side effects occur, and precautions for each drug

Understands and can implement measures to reduce the occurrence of problems caused by decreased activity

Understands use of adaptive devices

Understands and can implement specific treatments to be used at home

Understands therapeutic and restricted activities and can implement therapeutic ones

Understands and can implement any necessary wound care

Understands need for regular rest periods

COMPLICATIONS

Drug reaction
Inflammation
Large joint instability or deformity
Rheumatoid vasculitis
"Swan neck" finger deformity
Synovitis
Thrombophlebitis
Wound infection

Arthritis of spine, degenerative (Code: 713.1)

CONCURRENT CRITERIA
Identification of patient's physical and psychosocial needs and/or concerns

Relief from pain, malaise, anemia, and fatigue and inability to bear weight

Understanding of disease as related to its course, medical or surgical treatment, and nursing management, so that realistic health maintenance plans can be made for after discharge

Protective measures against injury and problems resulting from immobility

Anxiety over increased dependency and change in body image, role, life-style

Rehabilitative measures to maintain or reach optimal level of function within restrictions of disease

Recommended nursing action consistent with diagnosis
Nursing services

Implement measures to reduce pain; maintain adequate hydration, nutrition, and elimination; and maintain proper alignment

Implement specific measures consistent with medical management, such as providing adequate rest during acute phase, being sure that bedboards are in place, and applying cervical collars; implement measures to reduce or avoid emotional strain, which increases muscle tension and joint strain, to reduce trauma and further degenerative changes of joints by use of back-strengthening exercises when acute phase is over, to assist patient in losing prescribed amount of weight, to restrict activities that include lifting heavy objects or overhead reaching, to teach use of proper body mechanics and postural exercises, to prevent problems from immobility, to teach safety measures during ambulation and proper crutch, walker, or cane usage, and to aid the patient/family members in coping with role changes, changes in body image and life-style, and increased dependency of patient; implement diversional activities; observe therapeutic results from antiarthritic drugs with prompt nursing intervention should side effects occur

Implement nursing measures consistent with spinal fusion, including pain-reducing measures preoperatively and postoperatively; maintain proper alignment and positioning to reduce contractures, deformities, and strain on spine preoperatively and postoperatively; maintain adequate hydration, nutrition, and elimination preoperatively and postoperatively; prevent problems from immobility preoperatively and postoperatively; explain surgical procedure, recovery room, deep-breathing exercises, turning procedure (log fashion), measures to be used to reduce pain after surgery, and estimated period of hospitalization; prepare patient physically for surgery; implement measures to prevent wound infection and to strengthen joint-supporting muscles; teach safety measures during ambulation; assist patient in learning to use crutches, canes, or walker

Health education

Instruct as to name of each discharge medication and the purpose, dosage, frequency, side effects, action to take if side effects occur, and precautions for each

Explain therapeutic and restricted activities

Teach proper use of canes, walkers, or crutches and adaptive measures to activities of daily living

Explain diet to correct anemia and importance of regularly scheduled rest periods

Teach pain-reducing measures, necessary wound care, and measures to reduce the occurrence of problems caused by decreased activity

Indicators for discharge
Adaptation to health status

Condition stable
Complications not evident
Health teaching completed
Referrals made

Examples of community resources

Visiting Nurse Association or public health nurse
Social services
Orthopedic clinic for physiotherapy

RETROSPECTIVE CRITERIA
Health

Condition stable and wound healing
Complications not evident

Activity

Ambulatory
Able to use cane, walker, or crutches correctly

Knowledge

Knows the name of each discharge medication and understands the purpose, dosage, frequency, side effects, action to take if side effects occur, and precautions for each

Understands therapeutic and restricted activity and can implement therapeutic ones

Understands and can implement any necessary wound care

Understands and can implement safety measures

Understands and can implement proper diet

Understands importance of regularly scheduled rest periods

Understands and can implement pain-reducing measures

Understands and can implement measures to reduce the occurrence of problems caused by immobility or decreased activity

Understands and can implement adaptive measures to activities of daily living

COMPLICATIONS

Anemia

Drug reaction

Inflammation

Joint instability

Thrombophlebitis

Wound infection

Asthma, acute (Code: 493)

CONCURRENT REVIEW CRITERIA
Identification of patient's physical and psychosocial needs and/or concerns

Relief from acute respiratory distress, especially dyspnea, wheezing, tachypnea, shortness of breath, orthopnea and hard, dry cough

Apprehension with sympathetic nervous system symptoms

Relief from altered level of consciousness, skin color changes, tachycardia, fatigue, hyper- and hypotension

Relief from water and/or fluid deficit

Recommended nursing action consistent with diagnosis
Nursing services

Maintain adequate ventilation by drug therapy with epinephrine, oxygen, bronchodilators, or steroids and by positioning in high Fowler's position; check lungs for expiratory wheeze; evaluate tissue perfusion status as indicated by mental status and blood gases; keep environment free of all allergens

Decrease patient's anxiety by maintaining quiet environment and emotional support; give sedatives, and tranquilizers as ordered, avoid respiratory depressants; provide rest and sleep; anticipate patient needs

Observe for level of consciousness change, pallor, cyanosis, hypertension (early hypoxia), hypotension, tachypnea, and tachycardia; give oxygen as indicated

Maintain rest periods correlated with degree of hypoxia; avoid overtiring by prescribed rest periods and small, high caloric feedings; keep pulse in range of 60 to 100

Check skin turgor; maintain adequate fluid status and report oliguria if 20 ml per hour or below; report temperature of 100° F or above, tachycardia below 100, sensorium changes, hematocrit greater than 50% or sodium below 148

Health education

Instruct parents about precipitating causes and emergency treatment

Teach importance of avoiding asthma attacks and of controlling stressful situations

Instruct about the name, dosage, frequency, side effects, and actions to take if side effects occur for each medication

Indicators for discharge
Adaptation to health status

Absence of respiratory distress symptoms

Mental status calm; coping mechanisms functioning

Examples of community resources

Crippled Children Commission
American Respiratory Association
Medic Alert
Public health department

RETROSPECTIVE REVIEW CRITERIA
Health

Absence of respiratory symptoms, such as shortness of breath and wheezing
Afebrile
Free of cough

Activity

Ambulatory
Activity resumed as tolerated

Avoid physical and stressful situations

Knowledge

Knows cause of and importance of avoiding acute episodes
Understands need to avoid stressful situations
Understands need for outpatient care
Understands purpose and name of each discharge medication, as well as the dosage, frequency, side effects, and action to take if side effects occur for each

COMPLICATIONS

Atelectasis
Cor pulmonale
Drug reaction
Oliguria
Respiratory infection
Respiratory insufficiency
Status asthmaticus

Atrial fibrillation (Code: 427.4)

CONCURRENT CRITERIA
Identification of patient's physical and psychosocial needs and/or concerns

Fear and concern about dysrhythmia, heart palpitations, and interrupted lifestyle
Relief from chest pain, arm pain, dyspnea, syncope, fatigue, nausea, and vomiting
Relief from hypertension

Recommended nursing action consistent with diagnosis
Nursing services

Begin cardiac monitoring within 5 minutes of admission
Examine extremities for signs and symptoms of embolization (by pulse, edema, color of skin) and vital signs for baseline

Initiate delegated medical direction immediately
Record and document rhythm strips (EKG)
Reassure patient of safe environment and expert care

Health education

Explain purpose of techniques and procedures, such as drugs, pacemaker, if indicated, or cardioversion
Instruct on permitted and restricted physical activities, including sexual activity
Instruct on diet, discharge medication, medical follow-up, and importance of following recovery plan
Explain contributory risk factors
Explain arrhythmia, what it means and why it occurs

Indicators for discharge
Adaptation to health status

Pain, syncope, and dyspnea absent
Pulses in extremities palpable
Activity tolerated without signs and symptoms of cardiac stress
Acceptance of diagnosis verbalized
Knowledge of restriction on activity verbalized

Examples of community resources

Visting Nurse Association or public health nurse

RETROSPECTIVE CRITERIA
Health

Chest pain absent
Heart rate within normal range

Activity

Ambulatory without fatigue
Capable of self-care

Knowledge

Patient and/or significant other verbalizes understanding of diagnosis, risk factors, diet, drugs, importance of medical follow-up

COMPLICATIONS

Digitalis toxicity
Drug reaction
Infection

Behavioral disorders of childhood or adolescence (Code: DSM II 308)

CONCURRENT REVIEW CRITERIA
Identification of patient's physical and psychosocial needs and/or concerns

Identification of exact nature of child's or adolescent's behavior that necessitates hospitalization, including primary potential and/or history of self, other, or property destruction
Evaluation of child's or adolescent's state of physical health
Expression by child or adolescent of beliefs and attitudes about own behavior and hospitalization
Documentation of family's attitudes, beliefs, and expectations of child or adolescent, treatment facility, and staff
Determination of chronology of child or adolescent and family development

Recommended nursing action consistent with diagnosis
Nursing services

Assess child or adolescent, including family and community, within 7 days of admission

Observe and assess ongoing behavior of child or adolescent within 8 hours of admission
Implement behavior-specific interventions, such as life-space interview and seclusion, and evaluation of same
Assist in development and implementation of after-care plans and family-specific intervention
Implement and/or assist with physical therapies, such as drugs or diagnostic procedures

Health education

Explain to patient/family ward procedures and milieu
Discuss with patient/family treatment goals and therapeutic modalities
Teach family to use specific therapeutic modalities, such as principles of behavior modification, behavior dynamics, or communication
Discuss and explain any medication, including purpose, use, dosage, side effects, and actions to take should side effects occur

Indicators for discharge
Adaptation to health status

Decreased incidence of behavior that led to hospitalization, such as aggressive behavior, verbalization of self-destructive wishes, or property destruction

Evidence of beginning reintegration into family and community

Completion of planned medical evaluation and of outpatient care plan

Patient/family demonstration of self-care capability in areas of limit-setting, medication administration, and help-seeking

Examples of community resources

Outpatient psychiatric nurse
School Nurse
Visiting Nurse Association or public health nurse

RETROSPECTIVE REVIEW CRITERIA
Health

No physical illness or problems
Regular sleep pattern

Activity

No limitations

Resumption of activities consistent with age and developmental level

Decrease in destructive behavior

Interaction with peers and adults at appropriate age level

Knowledge

Knows what treatment goals were accomplished and are to be followed after discharge

Knows purpose of medication, dosage, side effects, actions to take should side effects occur, and what to report to physician

COMPLICATIONS

Adverse reactions to diagnostic or therapeutic modalities

Exacerbation of clinical signs and/or symptoms

Failure of family and/or social support system

Bunion (Code: 730)

CONCURRENT CRITERIA
Identification of patient's physical and psychosocial needs and/or concerns

Relief from pain and restricted activity

Understanding of diagnostic and surgical procedure as well as nursing management

Rehabilitative measures to regain ambulatory status

Preventive measures against problems of immobility

Concern over loss of time from work or school

Recommended nursing action consistent with diagnosis
Nursing services

Implement preoperative teaching and care, including explanation of surgical

procedure, recovery room, type of dressing afterward, such as a large bulky dressing with splint and drain or a cast in the case of McBride's procedure, importance of frequent change of position and deep-breathing and coughing exercises, the use of crutches, and active and passive exercises; physically prepare patient for surgery

Implement postoperative nursing care, including measures to reduce pain and maintain adequate hydration, nutrition, and elimination: instruct about crutch-walking techniques, cast care (when appropriate), how to prevent wound infection, decubitus ulcers, pneumonia, urinary tract infections, and thromboembolic complications

Closely observe for impairment of circulation via constrictive dressing or cast or dependent edema; implement prompt nursing intervention should signs of complications occur

Implement safety measures

Health education

Instruct about wound care and application of bunion pads or splints, if necessary, or about cast care, if patient is discharged with cast

Instruct on crutchwalking and type of shoes to wear, such as open-toed sandals or tennis shoes, during convalescence

Instruct patient on methods of reducing discomfort and dependent edema and about transient numbness of joint (associated with Keller's procedure)

Instruct patient on therapeutic and restricted activities and flexion and extension exercises of the great toe (if soft dressings are used, this can be started immediately; if cast is used, the exercises may be started from 3 to 14 days)

Instruct on name of each discharge medication and the purpose, dosage, frequency, side effects, action to take if side effects occur, and precautions for each

Indicators for discharge
Adaptations to health status

Condition stable
Complications not evident
Health teaching completed
Referrals made

Examples of community resources

Orthopedic clinic
Visiting Nurse Association
Social services

RETROSPECTIVE CRITERIA
Health

Condition stable; wound healing
Complications not evident

Activity

Ambulatory (if crutches are prescribed, able to use crutches properly)

Knowledge

Knows the names of each discharge medication and the purpose, frequency, dosage, side effects, action to take if side effects occur, and precautions for each drug

Understands and can do flexion and extension exercises

Understands therapeutic and restricted activities

Understands about transient numbness associated with Keller's procedure

Understands and can implement wound care, if any necessary

Understands and can implement measures to reduce pain and dependent edema

Understands and can implement cast care, if discharged with a cast

Understands when and why it is necessary to return to clinic or physician's office for follow-up visit

COMPLICATIONS

Decubitus ulcers
Dependent edema
Hemorrhage
Impairment of circulation
Infective or septic bursitis
Pneumonia
Thromboembolism
Urinary tract infection
Wound infection

Carcinoma of breast with metastasis (Code: 174)

CONCURRENT CRITERIA
Identification of patient's physical and psychosocial needs and/or concerns

Expression of concern about body image and relationship with spouse
Assessment of wound and arm function
Expression of feelings about treatment and prognosis
Indication of presence or absence of generalized discomforts and/or pain
Adjustment to diagnosis of cancer and fear of dying

Recommended nursing action consistent with diagnosis
Nursing services

Observe wound
Care for wound, if indicated
Monitor pain status
Assess mobility of affected limbs
Provide emotional support

Health education

Explain activity limits and goals
Explain methods of preventing infections
Acquaint with available resources and sources of rental of hospital equipment for home use
Explain rationale to treatments and medications
Instruct about consulting physician

Indicators for discharge
Adaptation to health status

Treatment goals of inpatient hospitalization reached

Plan for appropriate care and follow-up after discharge implemented
Disease and specific treatment goals understood

Examples of community resources

Public health nurse or Visting Nurse Association
Reach to Recovery
American Cancer Society

RETROSPECTIVE CRITERIA
Health

Pain controlled
Patient/family understand wound care

Activity

Maximum level of mobility reached

Knowledge

Patient/family understanding of appropriate follow-up care and resources
Patient/family understanding of diagnosis

COMPLICATIONS

Hypercalcemia
Mental depression
Spinal cord compression resulting from tumor
Wound infection

Carcinoma of cervix, clinically invasive, with radiation and/or chemotherapy (Code: 180.1)

CONCURRENT CRITERIA
Identification of patient's physical and psychosocial needs and/or concerns

Understanding of purpose, procedure, and side effects of radiation and/or chemotherapy

Understanding of nursing measures used to reduce side effects of therapy

Guilt, hostility, grief, fear of death, and/or anxiety over changing role and body image as related to disease and/or treatment

Preventive measures against secondary infection and/or bleeding caused by bone marrow depression

Maintenance of adequate nutrition, hydration, and elimination

Recommended nursing action consistent with diagnosis
Nursing services

Implement measures to reduce pain caused by the disease or discomforts as related to side effects of therapy

Implement measures to aid the patient in dealing with possible death, change in role or body image as related to disease and/or treatment, including encouraging the patient to ventilate feelings, providing realistic hope, suggesting the use of scarves or wigs when alopecia is present and cosmetics to hide changes in skin pigmentation (when this will not interfere with therapy); use diversional therapy; maintain patient's activities of daily living as much as possible; support family members so they, in turn, can support the patient; and secure necessary assistance in the home for health care and/or family care through social service

Implement measures to maintain proper nutrition, hydration, and elimination, including withdrawal of drug when uncontrolled diarrhea, mucositis, nausea, and vomiting occur; administer antidiarrhea and antiemetic drugs as ordered; provide oral hygiene with hydrogen peroxide three times daily, using nonabrasive cleaning materials; apply topical anesthetics to mucous membranes; instruct patient to avoid irritating foods and fluids, alcoholic beverages, and smoking; administer parenteral fluids according to type and amount ordered per 24 hours; suggest tube feedings or hyperalimentation; provide small frequent feedings of high-protein, high-carbohydrate, low-residue, bland foods with 6 to 8 feedings daily; force fluids to 2,800 to 3,000 ml daily; maintain intake and output; monitor and report blood chemistries daily; provide foods to correct constipation; establish bladder control program and, if unsuccessful, insert Foley catheter

Implement measures to prevent bleeding or secondary infection caused by bone marrow depression, including daily monitoring of leukocyte, erythrocyte, and platelet counts; report findings to physician daily; withhold drug until further orders if leukocytes fall below 1,200; implement reverse isolation; administer appropriate antibiotics; observe closely for bleeding and report signs of bleeding to physician, stating type and amount and presence of petechiae, bruises, or frank bleeding; administer replacement therapy for blood loss, if necessary, and prepare patient for packing, cauterization, or ligation, as may be necessary; take vital signs, including temperature, every 4 hours or more often if patient's condition warrants it; implement measures to reduce skin breakdown as a source for infection and promote incisional healing

Initiate discharge planning and referrals; give emotional support to patient/family

Health education

Instruct as to name, purpose, dosage, frequency, side effects, action to take if side effects occur, and precautions of each discharge medication

Instruct about diet, care of skin as related to radiation therapy, and measures to reduce side effects and discomforts of therapy

Explain wound care, if necessary (operational or as related to arterial infusion)

Instruct as to therapeutic and restricted activities

Explain when to return to clinic or physician's office for follow-up medical care

Indicators for discharge
Adaptation to health status

Condition stable
Complications not evident
Health teaching completed
Referrals made

Examples of community resources

American Cancer Society
Visting Nurse Association or public health nurse
Cancer clinic
Social services

RETROSPECTIVE CRITERIA
Health

Condition stable
Complications not evident

Activity

Ambulatory
Able to implement wound care properly
Understands therapeutic and restricted activities and can implement therapeutic ones properly
Able to give proper skin care as related to therapy
Able to implement measures to reduce side effects of therapy

Knowledge

Knows the name and understands the purpose, dosage, frequency, side effects, action to take if side effects occur, and precautions as related to each discharge medication
Understands diet
Knows when to return to clinic or physician's office for follow-up care
Aware of community resources available

COMPLICATIONS

Chemotherapy complications
Hemorrhage
Hydronephrosis
Hydroureter
Impaired kidney function
Incontinence of urine and feces
Infection
Mental depression
Metastasis to regional lymph nodes
Pain in back
Pelvic infections
Pneumonia
Uremia
Vaginal fistulas to the gastrointestinal and urinary tracts
Vascular and/or lymphatic stasis

Carcinoma of cervix, clinically invasive, with surgical intervention
(Code: 180.1)

CONCURRENT CRITERIA
Identification of patient's physical and psychosocial needs and/or concerns

Relief from leukorrhea, irregular vaginal bleeding, or pain

Understanding of medical, surgical, and nursing management of condition, so that realistic plans for health maintenance after discharge can be made

Fear of dying, concern over changes in body image or sexual role, and depression over diagnosis of cancer

Preventive measures concerning problems of immobility and postoperative complications

Recommended nursing action consistent with diagnosis
Nursing services

Implement preoperative nursing care and patient teaching, including assisting patient in dealing with fears of dying, relieving discomforts, providing adequate hydration, nutrition, and elimination, and explaining surgical procedure, recovery room, estimated period of hospitalization, methods that will be used postoperatively to reduce pain, deep breathing, turning, exercises, graduated steps to ambulation, presence and duration of Foley catheter, possibility of nasogastric tube, duration of order for nothing by mouth and intravenous therapy, dressings, or discharges

Physically prepare patient for surgery

Implement postoperative nursing care, including prevention of and observation for complications; administer prompt nursing intervention should signs of complications occur

Initiate discharge planning and referrals

Health education

Instruct on the name, purpose, dosage, frequency, side effects, action to take if side effects occur, and precautions concerning each discharge medication

Give diet instruction about food restrictions, if any, as well as foods included in special diet, if ordered; cooking methods; frequency of meals; measures to reduce nausea and to increase retention of foods, if this has been a past problem or is an anticipated problem

Instruct patient on therapeutic and restricted activities

Instruct patient on any necessary wound care

Instruct patient when and why it is necessary to return to clinic or physician's office for follow-up medical care

Indicators for discharge
Adaptation to health status

Condition stable
Complications not evident
Health teaching completed
Referrals made

Examples of community resources

Cancer clinic or surgical clinic
Visiting Nurse Association or public health nurse
Social services
American Cancer Society

RETROSPECTIVE CRITERIA
Health

Condition stable
Complications not evident

Activity

Ambulatory
Able to administer necessary wound care correctly
Independent in activities of daily living

Knowledge

Understands name, purpose, dosage, frequency, side effects, action to take if side effects occur, and precautions of each discharge medication

Understands therapeutic and restricted activities and can implement therapeutic ones

Understands and can implement diet

Understands and can implement correct techniques of wound care

Knows when to return to clinic or physician's office for follow-up care

COMPLICATIONS

Alterations in sex role
Arrhythmias
Atelectasis
Drug reaction
Hemorrhage
Incontinence of urine and feces
Metastasis to regional lymph nodes
Pelvic infections
Pneumonia
Pulmonary embolism
Respiratory embarrassment
Shock
Temperature of 100° F or over at time of discharge
Thrombophlebitis
Urinary incontinence
Urinary infections
Urinary retention
Vaginal fistulas to gastrointestinal and urinary tracts
Vascular and/or lymphatic stasis
Wound infection

Carcinoma of colon with metastasis (Codes: 153-153.8)

CONCURRENT CRITERIA
Identification of patient's physical and psychosocial needs and/or concerns

Expression of concern about body image
Expression of feelings about treatment and prognosis
Maintenance of body functions
Indication of presence or absence of generalized discomforts and/or pain

Recommended nursing action consistent with diagnosis
Nursing services

Assess level of pain and provide relief
Provide emotional support to patient and family
Assess bowel function and treat appropriately
Observe and assess laboratory tests and diagnostic procedures
Improve and/or maintain all body functions

Health education

Teach plan of bowel care to patient and/or family

Explain disease process and effects on body systems
Acquaint patient with available resources
Explain rationale to treatment and medications
Explain indicators about which to consult physician after discharge

Indicators for discharge
Adaptation to health status

Patient/family knowledge of disease and specific treatment goals
Treatment goals of inpatient hospitalization reached
Plan for appropriate care and follow-up after discharge implemented

Examples of community resources

American Cancer Society
Public health nurse or Visiting Nurse Association
Ostomy specialist

RETROSPECTIVE CRITERIA
Health

Pain controlled

Bowel program established and understood by patient and family

Activity

Maximum level of activity reached

Knowledge

Patient/family understand appropriate follow-up care and resources

COMPLICATIONS

Chemotherapy complications
Hemorrhage
Local recurrence of carcinoma in anastomotic suture line
Lymphatic or blood vessel invasion
Pneumonia
Skin irritation
Wound infection

Carcinoma of lung with metastasis (Code: 162.2-162.9)

CONCURRENT CRITERIA
Identification of patient's physical and psychosocial needs and/or concerns

Maintenance of adequate respiratory function

Maintenance of maximum comfort

Expression of concerns over disease process and treatment and fear of death

Maintenance of activity level appropriate to retain strength

Recommended nursing action consistent with diagnosis
Nursing services

Observation of respiratory status with measures to correct deficiencies

Observation of pain status with appropriate pain control

Assessment of activity tolerance with appropriate limit setting

Emotionally supportive care for patient and family

Health education

Help patient determine activity tolerance and set goals

Instruct as to prevention of infections

Explain rationale for treatment and medications

Acquaint patient with availability of community resources

Indicators for discharge
Adaptation to health status

Patient able to perform activities of daily living

Patient able to maintain maximum comfort

Patient has reached treatment goals of hospitalization

Patient/family have sufficient knowledge of disease process, treatment, and goals

Appropriate discharge planning completed

Examples of community resources

Visiting Nurse Association or public health nurse

American Cancer Society

RETROSPECTIVE CRITERIA
Health

Pain controlled
Afebrile

Activity

Maximum activity tolerance reached and understood by patient/family

Knowledge

Patient/family understand diagnosis, treatment, and medications

Patient/family aware of available resources

COMPLICATIONS

Atelectasis
Empyema
Hemoptysis
Lung abscess
Pleural effusion
Pneumonia
Pneumothorax
Septicemia

Carcinoma of ovary with metastasis (Code: 183)

CONCURRENT CRITERIA
Identification of patient's physical and psychosocial needs and/or concerns

Concern about change of body and self-image and of diagnosis of cancer; fear of death
Understanding of needs concerning progress, treatment, family perception, and spiritual contentment
Relief of pain
Observation for further symptoms of metastasis

Recommended nursing action consistent with diagnosis
Nursing services

Provide emotional support
Relieve discomfort
Observe and treat wound, if indicated
Monitor symptoms for further possible metastases

Health education

Explain disease process, progress, and treatments, available resources, activity limits and goals, indicators about which to consult the physician, methods of prevention of infection and other complications, and reassurance that complications are manageable

Indicators for discharge
Adaptation to health status

Treatment goals of inpatient hospitalization reached
Plans for appropriate care and follow-up after discharge made
Patient/family understand disease and specific treatment goals

Examples of community resources

American Cancer Society
Visiting Nurse Association or public health nurse

RETROSPECTIVE CRITERIA
Health

Pain controlled

Activity

Ambulatory

Knowledge

Knowledge of disease process, treatments, prognosis, symptoms of complications

COMPLICATIONS

Chemotherapy complications
Hemorrhage
Infections
Pneumonia

Carcinoma of pancreas with metastasis (Code: 157.9)

CONCURRENT CRITERIA
Identification of patient's physical and psychosocial needs and/or concerns

Relief of dull, steady, aching pain by supportive measures such as ordered medication and positioning

Modification to a bland, fat-free, controlled calorie diet, since pancreatic enzymes are not present for food digestion

Establishment of a diabetic regime for administration of insulin if pancreatic beta cells are affected and for glucagon if pancreatic alpha cells are affected

Concern over altered body image and lifestyle

Care in transferring to avoid the possibility of pathological fractures

Recommended nursing action consistent with diagnosis
Nursing services

Watch for signs of common bile duct obstruction (jaundice, dark, tea-colored urine, clay-colored stools with positive guaiac test, ascites) and other complications

Observe for hypo- or hyperglycemia by Clinitest and Acetest

Monitor vital signs every 4 hours

Observe and auscultate abdomen; measure girth daily

Health education

Teach administration of insulin and glucagon

Have dietician explain bland, low-fat, controlled-calorie diet for diabetic maintenance

Teach restrictions of activity and diet, and side effects of medications

Teach how to transfer from bed to chair (and vice versa) safely to prevent falls and fractures

Indicators for discharge
Adaptation to health status

Afebrile

Able to tolerate pain and effects of radiation and chemotherapy

Ambulatory

Able to tolerate bland, low-fat, controlled calorie diet and to utilize these foods

Examples of community resources

Visiting Nurse Association
Public health nurse
American Cancer Society

RETROSPECTIVE CRITERIA
Health

Afebrile
Pain controlled

Activity

Ambulatory
Administers own insulin, if indicated

Knowledge

Patient/family understand follow-up care, diagnosis, medication, diet, and chemotherapy

COMPLICATIONS

Chemotherapy complications
Diabetes as result of surgical removal of pancreas
Hemorrhage
Infection
Thrombophlebitis in legs

Carcinoma of prostate with metastasis (Code: 185)

CONCURRENT CRITERIA
Identification of patient's physical and psychosocial needs and/or concerns

Feelings of despair, depression, anger, fear, and rejection

Concern about treatment and prognosis

Concern about change in body function and image and about presence of generalized pain

Recommended nursing action consistent with diagnosis
Nursing services

Provide perineal, retropubic, or suprapubic wound care as indicated after radical prostectomy through open wound surgical approach

Observe for progress in healing and signs of disturbances in healing

Watch for hemorrhage, oliguria (uremia), or anuria (metastasis to kidney); note and record color of urine and intake and output

Note pain status, location, duration

Provide supportive care; assess activity level

Health education

In case of urinary and fecal incontinence from surgery, help patient regain fecal control through perineal exercise, contracting and relaxing gluteal muscles

Teach patient how to keep dry and odor free; make self-care simple and routine

Include family of patient in teachings; explain reason for procedures and medications prescribed

Teach principles of cleanliness to prevent infections

Inform patient and family of agencies available for assistance

Indicators for discharge
Adaptation to health status

Inhospital goals completed

Nature of disease understood by family, who will provide patient with appropriate follow-up and outpatient treatments

Discharge environment suitable and appropriate

Examples of community resources

American Cancer Society

Social worker or clergyman

Public health nurse or Visiting Nurse Association

RETROSPECTIVE CRITERIA
Health

Pain controlled

Suitable discharge environment available

Output at least 1,000 ml per day

Activity

Maximum level reached

Knowledge

Patient/family understanding of diagnosis, follow-up care, and medications

COMPLICATIONS

Hemorrhage

Infection

Low back pain with metastases to bones of pelvis and spine

Pathological fractures

Pneumonia

Radiotherapy complications

Renal damage

Renal insufficiency

Urinary obstruction

Carcinoma of stomach with metastasis (Code: 151.9)

CONCURRENT CRITERIA
Identification of patient's physical and psychosocial needs and/or concerns

Relief of dyspepsia
Relief of pain and/or other discomforts if present
Necessity of surgery (gastric resection, gastrectomy, gastrostomy)
Concern over treatment and prognosis

Recommended nursing action consistent with diagnosis
Nursing services

Explain operative procedure and possible outcome, if applicable
Be alert for signs of complications
Offer emotional support to patient and family
Observe and control pain and other discomforts

Health education

Explain diet instructions, disease process, treatment, rationale, wound care (if applicable), use of available resources, and prevention of infection or other complications

Indicators for discharge
Adaptation to health status

Adequate nutritional state; following proper diet
Plans for appropriate care and follow-up after discharge

Recognition of symptoms that require professional care
Patient/family understanding of disease and specific treatment goals

Examples of community resources

Public health nurse
American Cancer Society
Visiting Nurse Association

RETROSPECTIVE CRITERIA
Health

Free of pain or pain controlled by medications
Able to eat and drink without nausea and vomiting

Activity

Ambulatory

Knowledge

Patient/family understand follow-up care, diagnosis, and medications
Patient/family understand and can implement proper diet

COMPLICATIONS

Chemotherapy complications
Hemorrhage
Infection
Nausea and vomiting
Physical deterioration

Carcinoma of uterus with metastasis (Code: 182.9)

CONCURRENT CRITERIA
Identification of patient's physical and psychosocial needs and/or concerns

Feelings regarding treatment, prognosis, and sexuality

Relief of pain and/or generalized discomforts

Understanding of emotional sensitivity resulting from hormonal changes

Assessment of body function status

Recommended nursing action consistent with diagnosis
Nursing services

Provide emotional support to patient and family

Observe for signs of infection and/or vaginal discharge, including hemorrhage; note color, consistency, and amount

Observe and control pain and other discomforts

Monitor symptoms indicating metastasis

Health education

Explain physical activity limitations, including sexual activity

Explain effect of hormonal changes on all phases of reproductive process and emotions

Explain rationale to treatment

Explain indicators about which to consult physician, such as discharge; explain prevention of infection, including use of tampons and douching

Indicators for discharge
Adaptation to health status

Treatment goals of inpatient hospitalization reached

Plans for appropriate care and follow-up after discharge made

Disease and specific treatment goals understood by patient and family

Examples of community resources

American Cancer Society
Public health nurse
Visiting Nurse Association

RETROSPECTIVE CRITERIA
Health

Pain controlled
Afebrile

Activity

Ambulatory

Knowledge

Patient/family understanding of disease, prognosis, treatment, follow-up care, and medications

COMPLICATIONS
Back pain
Chemotherapy complications
Edema of legs
Hydronephrosis
Hydroureter
Impaired kidney function
Pelvic infections
Septicemia
Vascular and lymphatic stasis
Wound infection

Carcinomatosis (Code: 199)

CONCURRENT CRITERIA
Identification of patient's physical and psychosocial needs and/or concerns

Relief of generalized discomfort
Feelings about prognosis and treatment
Maintenance of self-worth
Maintenance of body functions
Emotional support for coping with death and dying

Recommended nursing action consistent with diagnosis
Nursing services

Observe laboratory work
Assess level of pain; provide relief
Provide emotional support
Provide safe environment
Maintain and/or improve present strengths and physical condition

Health education

Instruct on activity limitations and goals
Teach prevention of infections
Acquaint with available resources
Explain rationale to treatments and medications
Teach indications about which to consult physician

Indicators for discharge
Adaptation to health status

Treatment goals of inpatient hospitalization reached
Plan for appropriate care and follow-up after discharge implemented

Examples of community resources

American Cancer Society
Public health nurse or Visiting Nurse Association
Social services

RETROSPECTIVE CRITERIA
Health

Pain controlled

Activity

Assistance in activities of daily living
Assistance in ambulation

Knowledge

Patient and family understand appropriate follow-up care and resources

COMPLICATIONS

Drug reaction
Infections
Mental depression
Pain
Physical deterioration

Cardiac arrhythmias in children (Codes: 427.2 to 427.9)

CONCURRENT CRITERIA
Identification of patient's physical and psychosocial needs and/or concerns

Fear of monitoring equipment, limited mobility associated with monitoring devices, and possible rejection by parents because of machinery-induced image change
Necessary corrective treatment for any cardiac arrhythmias

Relief from perfusion deficit that leads to decreased strength, level of consciousness, and mentation
Relief from reactions to medications such as digitalis

Recommended nursing action consistent with diagnosis
Nursing services

Document activity level that results in perfusion deficit

Encourage parents and child to participate in care, such as assisting in elec-
trode placement

Accurately observe and record cardiac
functioning and drug therapy and
report reactions to medications

Nurse or parent provides activity consistent with type of monitoring equipment
needed and cardiac functioning, such
as lap sitting for "bed rest" children:
use telemetry if possible

Provide appropriate play therapy to aid
patient in adapting to hospitalization

Health education

Instruct parents on desired drug effects,
possible side effects to be reported to
medical personnel, cause of disease (if
identifiable), course, treatment, and
prognosis, so realistic plans will be
made of the child

Identify alternative activities below the
perfusion deficit level

Discuss function of monitor with parents
and child

Instruct parents on importance of continuous, regular cardiac follow-up care

Indicators for discharge
Adaptation to health status

Presence of stable heart rhythm

Parents/child comfortable with information about diagnosis and prognosis and
willing for child to return home

Understanding by parents of drug regimen and effects

Child sleeping well

Weight not less than at admission

Examples of community resources

School nurse

American Heart Association

Visiting Nurse Association or public
health nurse

RETROSPECTIVE CRITERIA
Health

Presence of stable heart rhythm

Absence of heart failure

Activity

Ambulatory

Knowledge

Understand medication schedule

Recognize signs of digitoxin toxicity, if
taking this drug

Know how to take child's pulse

Understand importance of continuous,
regular cardiac follow-up care

COMPLICATIONS

Cardiac arrest

Congestive heart failure

Ventricular fibrillation

Ventricular tachycardia

Cardiac diagnostic testing (Codes: 427.2, 427.9)

CONCURRENT CRITERIA
Identification of patient's physical and
psychosocial needs and/or concerns

Adaptation to physical limitations
brought on by condition being diagnosed

Relief of pain, dyspnea, pallor, and weakness

Fear of diagnostic procedures and findings

Fear of death

Adjustment to possible alteration in body
image

Recommended nursing action consistent
with diagnosis
Nursing services

Maintain physical quiet with bed rest, if
necessary, 18 hours prior to testing

Permit nothing by mouth after midnight
prior to testing, if applicable

Acquaint patient with individuals who

will be caring for patient following testing

Report temperature above 99.6° F

Report cardiac dysrhythmias, changes in heart sounds

Health education

Give patient a detailed, matter-of-fact, chronological explanation of procedures, including administration of intravenous solution before/after, state of consciousness before/during/after, presence of breathing equipment during/after, presence of trusted members of health team before/during/after testing

Indicate specific waiting area for family members during/after testing; give broad estimates of length of time for procedure and time when visiting can resume

Explain reasons for each test and what results will show

Indicators for discharge
Adaptation to health status

Decrease in anxiety level

Patient/family understanding of and will-

ingness to comply with physical activity limitations, if any

Plans made to return for definitive treatment, if indicated

Examples of community resources

Occupational health nurse at place of employment

School nurse, if student

RETROSPECTIVE CRITERIA
Health

Reduced anxiety level

Activity

At or above admission level

Knowledge

Understands nature of procedure experienced

Understands prognosis, if known

Understands purpose and effects of medication

COMPLICATIONS

Cardiac dysrhythmias

Drug reaction

Severe reaction to x-ray contrast media

Cataract (Codes: 374.9, 744.3)

CONCURRENT CRITERIA
Identification of patient's physical and psychosocial needs and/or concerns

Relief of symptoms, including gradual blurring of vision, light scattering, double vision, other visual distortions, and progressive nearsightedness with senile cataract

Fear of dependency resulting from second-degree blindness or fear of surgery

Understanding of diseases progress, treatment, medical and nursing management, duration of hospitalization, expected outcomes, and use of corrective lens following discharge

Adjustment for postoperative period when eye patches will be used, including orientation to environment, communication, and methods of safe ambulation

Recommended nursing action consistent with diagnosis
Nursing services

Administer and observe reactions to medications such as osmotic diuretics or cycloplegic drugs

Listen to expressions of fear; reassure patient by explaining surgical procedure, recovery room, use of eye bandages, measures to prevent postoperative discomfort and/or nausea and vomiting

Implement preoperative nursing care, including measures to ensure nutrition, hydration, and elimination; physically prepare patient for surgery

Administer postoperative nursing care, including use of smooth rolling bed to move patient; orientate patient to darkness; provide communications; prevent nausea and vomiting; provide nutrition, hydration, and elimination; observe physiological response parameters

Plan discharge and identify person to continue eye care after discharge

Health education

Teach patient/family methods of instillation of eye medications, eye bandage care, prevention of contaminating eye medication, medication dosage, frequency, duration, and side effects to report to physician

Explain disease process, treatment, medical and nursing management, duration of hospitalization, expected outcomes, when to return for corrective lends, and symptoms to report to physician

Instruct in methods for safe ambulation and means of communication during use of eye bandages

Teach activity limitations and/or restrictions

Indicators for discharge
Adaptation to health status

Patient administers own medications and eye care, unless unassociated limitations exist

Planning with physician about securing cataract eyeglasses and about follow-up physician visits completed

Complications not evident

Health teaching completed

Examples of community resources

Visiting Nurse Association or public health nurse

RETROSPECTIVE CRITERIA
Health

Complications not evident

Cataract surgically removed

Activity

Safe ambulation within activity limitations

Activities of daily living with minimal assistance

Knowledge

Understands and can verbalize instructions about medication, eye care, discharge care, disease process, and symptoms to report to physician

COMPLICATIONS

Cystoid maculopathy (following hospitalization)

Intraocular hemorrhage

Postoperative intraocular infection

Shallow anterior chamber

Vitreous loss with retinal detachment or corneal damage

Cerebellar degenerative disease (ataxia, coordination disturbances)
(Code: 773.4)

CONCURRENT CRITERIA
Identification of patient's physical and psychosocial needs and/or concerns

Relief from symptoms, including dysmetria, dysdiadochokinesia, dysarthria, intention tremors, cerebellar nystagmus, hypotonia, loss of equilibrium, and/or sensory changes

Maintenance of adequate hydration, nutrition, and elimination

Anxiety over and assistance in coping with increased dependence and changes in body image and life-style

Understanding of medical and nursing management, course of disease, prognosis, and needs for home care in order to make realistic plans for the management of patient outside acute care setting

Recommended nursing action consistent with diagnosis
Nursing services

Implement measures to maintain proper nutrition, hydration, and elimination

Implement measures to prevent injury and problems caused by immobility

Implement measures designed to assist the patient and family in coping with increased dependence of the patient and changes in patient's body image and life-style

Implement measures designed to reduce severity of coordination problem, for example, the use of adaptive devices, such as weighted silverware, plate guards, plastic cups, and covered drinking glasses with straw holes

Observe for effectiveness of drug therapy and for side effects, with proper nursing intervention should any occur

Health education

Provide family/patient with activity education regarding measures to take to avoid fatigue, such as pacing techniques, scheduled rest periods, therapeutic and restricted activities

Instruct family/patient on diet-soft or regular diet, depending on disability; use of finger foods; need for small, frequent (2-hour) feedings; use of weighted eating utensils and plate guards, if patient can feed self; teach methods of feeding patient; instruct on daily fluid requirement and methods of achieving it

Instruct in the use of adaptive devices; range of motion, active and passive, flexor and extensor, and resistive exercises; the need and method of achieving good skin care, frequent turning, if bedridden, Foley catheter care, if the patient is discharged with one, and transfer techniques; and the use of safety measures and devices

Instruct regarding the name of each discharge medication and the dosage, frequency, side effects, action to take should side effects occur, purpose of medication, and precautions for each drug

Educate concerning community agencies available for assistance in care after discharge

Indicators for discharge
Adaptation to health status

Condition stable
Complications not evident
Referrals made

Examples of community resources

Multiple Sclerosis Association (ataxic conditions)

Visiting Nurse Association, public health nurse, home health aid program, and Meals on Wheels

Social services and physical or vocational rehabilitation centers (for family member or patient)

RETROSPECTIVE CRITERIA
Health

Condition stable
Complications not evident

Activity

Gait and coordination improved
Able to carry out activities of daily living with adaptive devices

Knowledge

Patient/family understands and can implement activity restrictions; pacing techniques; rest periods; therapeutic exercises (range of motion, active, passive, resistive); proper diet and methods for self-feeding or, when necessary, assisted feedings with proper quantity of intake; application and use of prosthetic devices or adaptive devices; skin care; frequent change of position and proper alignment; and Foley catheter care
Patient/family knows and understands the purpose and name of each discharge medication and the dosage, frequency, side effects, action to take should side effects occur, and precautions for each drug
Patient/family understands the role of community agencies available to assist them with care after discharge

COMPLICATIONS

Atelectasis
Bladder dysfunction
Bulbar or pseudobulbar palsy
Decubitus ulcer
Dysphagia
Injury from falling
Pneumonia

Cerebral palsy (Code: 343.9)

CONCURRENT CRITERIA
Identification of patient's physical and psychosocial needs and/or concerns

Control of symptoms, including vomiting, cyanosis; mental retardation; decreased muscle tone; spasticity of arms, trunk, or legs; incoordination; bizarre purposeless movements; rigidity of postural attitudes; ataxias; difficulty swallowing and chewing; visual, hearing, or speech impairments; and possibly emotional or behavioral disturbances, convulsions, and/or contractures
Maintenance of vital bodily functions and prevention of physical, mental, and social deterioration, including adequate nutrition, hydration, and elimination; protection from and prevention of trauma such as aspiration (respiratory distress); falls (fractures); seizures (fractures, aspiration, head injuries, respiratory distress, and emotional trauma); vomiting (aspiration and inanition); immobility (problems from circulatory stasis, such as emboli and decubitus ulcers, infections such as urinary infection and pneumonia); social isolation (behavioral disturbances); sensory deprivation (impairment of normal mental growth)
Ego supportive measures and discipline
Instruction in adaptive measures and methods by which to reach maximum potential
Understanding by family of nursing and medical management of child, so that realistic plans for care after discharge can be made

Recommended nursing action consistent with diagnosis
Nursing services

Ensure adequate nutrition, hydration, and elimination by encouragement of parental participation in feeding child under supervision; proper positioning of child for maximum eating ease; proper placement of food in child's mouth so that swallowing is facilitated and choking or vomiting is reduced; proper rest prior to feeding time so that child is not too tired to eat; teach child to feed self with adapted eating utensils; provide atmosphere conducive to self-feeding (and do not worry about a messy floor) by giving preferred foods, foods that the child can keep on a spoon, such as mashed potatoes, thick puddings, fruits that are thick in consistency, or finger foods, by eating with other children in the same age group when possible; implement use of prosthetic devices to control unwanted movements and to assist in coordination in older cerebral palsy patients; use consistency in approach to bladder and bowel control program

Implement safety measures, including parental participation in safety measures, selection of toys that with parental guidance are safe, use of helmets for ataxic children who fall easily, seizure precautions and care for convulsive children, proper positioning of children or infants for maximum comfort and breathing action; and use of suction machine to prevent respiratory distress, when necessary

Implement measures to assist family in coping with stresses of cerebral palsy

Implement rehabilitiative measures, including appropriate exercises to maintain muscle strength; proper alignment and use of supportive devices to prevent contractures; use of prosthetic devices, such as casts, braces, splints, to assist in the control of unwanted movements and to correct deformities; use of play techniques, such as pegboard games or puzzles to improve coordination; speech therapy and physiotherapy; vision correction if necessary; vocational guidance and rehabilitation; occupational therapy; methods for achieving activities of daily living; and adjustment measures to assist patient in adaptation of sexual role

Initiate appropriate referrals

Health education

Instruct physical care of child and application of prosthetic devices, use of adaptive devices, skin care, positioning, alignment techniques, exercises (physical and speech), feeding techniques, bladder and bowel control methods, and play techniques

Instruct parents in ego supportive measures and necessity to impose limits and discipline child

Instruct as to importance of regular medical and dental check-ups as well as surveillance for visual and hearing difficulties

Instruct as to patient's restrictions or limitation and capabilities as related to severity of cerebral palsy

Instruct about measures that promote maximum achievement of potential, including socialization, physical and mental stimulation, interaction with a normal environment, administration of medications to control tremors or spasticity (patient, if possible, and family should know the name of each drug and the dosage, frequency, purpose, side effects, actions to take if side effects occur, and precautions for each drug), development of problem-solving ability within limitations of disorder, and establishment of realistic short-term and long-term goals

Indicators for discharge
Adaptation to health status

Condition stable
Complications not evident
Necessary teaching completed
Referrals made

Examples of community resources

National Cerebral Palsy Association or social services
School nurse, exceptional child center, or rehabilitation centers (blind, deaf, physical, vocational, and speech)
Visiting Nurse Association or public health nurse

RETROSPECTIVE CRITERIA
Health

Condition stable; symptoms controlled
Complications not evident

Activity

Muscle function appropriate for age improved within limitations of disease
Coordination appropriate for age improved

Knowledge

Patient, when possible, and parents understand and are able to implement physical care, such as application of prosthetic devices, use of adaptive devices, skin care, positioning, alignment, exercises, and feeding techniques
Patient, when possible, and parents understand and know the name of each discharge medication and the dosage, frequency, purpose, side effects, action to take if side effects occur, and precautions for each drug

Parents understand and are able to provide ego supportive measures and discipline for child
Parents understand restrictions and capabilities as related to severity of cerebral palsy
Parents understand and can implement regular medical and dental check-ups and can provide surveillance for visual and hearing difficulties
Parents understand the importance of and can implement the following: socialization, physical and mental stimulation, development measures for problem-solving skills, and realistic short-term and long-term goals
Parents understand and can implement safety measures

COMPLICATIONS

Deafness
Decubitus ulcers
Dystonia
Joint contractures
Speech impairment

Cerebrovascular accident, acute (Codes: 331, 332, 332.1, 334.8)

CONCURRENT CRITERIA
Identification of patient's physical and psychosocial needs and/or concerns

Observation for alteration in condition, including changes in level of consciousness, behavior, vital signs, temperature, urinary output, and cardiovascular functioning
Maintenance of vital bodily functions, including adequate ventilation, elimination, normal body temperature, cardiovascular functioning, and adequate hydration and nutrition
Minimization of functional loss from initial accident; prevention of physical trauma and physical deterioration, such as contractures, fractures, circulatory problems from stasis, infections, sensory disturbances, or corneal ulcers; prevent aspiration of food and fluids; maintain nutrition and hydration
Restoration of motor functions—mobility, bowel and bladder control, communication, visual correction, activities of daily living—to optimal level possible
Assistance in adjusting to changes in body image; protection from mental trauma; prevention of intellectual regression

Recommended nursing action consistent with diagnosis
Nursing services

Implement and evaluate plan for acquiring mobility, improving motor function, and preventing complications
Implement and evaluate plan for providing adequate nutrition and hydration

and for preventing aspiration of foods and fluids

Implement and evaluate plan for controlling bowel and bladder

Implement and evaluate plan for improving communication and minimizing effects of visual disturbances

Implement and evaluate plan for modifying patient's life-style to fit needs or activities of daily living and restrictions imposed by condition

Health education

Explain to family/patient about medical and/or surgical management of patient

Explain to family/patient about nursing management of patient

Educate family concerning patient's emotional needs and behavior

Educate family concerning assisting health agencies, such as social services, Visiting Nurse Association, public health nurse, speech rehabilitation centers, and stroke centers

Indicators for discharge
Adaptation to health status

Condition stable

Motor, sensory, and mental status improved

Complications not evident

Family and/or responsible person assisting with care understands medical and/or surgical and nursing management

Necessary means and equipment for patient's discharge care available

Examples of community resources

Visiting Nurse Association or public health nurse

Speech and physical rehabilitation centers

Stroke clinic

RETROSPECTIVE CRITERIA
Health

Complications not evident
Condition stable
Discharge environment medically safe

Activity

Able to communicate needs to others
Shows progressive improvement in bowel and bladder control
Able to assume a degree of mobility in keeping with level of impairment

Knowledge

Patient/family understands diet, medications, speech rehabilitation program, vision correction program, bowel and bladder program, motor rehabilitation program, and patient's abilities and limitations

Aware of referral agencies that have been contracted to assist patient after discharge from acute care setting; understands purpose of these agencies

Patient/family expresses realistic plans for care after discharge

COMPLICATIONS

Aphasia
Atelectasis
Decubitus ulcers
Neurological deficit
Paralysis
Pneumonia
Pulmonary embolism
Shock
Subarachnoid hemorrhage
Urinary incontinence
Urinary infection
Urinary retention

Cerebrovascular accident, chronic (Code: 8)

CONCURRENT CRITERIA
Identification of patient's physical and psychosocial needs and/or concerns

Protection from mental trauma and the prevention of intellectual regression, including avoidance of sensory deprivation or overload and highly frustrating situations; avoidance of treatment as a nonperson, including invasion of privacy or delayed fulfillment of needs, provision of adequate time for patient response to directives, questions, and situations; explanation and instruction as to purpose of procedures, diagnostic studies, directives, and requests; explanations and instructions given very slowly; assistance in adjusting to changes in body image; assistance and encouragement in gaining and retaining motivation to improve

Protection from physical trauma and prevention of physical deterioration, including promotion of adequate nutrition and hydration, with 2,500 ml every 24 hours and 100 gm protein intake every 24 hours; prevention of further immobility from contractures, join dislocations, or fractures; prevention of problems of immobility, such as circulatory stasis, phlebitis, decubitus ulcers, thrombus, infections of urinary tract and respiratory system, inadequate elimination of urine or urinary or fecal incontinence or retention; prevention of sensory disturbances, such as hallucinations, confusion, loss of balance, and loss of awareness of body part positions; prevention of corneal ulcers, if eye muscle function has deteriorated; and prevention of aspiration of food and fluids, if swallowing ability has deteriorated

Restoration of motor function to optimal level within restrictions of neurological deficits, including promoting acquisition of mobility to highest level possible, promoting bowel and bladder control to highest degree possible, promoting nonverbal and/or verbal communications, minimizing effects of diplopia and/or hemianopia, and aiding in adapting and modifying life-style to permit activities of daily living to be carried out as normally as possible

Understanding of medical and nursing management and means by which further strokes can be averted

Understanding and support of family

Recommended nursing action consistent with diagnosis
Nursing services

Implement and evaluate plan for acquiring mobility, improving motor functions, and preventing contractures, joint dislocations, and fractures

Implement and evaluate plan for prevention of aspiration of food and fluids; promote adequate nutrition and hydration

Implement and evaluate plan for bowel and bladder control

Implement and evaluate plans for communication improvement and for minimizing effects of visual disturbances

Implement and evaluate plan for aiding patient in modifying life-style to fit restrictions in carrying out independent activities of daily living imposed by condition

Health education

Teaching family/patient about medical management of patient, including diet for promotion of healing, prevention of constipation and/or diarrhea, and provision of nutrients necessary for neurological function (if obesity is a problem, also teach principles of sound nutrition with decreased calories); fluid intake with adequate hydration for support of normal functioning and bladder control regime, including recommended amount of fluid intake to ensure desired daily output and methods by which desired intake can be achieved; teach name, purpose, desired effect, side effects, action to take if side effects occur, dosage, and frequency of medications; explain activity restrictions and schedule of prescribed activity, stressing importance of consistency in environment and activity for orientation purposes; emphasize importance of regular medical and nursing follow-up care and restrictions for foods, activities, and nicotine

Teach family/patient about nursing management of patient, including positioning techniques, maintaining good alignment, administering range of motion exercises, triceps and quadriceps strengthening exercises, and transfer techniques; teach use of prosthetic, safety, and adaptive devices to assist patient in dressing, eating, and moving about; teach bowel and bladder regime, communication improvement techniques, means by which visual disturbance effects can be minimized, and methods by which the home environment can be modified to meet the patient's needs

Teach family about patient's emotional needs and behavior

Teach family about health agencies available to assist with discharge care

Indicators for discharge
Adaptation to health status

Condition stable

Motor, sensory, and mental status improved

Complications not evident

Family and/or responsible person assisting with care understands medical and nursing management

Necessary equipment for patient's discharge care available

Examples of community resources

Visiting Nurse Association or public health nurse

Speech and physical rehabilitation centers

Stroke clinic

RETROSPECTIVE CRITERIA
Health

Bowel and bladder control progressively improved

Complications not evident

Environment for discharge medically safe

Activity

Able to assume optimal level of activity necessary for self-care

Able to assume a degree of mobility in keeping with level of impairment

Knowledge

Patient/family understands diet, medications, speech and motor rehabilitation programs, visual correction program, bowel and bladder program, patient's abilities and limitations, and program to help patient acquire a degree of independence

Aware of referral agencies that have been contacted to assist patient after discharge from acute care setting; understands purposes and functions of these agencies

COMPLICATIONS

Aphasia
Atelectasis
Decubitus ulcers
Joint contractures
Mental depression
Pneumonia
Pulmonary embolism
Subarachnoid hemorrhage
Urinary incontinence
Urinary infections
Urinary retention

Cerebrovascular disease with paralysis (Codes: 430.1, 431.1, 431.3, 432.1, 433.1, 434.1, 436.1, 438)

CONCURRENT CRITERIA
Identification of patient's physical and psychosocial needs and/or concerns

Adaptation to hemiplegia, hemisensory loss, and feeding limitations

Observation for and prevention of bowel and bladder incontinence, aphasia, visual/perceptual deficits, and decubitus ulcers

Understanding of emotional alteration or reaction

Relief from medical complications, such as hypertension and reactions to anticoagulant therapy

Recommended nursing action consistent with diagnosis
Nursing services

Provide special positioning of paralyzed extremities every 2 hours, skin care, relief of pressure, prevention of friction burns, inspection of bony prominences every 2 to 3 hours, and passive range-of-motion to active exercises every 6 hours

Establish a bowel program either daily or every 2 to 3 days and a voiding program of every 3 to 4 hours during waking period

Measure pulse and blood pressure daily; monitor medications and administer prescribed medications

Reassess every 3 weeks; implement home assessment and family involvement

Establish counseling sessions for alterations in life-style and adaptations in activities of daily living; teach program of activities of daily living (self care, mouth care, dressing, grooming, assistive devices) and program of safety and environment awareness for hemianopia and/or other perceptual problems; establish a program of sitting, standing, transferring, ambulation, and/or wheel-chair use and a communication program for aphasic patients

Implement communication program for aphasic patients

Health education

Teach patient/family adaptations to disability, activities of daily living, and mobility program

Teach patient/family about cerebrovascular disease, prevention program, and health maintenance program

Teach medication regime and side effects

Teach safety program

Indicators for discharge
Adaptation to health status

Activities of daily living and mobility goals attained

Medical condition and vital signs stable

Care, disease, and prevention program understood by patient/family

Alterations necessary for home scheduled or completed as necessary

Examples of community resources

Visiting Nurse Association, public health nurse as needed, home care program, and medical follow-up as needed

Rehabilitation center

RETROSPECTIVE CRITERIA
Health

Vital signs stable

Bowel and bladder program implemented

Full range of motion in all joints

Activity

Activites of daily living goals attained

Communication program for aphasic patient

Knowledge

Disease process and prevention program understood

Adaptive devices with used or without assistance

COMPLICATIONS

Acute chest pain
Decubitus ulcers

Hypertension
Joint contractures
Painful, swollen calf
Pulmonary embolism
Reaction to anticoagulant therapy
Temperature above 100.6° F
Thrombophlebitis
Urinary tract infection

Cervical pain syndrome (Codes: 357, 725, 728.2, 788.1, 847)

CONCURRENT REVIEW CRITERIA
Identification of patient's physical and psychosocial needs and/or concerns

Relief of severe persistent pain

Fear of motor deficits, sensory deficits, possible bladder and/or bowel dysfunction, loss of time from normal activities, or dependency

Understanding of condition, course, and treatment alternatives; medical and nursing management; expected outcomes; and duration of hospitalization

Psychological support to decrease anxiety and/or depression and to promote rest

Recommended nursing action consistent with diagnosis
Nursing services

Provide daily neurological assessment

Assess patterns of pain and/or spasms; develop nursing measures for intervention

Provide planned counseling sessions to focus on factors causing anxiety and/or depression

Review physical and emotional status every 3 days

Design activities of daily living program to minimize pain and/or fatigue

Health education

Teach proper body mechanics for physical activities

Teach critical signs of progressive neurological deficit involvement, such as muscle atrophy and/or weakness, decreased or altered sensations, change in bladder and/or bowel function

Explain course of condition and medical and nursing management

Instruct on medication, including name, dosage, frequency, duration, and side effects to report to physician

Indicators for discharge
Adaptation to health status

Pain absent or decreased to tolerable level

Neurological involvement not increasing

Anxiety or depression absent or controlled

Examples of community resources

Referral usually not indicated

RETROSPECTIVE REVIEW CRITERIA
Health

Pain absent or at a tolerable level
Neurological involvement not increasing

Activity

Independent in activities of daily living

Knowledge

Understands and can verbalize proper body mechanics, symptoms of progres-

sive neurological deficit, and what to
report to physician
Understands medication instructions

COMPLICATIONS

Anxiety or depression
Neurogenic bladder

Pulmonary embolism
Quadriparesis
Thrombophlebitis
Upper extremity nerve root compromise

Chemical injury to esophagus (Code: 947.2)

CONCURRENT CRITERIA
Identification of patient's physical and psychosocial needs and/or concerns

Prevention of dehydration
Maintenance of open airway
Emotional support for patient/family
Teaching about safety in environment
Instruction about gastrostomy, if needed

Recommended nursing action consistent with diagnosis
Nursing services

Give patient a clear or full liquid diet
until inflammation subsides
Observe rate and depth of respiration,
dyspnea; suction as needed
Give thorough mouth care to reduce
chances of infection of esophagus
Use therapeutic communication to help
relieve anxiety and possible guilt feelings of patient/family
Position patient on side with neck hyperextended

Health education

Discuss with patient and family procedures such as esophageal dilatation
that are carried out on long-term basis
Teach family about safety factors in home
environment that can prevent accidents
Instruct family about what should be
done in case another poisoning occurs
Teach family and patient about purpose
and care of the gastrostomy, if discharged with one

Indicators for discharge
Adaptation to health status

Vital signs stable, afebrile for 24 hours
prior to discharge
Full liquid diet via mouth or gastrostomy
tube tolerated
Teaching about gastrostomy, if present,
completed
Respiratory difficulty not evident
Teaching about safety in environment
completed

Examples of community resources

Home visit by public health nurse or
visiting nurse to assess safety hazards
and progress in care of the gastrostomy

RETROSPECTIVE CRITERIA
Health

Vital signs stable, afebrile for 24 hours
prior to discharge
Respiratory difficulty not evident
At least full liquid diet tolerated via
mouth or gastrostomy

Activity

Tolerating normal activity

Knowledge

Can verbalize knowledge learned about
providing a safe environment
Understands about care of gastrostomy, if
needed

COMPLICATIONS

Aerophagia
Anorexia
Dyspepsia
Epigastric fullness
Esophageal distention

Esophageal obstruction
Nausea
Odynophagia
Pneumonia
Respiratory depression
Retrosternal burning pain

Circumcision of redundant foreskin (phimosis) (Code: 605)

CONCURRENT REVIEW CRITERIA
Identification of patient's physical and psychosocial needs and/or concerns

Patient/family education regarding surgical procedure and postoperative care
Adaptation to hospitalization
Adequate urinary output postoperatively (800 to 1,000 ml per 24 hours)
Care of incision and promotion of wound healing

Recommended nursing action consistent with diagnosis
Nursing services

Closely observe for adequacy of voiding of 800 to 1,000 ml per day, quality of urinary stream, and presence of blood in urine
Assess and record condition of operative area every 2 to 8 hours depending on patient's condition; observe for signs of infection, such as swelling, redness, pus, or purulent discharge
Provide appropriate play therapy to aid patient in adaptation to hospitalization, if applicable
Keep operative site covered with petroleum gauze; observe for excessive bleeding

Health education

Educate patient/family regarding need to maintain cleanliness of operative area
Educate patient/family in application of petroleum gauze, with return demonstration

Educate patient/family regarding signs of infection or excessive bleeding

Indicators for discharge
Adaptation to health status

Afebrile and vital signs stable
Voiding normally
Healing of operative area
Parent education regarding postoperative care completed
Food and fluids tolerated

Examples of community resources

Referral usually not indicated

RETROSPECTIVE REVIEW CRITERIA
Health

Afebrile
Voiding normally
Wound healing

Activity

Alert
Movement not limited

Knowledge

Patient/family understands need to observe for excessive bleeding or infection
Patient/family knows when tub baths can be given

COMPLICATIONS

Postoperative bleeding
Wound infection

Colitis, chronic nonspecific ulcerative, with surgical intervention
(Code: 563.1)

CONCURRENT CRITERIA
Identification of patient's physical and psychosocial needs and/or concerns

Relief of symptoms, including bloody diarrhea with lower abdominal cramps; nocturnal diarrhea; rectal tenesmus; anal incontinence; anorexia; dyspeptic symptoms; malaise; weakness; fatigue; fever; weight loss; abdominal distention; or anemia

Understanding about disease process of unknown etiology, tendency to remissions and exacerbations, prognosis, medical and nursing management, potential complications, surgical procedure of colectomy and/or ileostomy

Avoidance of milk, milk products, and wheat

Control of pain and diarrhea

Fears about change in body image and/or bowel function, death, surgical invasion of body, dependency or loss of time from normal activities, and cancer

Recommended nursing action consistent with diagnosis
Nursing services

Control pain and diarrhea

Provide patient with opportunity to express feelings and fears

Provide preoperative nursing care and teaching, including adequate nutrition, hydration, and elimination; explanation about surgical procedure, recovery room, postoperative pain control, turning, coughing, deep breathing, and bowel function expectations; physically prepare patient for surgery

Provide postoperative nursing care, including assessment of physiological response parameters; maintain nutrition, hydration, and elimination; prevent wound or respiratory infections; provide emotional support

Assist in early self-care and progressive ambulation

Health education

Instruct on medications, including the name, dosage, frequency, duration, side effects, and what to report to physician for each drug

Instruct about diet, including restrictions and methods to avoid constipation

Teach rationale for postoperative turning, coughing, deep breathing; teach infection prevention, wound care, and self-care

Advise when and why it is important to return for follow-up medical care

Instruct about disease process and symptoms to observe and report to physician

Indicators for discharge
Adaptation to health status

Bloody diarrhea absent
Pain controlled
Normal physiological responses reestablished, including tolerating diet for 2 to 3 days prior to discharge
Wound healing
Complications not evident

Examples of community resources

Usually not indicated, unless complications occur, then refer to Visiting Nurse Association or public health nurse

RETROSPECTIVE CRITERIA
Health

Normal physiological responses reestablished
Wound healing
Pain controlled
Diet tolerated
Diarrhea and/or complications absent

Activity

Independent in activities of daily living

Knowledge

Understands wound care, activity level permissible, medication instructions, diet, and symptoms of disease process to report to physician

COMPLICATIONS

Abscess formation
Acute arthritis
Constipation
Hemorrhoids
Malabsorption and/or protein deficiency
Malignant degeneration
Pericolitis
Pneumonia
Ulcerative esophagitis

Colitis, chronic ulcerative, resulting in colostomy (Code: 563.1)

CONCURRENT CRITERIA
Identification of patient's physical and psychosocial needs and/or concerns

Relief of symptoms, including frequent liquid stools, abdominal pain and distention, loss of appetite, weight loss, fever, nausea, vomiting, weakness, depression, dehydration, electrolyte disturbance, or frank bleeding

Maintenance of vital body functions

Fear of cancer, concern over change in body image, concern over loss of time from work or school

Preventive measures for problems from decreased activity

Understanding of medical, surgical and nursing management, so that realistic plans for health maintenance after discharge can be made

Recommmended nursing action consistent with diagnosis
Nursing services

Implement measures to maintain vital body functions, including replacing fluids and restoring electrolyte balance to maintain cardiovascular functioning; give parenteral fluids if nothing by mouth allowed; ensure adequate ventilation, conservation of body heat; implement measures to relieve pain, promote rest, reduce anxiety, and prevent problems caused by inactivity

Implement measures to promote adequate hydration, nutrition, and elimination, including administration of low-residue, high-calorie, high-protein diet; restrict all spicy or gas-producing foods; restriction of milk; restriction of extreme temperatures; and administration of small frequent feedings; maintain intake and output; administer oral hygiene frequently; observe for adverse reaction to diet with prompt intervention; administer antispasmodics, steroid therapy, or antibiotics; implement nursing care consistent with surgical management

Provide preoperative teaching, including explanation of surgical procedure, recovery room type of dressing, intravenous solutions, nasogastric suction, estimated period of time of hospitalization, frequent vital sign checks, instruction and explanation of deep-breathing, coughing and turning exercises, explanation of postoperative pain reducing measures, expected gradual steps to ambulation; physically prepare patient for surgery

Implement postoperative nursing care for close observation of signs of deterioration by vital signs monitoring every 10 to 15 minutes, dressing checks every 2 to 4 hours, and bowel sounds assessment every 2 to 4 hours; observe for abdominal distention every 2 to 4 hours; check mental status; monitor urinary output with prompt nursing intervention should signs of complications occur

Provide colostomy rehabilitative care, including assisting patient in adjusting to changes in body image; teach patient to initiate colostomy care; prevent wound infection, excoriation of skin surrounding stoma, and stricture

Health education

Instruct about medications, including name of each discharge medication and the purpose, dosage, frequency, side effects, action to take if side effects occur, and precautions for each drug

Instruction diet, permitted and restricted foods, as well as cooking methods to be used and avoided: for nonsurgical patient—low residue, high-calorie, high-protein diet with avoidance of foods that tend to cause diarrhea or increased peristalsis; for colostomy patient—low-residue diet, avoiding gas-producing foods and those foods not tolerated well by the individual patient

Instruct about therapeutic and restricted activities

Instruct about measures to prevent excoriation of the skin in both medically and surgically managed patient; instruct patient with colostomy about needed equipment for home care (and where to purchase), techniques for irrigation, and for achieving and supporting regularity, such as avoidance of fatigue, stress, and changes in diet

Stress importance of continual follow-up medical care; instruct patient when to return to physician's office or clinic

Indicators for discharge
Adaptation to health status

Bowel function reestablished
Self-care of colostomy
Condition stable
Complications not evident
Health teaching completed
Referrals made

Examples of community resources

Ostomy club
Surgical or medical clinic
Visiting Nurse Association or public health nurse
Social services

RETROSPECTIVE CRITERIA
Health

Bowel function reestablished
Condition stable
Complications not evident

Activity

Ambulatory
Able to carry out activities of daily living
Able to carry out stoma care correctly (including skin care, irrigations, applications of bags)

Knowledge

Understands and can implement dietary regime, including proper cooking methods and permitted and restricted foods

Understands therapeutic and restricted activities and can implement therapeutic ones

Knows the name of each discharge medication, including the purpose, dosage, frequency, side effects, action to take if side effects occur, and precautions for each drug

Understands measures to protect skin from excoriation; if patient has a colostomy, understands and can correctly implement colostomy care

Understands the importance of continual medical follow-up care; knows when to return to physician's office or clinic

COMPLICATIONS

Atelectasis
Dehydration
Emotional problems
Fissures
Hemorrhage
Hemorrhoids
Malignant degeneration

Perforation
Perianal abscessess
Pericholangitis
Pericolitis
Pneumonia
Rectovaginal prolapse or rectovesical fistula

Retarded physical and sexual maturity, in disease starting in childhood
Shock
Skin irritation
Strictures
Wound infection

Coma (stupor) (Code: 770)

CONCURRENT CRITERIA
Identification of patient's physical and psychosocial needs and/or concerns

Close observation for changes in condition, such as level of consciousness (size, equality, reaction of pupils; presence or absence of spontaneous behavior; resistance to care; response to stimuli; presence of voluntary motion of extremities; changes in muscle tone or in position of body or head; changes in color of face, lips, extremities; absence or presence of gag, swallowing, blink reflexes, convulsions, speech); monitoring of vital parameters (rectal temperature every 2 hours; blood pressure, pulse, respiration every 15 minutes for 2 hours, then every 2 hours for 24 hours, then every 4 hours, observations to include character and quality of pulse and respiration and peripheral pulses; hourly urine output, arterial blood gases; central venous pressure); observation of signs and symptoms, such as nausea or vomiting

Maintenance of vital body functions, such as hydration, electrolyte balance, cardiopulmonary function, and elimination

Protection from trauma and/or physical deterioration complications

Family understanding of medical and nursing management, including the purpose and duration of special care units and possible home management care

Support for family—emotional, financial, and social

Recommended nursing action consistent with diagnosis
Nursing services

Establish and maintain adequate airway and measures to ensure proper ventilation (semiprone position, oral airway, suction, oxygen or IPPB, ventilator)

Assess level of consciousness and vital parameters and notify physician immediately when signs of deterioration are present

Implement measures to maintain adequate fluid and electrolyte balance

Implement measures to prevent injury to patient, such as the use of side rails and tongue blades and the assessment of sedative needs

Implement measures to prevent complications

Health education

Teach family about medical management and use of special care units

Teach family the cause, if known, course, prognosis, and residual disabilities of disorder

Teach family about nursing management, such as skin care, turning, suctioning, and catheter care

Educate family about community agencies available to assist them after patient's discharge

Indicators for discharge
Adaptation to health status

Condition stable
Conscious
Complications not evident

Examples of community resources

Mental health agencies; for example drug, suicide, or alcoholic centers (as indicated); social services

Diabetic clinic or kidney clinic

Public health department (industrial hazards, heavy metals)

Visiting Nurse Association

RETROSPECTIVE CRITERIA
Health

Conscious
Complications not evident
Precipitating cause under treatment

Activity

Able to carry out activities of daily living with minimal or no assistance
Ambulatory

Knowledge

Understands pathology of disorder, course, and prognosis

Understands medications; knows the name, side effects, desired effects, dosage, frequency, precautions, route, and method of administration for each drug

Understands special diet, if any, and other restrictions

Understands special nursing management as related to disability, that is, skin care and prevention of contractures, decubitus ulcers, and inanition

Understands community agency—purpose and method of contacting—that is needed postdischarge

COMPLICATIONS

Aspiration
Bruises
Corneal ulceration
Decubitus ulcers
Dehydration
Fractures
Hematemesis
Joint contractures
Oliguria
Oversedation
Paralysis
Pneumonia
Respiratory distress
Seizure activity
Thrombophlebitis
Trauma
Urinary incontinence
Urinary retention
Urinary tract infections

Concussion (Code: 850)

CONCURRENT CRITERIA
Identification of patient's physical and psychosocial needs and/or concerns

Relief of symptoms, such as headache, dizziness, amnesia, confusion, unsteadiness of gait

Close observation for deterioration in condition; immediate intervention should signs of deterioration appear, such as changes in vital signs, pupil characteristics, level of consciousness, motor function, the appearance of convulsions or otorrhagia

Concern and anxiety over amnesia

Understanding of pathology, course, and prognosis of injury

Understanding of medical and nursing management, such as frequent neurological checks, bed rest, avoidance or restriction of analgesics and sedation, and intravenous fluids, if vomiting

Recommended nursing action consistent with diagnosis
Nursing services

Observe for signs of deterioration in condition; notify physician should any occur

Promote comfort; decrease dizziness; promote rest

Reduce anxiety; promote orientation

Promote safety; prevent injury

Health education

Instruct patient/family, if discharged, concerning signs and symptoms of increased intracranial pressure and need to return to hospital should these signs occur: dizziness, vomiting, drowsiness at odd times, or double vision

Instruct about activity restrictions while convalescing at home

Teach measures to promote comfort and rest while convalescing at home

Teach wound care, if there is a laceration

Teach drug names and the desired effects, side effects, dosage, frequency, and precautions of each

Indicators for discharge
Adaptation to health status

Vital signs and neurological status normal; no neurological deficits evident

Medical and nursing management for convalescing period at home understood, such as signs of deteriorating condition, avoidance of sedation, comfort measures, activity restrictions, and wound care (if there is a laceration)

Amnesia absent or decreasing; orientation improved

Examples of community resources

Referral not usually indicated

RETROSPECTIVE CRITERIA
Health

Condition stable

Amnesia absent or decreasing

Orientation improved

Activity

Able to carry out activities of daily living with minimal or no assistance

Knowledge

Understands any activity restrictions while convalescing at home

Understands and is able to utilize comfort and rest promoting measures

Understands and can demonstrate method of wound care, if laceration is present

Understands and knows drug name(s), dosage, frequency, desired effects, side effects, and precautions

Understands signs and symptoms which should prompt him to seek medical attention as related to increased intracranial pressure

COMPLICATIONS

Anxiety

Convulsions

Disorientation

Dizziness

Double vision

Increased intracranial pressure

Otorrhagia

Subarachnoid hemorrhage

Vomiting

Wound infection, if applicable

Convulsive disorders (Code: 780.2)

CONCURRENT REVIEW CRITERIA
Identification of patient's physical and psychosocial needs and/or concerns

Seizure control, including maintaining clear airway and avoiding excessive environmental stimuli

Aid in obtaining acceptance of disorder by self and others

Understanding of disorder, including cause, chronicity, restrictions, and legal implications

Understanding of medical and nursing management

Support of family and community

Recommended nursing action consistent with diagnosis
Nursing services

Closely observe characteristics of seizures

Protect from psychological trauma

Protect from bodily harm during and immediately after seizure

Observe for desired and toxic effects of drug therapy

Explain purpose, preparation, and outcome of diagnostic and therapeutic procedures

Health education

Instruct on medication—desired and toxic effects, the name, dosage, and frequency for each drug; and need for maintaining a therapeutic blood level and follow-up medical supervision

Teach to recognize signs and symptoms of aura, if present, and correct action to take

Design plan for moderate activity for purpose of deterring seizures

Design plan for avoiding excessive fatigue, emotional stress, physical excitement, and alcohol (if appropriate)

Explain importance of wearing a medical tag or having information on person indicating medications being taken

Indicators for discharge
Adaptation to health status

Toxic effects from medications not evident

Convulsions absent for 3 to 5 consecutive days prior to discharge

Discharge environment suitable

Previous referral initiated and contact made for follow-up visits

Examples of community resources

Visiting Nurse Association or public health nurse

National Association to Control Epilepsy or Alcoholics Anonymous (if appropriate)

Bureau of Vocational Rehabilitation (if appropriate)

RETROSPECTIVE REVIEW CRITERIA
Health

Seizures under control
Afebrile
Drug toxicity not evident
Complications not evident

Activity

Ambulatory
Able to perform activities of daily living
Able to go back to previous employment

Knowledge

Understands dosage, toxic effects, name, and frequency of medication

Understands need for maintaining therapeutic blood sugar level and for following up with medical supervision

Knows signs to report to physician

Family knows and can implement emergency care during seizure

Understands reasons for avoiding excessive fatigue, emotional stress, physical excitement, and alcohol

COMPLICATIONS

Automatisms
Disorientation
Drug reaction
Erratic behavior
Fracture
Hallucinations
Incoherent speech
Irritability
Mental dullness
Mental or emotional changes
Soft tissue injury

Convulsive disorders, idiopathic seizures, in children
(Codes: 345, 761, 770, 773)

CONCURRENT REVIEW CRITERIA
Identification of patient's physical and psychosocial needs and/or concerns

Relief from symptoms—either very listless or irritable and restless
Soothing of fears and confusion
Protection from excessive environmental stimuli
Maintenance of a patent airway
Emotional support to patient and family

Recommended nursing action consistent with diagnosis
Nursing services

Observe for desired and toxic effects from drug therapy
Tape padded tongue blade and/or airway at head of bed; provide safe, quiet environment, suction equipment, and oxygen at bedside
Observe closely for any seizures; describe seizures in detail; evaluate neurological status and vital signs hourly
Understand parents fears; assist them toward a realistic attitude about child's condition
Prepare patient/family emotionally for scheduled tests

Health education

Teach parents techniques to maintain a clear airway until medical assistance is available should a seizure occur
Instruct parents in importance of giving anticonvulsive medication properly and daily
Stress importance of having child wear medical alert information, including condition and medication for emergency situation

Indicators for discharge
Adaptation to health status

Seizures under control
Afebrile
Ambulatory

Parents ready to accept responsibility of child
Side effects from convulsive medications not evident

Examples of community resources

National Association to Control Epilepsy
Visiting Nurse Association or public health nurse
School nurse

RETROSPECTIVE REVIEW CRITERIA
Health

Afebrile
Seizures under control
Anticonvulsive medications tolerated

Activity

Ambulatory
Able to perform activities of daily living

Knowledge

Parents understand importance of giving anticonvulsive medication and keeping child on it until physician discontinues it
Parents understand need for continued medical follow-up care
Parents acquainted with appropriate referral agencies, if further aid is necessary after discharge
Parents understand legal implications of convulsive disorder

COMPLICATIONS

Automatisms
Disorientation
Drug reaction
Erratic behavior
Fractures
Hallucinations
Incoherent speech
Irritability
Mental dullness
Mental or emotional changes
Soft tissue injury

Craniostenosis (Code: 743.9)

CONCURRENT CRITERIA
Identification of patient's physical and psychosocial needs and/or concerns

Correction of defect and relief or control of symptoms, including abnormal head shape caused by premature closure of one or more cranial sutures, vomiting, lethargy, developmental retardation, or visual deficits

Understanding by parents of cause, if known, treatment, course, prognosis, medical and nursing management, and the possibility of future multiple surgeries, so that realistic plans can be made for care of the child

Assistance for parents in coping with a defective child

Understanding by parents of importance of continuous regular medical checkups and evaluation (physical, mental, and emotional) as child matures

Understanding by parents of community agencies available to assist them after child's discharge

Recommended nursing action consistent with diagnosis
Nursing services

Implement preoperative and supportive nursing measures, including implementation of measures to protect child from trauma resulting from convulsions and infections caused by exposure to drafts and personnel with infections; observe child's behavior and reactions to care daily for signs of deterioration as related to increased intracranial pressure by checking color, temperature, quality and rate of pulse and respiration; watch for increased drowsiness, apathy, vomiting, convulsions; take daily measurements of head, since hydrocephalus is frequently associated with craniostenosis or is a complication of corrective surgery for craniostenosis; implement measures to maintain adequate hydration and nutrition, to prepare child physically for surgery, and to prepare parents psychologically and emotionally for surgery of child by explaining special care units, procedures, expected outcomes, and general care

Implement postoperative nursing measures, including close observation for signs of shock, meningitis, encephalitis, pneumonia, fever, decubitus ulcers, impairment of motor function, spasticity, or contractures by checking color, temperature, quality and rate of respiration and pulse; watch for increased drowsiness; ensure adequate hydration and nutrition; implement measures to prevent increased intracranial pressure by elevating head 20 to 30 degrees and possibly restricting fluids, as ordered; prevent decubitus ulcers by frequent repositioning of child with proper supports and "props" to maintain position and alignment; prevent wound infection and hypostatic pneumonia; consult with parents about planning for emotional support and development of child

Initiate appropriate referrals

Implement measures to assist parents in adjusting to having a deformed child

Health education

Instruct parents in physical and emotional care of the child, such as skin care, hydration, nutrition, emotional security, mental stimulation, ego support, the necessity of imposing limits on the child, and measures to prevent infection and problems from immobility

Instruct parents as to the importance of regular medical checkups and psychological testing at prescribed intervals in order to determine realistic long-range and short-term goals

Instruct parents as related to safety of child with convulsions, neurological deficits (sensory, motor, visual), and mental retardation if such is the case

Teach measures to assist the child in reaching maximum potential as related to exercise and mental stimulation for growth

Instruct parents as related to the name, purpose, dosage, frequency, side effects, actions to take should side effects occur, and precautions for each medication and to duration of drug therapy

Indicators for discharge
Adaptation to health status

Condition stable

Signs of increased intracranial pressure absent

Necessary health teaching completed

Referrals made

Examples of community resources*

National Cerebral Palsy Association

School nurse or exceptional child center

Visiting Nurse Association or public health nurse

Rehabilitation center

Social services

RETROSPECTIVE CRITERIA
Health

Condition stable

Hydration and nutrition adequate

Intracranial pressure signs absent

Surgical grafts allowing for head expansion completed

Complications not evident

Activity

Activity according to medical expectations and appropriate for age

---

*Agencies may not be appropriate for age of child at this time, but parents should be made aware of need for contact with referral agencies at early stage.

Knowledge

Parents understand and can implement necessary physical care of child, including skin care, adequate hydration and nutrition, measures to promote emotional security, and measures to prevent infection

Parents understand and can implement ego supportive measures and can set necessary limits on child as child grows older

Parents understand the importance of frequent regular medical checkups and psychological testing of child; parents have the financial means by which to secure this type of health surveillance

Parents understand and know the name, dosage, frequency, purpose, side effects, action to take if side effects occur, and precautions for each discharge medication

Parents understand and can implement care as related to residual permanent neurological deficits

COMPLICATIONS

Acrobrachycephaly

Craniofacial dysostosis
  Exophthalmos
  Optic atrophy
  Papilledema
  Strabismus
  Underdeveloped face
  Underdeveloped upper jaw

Oxycephaly
  Blindness
  Exophthalmos
  Mental retardation
  Optic atrophy
  Papilledema
  Strabismus

Scaphocephaly
  Blindness
  Increased intracranial pressure
  Optic atrophy

Cystic fibrosis (Code: 273)

CONCURRENT CRITERIA
Identification of patient's physical and psychosocial needs and/or concerns

Adequate ventilation for comfort and ease in performance of activities of daily living

Freedom from digestive and elimination disorders that cause discomfort, such as nausea, spasmodic coughing with vomiting, distention, diarrhea, and abdominal pain and appropriate nutrition to permit strength and energy for normal daily activities

Assistance in separating from parent and adjustment to hospital

Parental knowledge of disease condition, including treatment, prognosis, and genetic implications

Patient knowledge of reasons for and nature of dietary and activity restrictions, as age permits

Recommended nursing action consistent with nursing diagnosis
Nursing services

Maintain adequate ventilation through positioning, postural drainage, percussion, and inhalation therapy; prevent infection through proper room and bed placement; administer antibiotics as ordered; continuously monitor and record respiratory status with intervention to reduce stress; contact physician when patient's condition is critical

Maintain adequate nutrition and elimination to promote growth and development through planned individualized diet served at time and in manner most conducive to consumption; administer pancreatic extracts and other medication as ordered; implement daily monitoring of dietary intake and elimination with adjustment as appropriate; monitor weight

Provide daily schedule that promotes activity and rest periods compatible with disease status and normal developmental level of patient

Provide emotional support to parents for coping with child's condition

Health education

Teach parents nature of disease and priorities of care, including specific methods of treatment for respiration; nutrition; and purpose, dosage, and mode of administration of medication; importance of activity control and prevention of infection; and genetic implications of disease

Depending on age and level of understanding, teach child reasons for and method of assistance in maintaining adequate ventilation, nature of diet, and reasons for hospitalization; introduce to staff

Provide information regarding services and financial assistance available through national or local Cystic Fibrosis Foundation

Indicators for discharge
Adaptation to health status

Afebrile with vital signs stable

Improved respiratory status, including decreased rate, no dyspnea, orthopnea, or retractions

Improved absorption and digestion as evidenced by toleration of diet without distention, pain, or other abdominal distress

Beginning weight gain relative to length of hospitalization

Resumption of normal activities including sleeping and eating patterns

Referrals completed

Examples of community resources

Public health nurse or Visiting Nurse Association

Cystic Fibrosis Foundation

Cystic fibrosis center

RETROSPECTIVE CRITERIA
Health

Afebrile

Stable vital signs within normal limits

Adequate respiratory status, including rate within normal limits, and no evidence of dyspnea, orthopnea, or retractions

Potential for adequate nutrition and toleration of prescribed diet with no evidence of distention or diarrhea

Beginning weight gain

Activity

Normal activity schedule resumed, including sleeping patterns, consistent with age and developmental level

Knowledge

Parent able to give verbal evidence of understanding disease condition and implications for care, as well as genetic implications

Parent understands respiratory care necessary and can demonstrate positioning, postural drainage, percussion, and administration of medication and aerosol or nebulizer as ordered

Parent has written dietary plan and can explain plans for implementation

Parent gives verbal evidence of knowledge of how to prevent infection

COMPLICATIONS

Bronchitis
Diabetes mellitus
Excessive sodium chloride loss in sweat
Heat exhaustion in hot weather
Heart failure or cor pulmonale
Malnutrition
Pancreatic insufficiency
Pulmonary infection
Steatorrhea
Viscid sputum

Dementia (organic brain syndrome) (Pick's disease, Alzheimer's disease, and senile dementia) (Code: 309.9)

CONCURRENT CRITERIA
Identification of patient's physical and psychosocial needs and/or concerns

Control of symptoms, including impairment of memory, loss of orientation, shallowness of affect, impairment of intellectual function, impairment of judgment, irritability, anger, rage as predominant mood, rigidity, stubborn behavior, garrulousness, and narrowed interest

Patient/family understanding of nature of disease process, course, prognosis, progression, and use of tranquilizers to increase patient manageability

Prevention of trauma (physical, social, psychological) caused by impaired mental functioning

Assistance to family in coping with changes in role and life-style

Family understanding of community

agencies available for assistance in care of patient after discharge

Recommended nursing action consistent with diagnosis
Nursing services

Implement safety measures to protect patient from injury, through supervision of smoking, supervision of movements, supervision of financial matters, use of side rails at night because of disorientation

Implement measures to assist with orientation, including clocks, calendars, referrals to events, persons, or times

Adhere to plan of care and routines according to established schedule to provide consistency in environment

Observe for therapeutic effects and side effects of medication with prompt nursing intervention should side effects occur

Implement measures to assist family in coping with change in roles and lifestyle

Health education

Explain medications, including the name, dosage, frequency, purpose, side effects, actions to take if side effects occur, and precautions for each discharge medication

Teach safety measures as related to deterioration of mental functioning

Explain the need and means of achieving consistency in routine of home care and environment for aiding in manageability and orientation

Recommend community agencies available for assisting with care after discharge

Indicators for discharge
Adaptation to health status

Manageable
Suitable discharge environment
Symptoms under control

Examples of community resources

Social services
Visiting Nurse Association or public health nurse
Convalescent home

RETROSPECTIVE CRITERIA
Health

Patient manageable
Condition stable
Discharge environment suitable

Activity

Ambulatory
Able to complete activities of daily living with supervision

Knowledge

Family understands need for and can implement consistency in daily routine

Family understands and knows the name, dosage, purpose, frequency, side effects, action to take should side effects occur, and precautions for each discharge medication

Family understands and is able to implement safety measures

Family understands function of community agency that can best aid in care of patient after discharge

COMPLICATIONS

Decubitus ulcers
Paralysis
Persistent fever
Severe drug reaction
Shock as adverse reaction to x-ray contrast media

Diabetes mellitus (Code: 250)

CONCURRENT CRITERIA
Identification of patient's physical and psychosocial needs and/or concerns

Relief from increased thirst, polyuria, increased appetite, weight loss, fatigue, skin infection, diabetic acidosis, or insulin reactions

Understanding of cause, prognosis, and medical and nursing management, so that realistic plans for health maintenance can be made

Fear of death, invalidism, or rejection and assistance in dealing with problems related to changes in body image or fears of death or rejection

Understanding of community services available after discharge

Recommended nursing action consistent with diagnosis
Nursing services

Ensure proper nutrition, hydration, and elimination for proper control of diabetic condition

Survey patient's responses to medical management by testing urine regularly for sugar and acetone, preparing patient properly for fasting blood sugars, coordinating all diagnostic tests so that prolonged periods of fasting do not interfere with insulin administration and diet control of the disease

Administer hypoglycemic agent according to orders with close observation for side reactions, hypoglycemic shock, or coma; implement prompt nursing intervention should any of the above occur

Maintain activity requirements and prevent infection

Assist patient and family in accepting the diagnosis

Health education

Instruct on signs and symptoms of insulin shock, hypoglycemic shock, and diabetic acidosis and on the appropriate actions to take should any occur

Provide dietary instruction

Instruct on methods of preventing skin infections and irritations and carrying out good general skin hygiene; stress regular medical and dental visits, prompt attention to minor cuts, bruises, or symptoms of systemic or localized infections, such as sore throats and flu

Instruct on sterilization of insulin injection equipment, technique of drawing up proper dosage, the importance of rotating sites of injection, proper technique for administering insulin, name of insulin or hypoglycemic agent, dosage, frequency, side effects, actions to take if side effects occur, and precautions; instruct on relationship of activity to diet to hypoglycemic agent to diabetic control

Stress the importance of continual follow-up medical care

Indicators for discharge
Adaptation to health status

Blood sugar decreasing
Symptoms controlled
Weight being gained

Complications not evident
Health teaching completed
Referrals made

Examples of community resources

Diabetic clinic
Visiting Nurse Association or public health nurse
Diabetes Association of America
Social services

RETROSPECTIVE CRITERIA
Health

Blood sugar approaching normal range
Symptoms controlled
Diet tolerated
Urine free of sugar and acetone
Complications not evident

Activity

Able to administer hypoglycemic agent correctly; when agent is insulin, able to sterilize equipment properly, to maintain sterility of equipment correctly while administering insulin, and to carry out proper technique of injection; able to test urine for sugar and acetone

Able to plan meals correctly in accordance with diet

Wears medic alert identification

Knowledge

Understands signs and symptoms of hypoglycemic shock and diabetic coma and knows appropriate action to take

Understands the purpose, dosage, frequency, side effects, action to take should side effects occur, and precautions for each medication

Understands the relationship of activity to diet, to hypoglycemic agent, and to control of disease

Understands the importance of and means of preventing and managing infection, in terms of diabetic control

Understands the importance of regular medical follow-up care and when to return to physician's office and/or clinic

COMPLICATIONS

Degenerative vascular diseases
Dehydration
Diabetic ketosis, acidosis, and coma
Infection
Insulin allergy
Insulin reactions
Intercapillary glomeruloslerosis
Muscular atrophy
Ocular disorders

Diabetes mellitus, cellulitis, chronic complications (Code: 250)

CONCURRENT CRITERIA
Identification of patient's physical and psychosocial needs and/or concerns

Relief from symptoms such as pain, swelling, inflammation, weeping, or drainage
Concern over possible scarring
Understanding of medical and nursing management
Reinforcement of diabetic teaching

Recommended nursing action consistent with diagnosis
Nursing services

Observe for therapeutic effect as well as side effects of antibiotic treatment; implement prompt nursing intervention should side effects occur
Implement measures to reduce pain and general discomfort
Implement nursing measures to ensure proper nutrition, hydration, and elimination in keeping with dietary prescription for diabetic control
Reinforce diabetic teaching
Implement measures to prevent further spreading of existing infection, as well as to prevent other secondary infections

Health education

Instruct on the name, purpose, dosage, frequency, side effects, action to take if side effects occur, and precautions regarding all discharge medications
Instruct as to therapeutic and restricted activities
Instruct as to wound care, if any

Instruct as to means of preventing infection
Instruct as to when to return to clinic or physician's office for follow-up medical care

Indicators for discharge
Adaptation to health status

Blood sugar in acceptable range
Complications not evident
Health teaching completed
Referrals made

Examples of community resources

Visiting Nurse Association or public health nurse
Diabetic clinic

RETROSPECTIVE CRITERIA
Health

Blood sugar in acceptable range
Urine free of sugar and acetone
Wound healing
Complications not evident

Activity

Ambulatory
Able to carry out wound care properly
Able to carry out diabetic control regime
Able to carry out activities of daily living

Knowledge

Knows the name, purpose, dosage, frequency, side effects, action to take if side effects occur, and precautions of all discharge medications

Understands and can implement therapeutic and restricted activites

Understands and can implement measures to prevent infection

Understands when and why it is necessary to return to physician's office or clinic for follow-up care

COMPLICATIONS

Acute or progressive renal failure
Amputation
Blindness
Septicemia

Diabetes mellitus, coma and precoma (Code: 250)

CONCURRENT CRITERIA
Identification of patient's physical and psychosocial needs and/or concerns

Relief from symptoms of increased thirst, hunger, frequency of urination, loss of appetite, nausea, vomiting, abdominal pain, drowsiness, distorted vision, behavioral changes, Kussmaul's respirations, acetone or fruity odor to breath, dehydration, or unconsciousness

Understanding of condition in terms of diabetes, course, prognosis, and medical and nursing management, so that realistic plans for health maintenance can be made for after discharge

Fear of death or invalidism

Adequate hydration, nutrition, and elimination as related to general health and diabetic control

Understanding of community agencies available for assistance after discharge

Recommended nursing action consistent with diagnosis
Nursing services

Implement nursing measures to restore fluid and electrolyte balance and to maintain proper nutrition and hydration consistent with diabetic diet; administer parenteral fluids and insulin according to orders; maintain strict intake and output; supervise dietary intake with appropriate administration of "weigh back" supplemental feedings; restrict unauthorized snacks that may be provided by family; make frequent urine checks for sugar and acetone; implement surveillance of ordered laboratory studies with appropriate action in the event of omission, abnormal reports, or delays that interfere with regularity of diet or insulin administration; administer appropriate drugs to correct infection, nausea, and vomiting, as ordered, such as antibiotics or antiemetics

Implement measures to assist the patient in dealing with fears of death or invalidism or in accepting diabetes

Initiate proper referrals

Health education

Instruct patient on importance of adherence to dietary regime; supervise patient in planning three separate meals in accordance to diabetic allowance and food exchange system; maintain instruction until patient shows understanding by planning meals correctly; instruct patient on correct techniques of monitoring insulin needs by testing urine for sugar and acetone; maintain instruction until patient can monitor this correctly; instruct patient on the method and importance of keeping daily records for medical surveillance

Instruct patient on the importance and method of preventing infection, as well as on the appropriate action to take should signs of one occur

Instruct patient on the importance of maintaining activity level as relates to diabetic control

Instruct patient on the name, purpose, dosage, frequency, side effects, action to take if side effects occur, route of administration, proper technique for administration, and precautions for each discharge medication; in the case of insulin, patient should know how to sterilize equipment, how to maintain sterility, and the importance of rotation of sites of injection; maintain instruction until patient shows understanding and ability to administer medications correctly

Instruct patient on when and why it is necessary to return to clinic or physician's office for medical follow-up

Indicators for discharge
Adaptation to health status

Blood sugar within acceptable range
Urine free of sugar and acetone
Complications not evident
Health teaching completed
Referrals made

Examples of community resources

Social services
Visiting Nurse Association or public health nurse
Diabetic clinic
Diabetes Association of America

RETROSPECTIVE CRITERIA
Health

Blood sugar within acceptable range
Urine free of sugar and acetone
Conscious
Complications not evident

Activity

Wears medic alert identification
Ambulatory
Able to administer hypoglycemic agent correctly
Able to plan diabetic meals correctly
Able to test urine correctly
Can identify precipitating event

Knowledge

Understands importance of adhering to diet to control disease and how to plan meals correctly
Understands method and importance of checking urine regularly
Understands importance of taking the hypoglycemic agent according to prescription
Understands therapeutic and restricted activities and can implement therapeutic ones
Understands and can implement measures to prevent infection
Knows when and why it is necessary to return to clinic or physician's office for follow-up medical care

COMPLICATIONS

Aspiration
Degenerative vascular disease
Dehydration
Drug reaction
Infection
Ocular disorders
Pneumonia
Respiratory distress
Urinary incontinence
Urinary infections
Urinary retention

Diabetes mellitus, juvenile (Codes: 250, 250.3, 250.4)

CONCURRENT REVIEW CRITERIA
Identification of patient's physical and psychosocial needs and/or concerns

Relief from increased thirst, polyuria, increased appetite, weight loss, fatigue, skin infection, diabetic acidosis, or insulin reaction

Family/patient understanding of cause, prognosis, and medical and nursing management, so that realistic plans for health maintenance can be made

Family/patient dealing with guilt feeling, problems related to changes in body image, fears of death or incapacitation, and feeling of rejection

Maintenance or increase of independence of child through self-care of condition

Family/patient understanding of community services available after discharge

Recommended nursing action consistent with diagnosis
Nursing services

Implement nursing measures to ensure adequate hydration, nutrition, and elimination; observe type and amount of food intake; implement carbohydrate restriction; observe therapeutic action of patient's diet in terms of growth needs, activity, and diabetic control; report any adverse effects to physician; encourage adherence to ordered diet by making appropriate substitutions from exchange list when necessary to include food preferences; incorporate child's normal dietary habits to facilitate diet adherence

Survey patient's response to medical management, including testing urine for sugar and acetone, preparing for fasting blood sugars, and coordinating all diagnostic tests to prevent prolonged period of fasting from interfering with insulin administration and diet control of disease

Administer insulin according to orders with close observation for insulin shock or coma; implement prompt nursing intervention should either occur

Maintain activity requirements and prevent infection

Provide emotional support to family/patient as necessary for acceptance of diagnosis and treatment regime

Health education

Instruct on signs and symptoms of insulin shock, diabetic acidosis, and appropriate actions to take should either occur

Explain dietary instructions and restrictions

Instruct on methods of preventing skin irritation, infections, and skin hygiene; stress immunizations and dental care

Instruct on sterilization of insulin injection equipment; technique of drawing up proper dosage; proper technique for administering insulin; name, dosage, and frequency of insulin; importance of rotating sites of injection; and relationship of activity to diet to insulin in diabetic control

Stress importance of continual follow-up medical care

Indicators for discharge
Adaptation to health status

Blood sugar within acceptable range
Urine free of sugar and acetone
Symptoms controlled
Parent/child able to cope with disease and treatment regime
Complications not evident
Health teaching completed
Referrals made

Examples of community resources

Juvenile Diabetic Association
Visiting Nurse Association or public health nurse

Diabetic clinic
School nurse

Health

Condition stable, including acceptable limits for blood sugar and for urine testing of sugar and acetone

Complications not evident

Parents/child can cope with diagnosis and treatment

Activity

Parents/child can give insulin injections correctly, including use of proper dosage and technique

Parents/child have made appropriate and correct food selection for three separate meals to meet calorie, protein, fat, and carbohydrate needs from exchange list; can plan meals according to dietary prescription

Can sterilize equipment for insulin injections and can maintain sterility in administration of insulin

Ambulatory

Able to perform activities of daily living

Able to test urine for sugar and acetone correctly

Knowledge*

Knows the name of each medication and the purpose, dosage, frequency, route,

---

*If patient is unteachable and there is no family, the responsible party assuming health care supervision is required to know the above, and this must be documented in the nurse's notes.

side effects, action to take if side effects occur, and precautions for each

Understands signs and symptoms of insulin shock and diabetic coma and knows appropriate action to take

Understands importance of diet in control of diabetes mellitus; can correctly plan meals according to prescribed diet

Understands importance of avoiding and treating infections energetically and promptly

Understands relationship of activity to diet and control of diabetes

Understands importance of continuous follow-up medical care; knows when to return to physician's office or diabetic clinic

COMPLICATIONS

Degenerative vascular disease
Dehydration
Electrolyte imbalance
Emotional disturbances
Infections, including urinary tract infections, gram negative rod bacteremia, soft tissue infections, tuberculosis, and fungous infections
Insulin allergy
Insulin reaction
Ketoacidosis
Ocular disorders

Diabetes mellitus, nephropathy (nephrotic syndrome, uremia), chronic complications (Code: 250)

CONCURRENT CRITERIA
Identification of patient's physical and psychosocial needs and/or concerns

Relief from symptoms, such as weight loss from dehydration, weight gain

from edema, anorexia, nausea, vomiting, diarrhea, hemorrhage, elevated blood pressure, insulin shock, diminished urinary output, twitching, mental dullness, personality changes, convulsions, itching, stupor, coma, or septicemia

Understanding of nature of condition in terms of chronicity, prognosis, diabetic relationship, medical and nursing management

Fear of death or death wish

Maintenance of vital body functions

Preventive measures against problems caused by immobility

Recommended nursing action consistent with diagnosis
Nursing services

Implement nursing measures to assist patient and family in coping with chronicity of condition, possible need for continual dialysis, fear of death, and suicidal expressions by patient or in securing financial assistance

Implement measures to maintain vital body functions—provide adequate ventilation by positioning to facilitate respiration, administering oxygen as required, suctioning as required, maintaining patent airway, limiting fluids if edematous (and interfering with respiration), changing position every 2 hours to prevent hypostatic pneumonia, and implementing chest physiotherapy; maintain adequate cardiovascular functioning by limiting fluid intake as related to congestive heart failure, maintaining administration of parenteral fluids as ordered, if dehydration or hemorrhage has occurred, conserving body heat, administering antihypertensive drugs as appropriate, checking vital signs and apical pulse every 2 hours; implement cardiac monitoring in the presence of hyper- or hypokalemia, observing closely for bleeding, administering vasopressors as ordered, applying pressure to needle injection sites, and administering vitamin K as ordered; implement safety measures, such as checking mental status every 2 hours, maintaining side rails, providing measures to assist orientation, and implementing seizure precautions;

maintain adequate hydration, nutrition, and elimination by maintaining strict intake and output, maintaining prescribed diet (sodium, protein, potassium may be restricted for uremia), observing and intervening should insulin shock occur (frequently need for insulin decreased when in renal failure; activity also diminished; appetite poor), maintaining caloric needs to maintain diabetic control via small frequent feedings, consulting dietician, administering measures to control nausea, vomiting, and diarrhea, maintaining good oral hygiene, and administering diuretics

Implement nursing measures for hemodialysis as may be needed, including maintaining patency of external cannula, preventing dislodging of cannula, and preventing infection; implement plan to prevent arteriovenous fistula spasms or bleeding from fistula and measures supportive of dietary adherence by the dialyzing patient who is also a diabetic; monitor weight, temperature, pulse, blood pressure, food and/or fluid intake, and clotting time for dialysis during and following the procedure; observe for signs of adverse reactions, such as cerebral abnormality (agitation), twitching, confusion, seizures (called dialysis disequilibrium syndrome), hypotension, arrhythmias (usually only occurring during dialysis when potassium is reduced and patient has been taking digitalis), chest pain, muscle cramping; intervene should any signs occur by administering phenytoin, tranquilizers, and vasopressors, slowing rate of blood pumping, positioning patient to facilitate blood return, conserving body heat, applying heat and massage; implement measures to assist the patient in coping with "life via machine"

Implement measures to prevent infection from diabetic condition or renal condition; explain importance of avoiding respiratory infections, flu, and skin injuries; getting prompt medical attention for "minor" infections; giving adequate attention to cuts, irritations, and pressure areas; maintaining good perineal care and skin hygiene

Initiate appropriate referrals

Health education

Provide diet instruction, reinforcing teaching of diabetic diet in keeping with diet for control of renal failure (usually, low-protein and low-sodium diet and restricted fluid intake)

Explain therapeutic and restricted activities

Teach measures to prevent infection, by explaining shunt care, care of external cannulas, and low resistance from renal problem

Explain the name, purpose, dosage, frequency, side effects, action to take if side effects occur, and precautions for each discharge medication

Explain importance of maintaining records (including urine test for sugar and acetone, daily weights, and daily intake and output records) and keeping regular medical appointments for follow-up care

Indicators for discharge
Adaptation to health status

Intake and output within acceptable range

Blood sugar controlled

Urine free of sugar and acetone

Dialysis completed, if indicated

Complications not evident

Health teaching completed

Referrals made

Examples of community resources

Visiting Nurse Association or public health nurse

Kidney clinic

Social services

RETROSPECTIVE CRITERIA
Health

Blood sugar within acceptable range

Urine free of sugar and acetone

Intake and output within acceptable range

Complications not evident

Activity

Ambulatory

Able to carry out activities of daily living

Able to implement renal and diabetic diet correctly

Able to administer medications correctly

Able to implement cannula and/or shunt care, if indicated

Knowledge

Knows the name, purpose, dosage, frequency, side effects, action to take if side effects occur, and precautions for each discharge medication

Understands diet and can plan meals correctly

Understands therapeutic and restricted activities and can implement therapeutic ones

Understands and can implement measures to prevent infection

Understands the importance of keeping daily records as early means of detecting changes in health; can implement record-keeping correctly

Understands when and why it is necessary to return to clinic or physician's office

Understands process of dialysis, frequency, shunt care, and signs to report to physician

COMPLICATIONS

Acute or progressive renal failure

Blindness

Degenerative vascular disease

Ocular disorders

Septicemia

Uremia

Diabetes mellitus, neuropathy (persistent pain, visceral), chronic complications (Code: 250)

CONCURRENT CRITERIA
Identification of patient's physical and psychosocial needs and/or concerns

Relief from pain, paresthesia, muscle weakness, paralysis, nausea, vomiting, heartburn from delayed gastric emptying, atonic urinary bladder

Understanding of course of disease, medical and nursing management, and prognosis, so that realistic plans for health maintenance can be made for after discharge

Fear of death or anxiety over changes in body image

Prevention of problems caused by immobility

Understanding of community agencies available for assistance after discharge

Recommended nursing action consistent with diagnosis
Nursing services

Implement pain-reducing measures

Implement measures to maintain adequate hydration, nutrition, and elimination, by monitoring intake and output; administering antiemetics; providing smaller, more frequent feedings consistent with retention and meeting diabetic needs; administering supplementary vitamins; positioning patient as related to retention of food and comfort; including foods to facilitate elimination and adequate fluid intake to assist in the prevention of urinary infection, calculi, or retention

Implement measures to maintain or improve muscle tone as well as to prevent problems related to immobility by instigating range of motion exercises, quadriceps exercises, frequent change of position, maintaining proper alignment, and use of supportive devices

Implement diabetic control-reinforcement program, such as reteaching dietary control and meal planning, explaining purpose of diet control, proper techniques for administration of hypoglycemic agent, purpose, dosage, frequency, and side effects of hypoglycemic agent, reemphasizing need for urine testing and for regular activities without skipping meals; closely observe for therapeutic effect of diabetic regime; implement prompt nursing intervention should signs of diabetic deterioration occur

Implement measures to assist patient in dealing with fears of death or anxiety over changes in body image

Health education

Instruct patient/family on the name, purpose, dosage, frequency, side effects, action to take if side effects occur, and precautions for each medication

Instruct patient/family on diet, including meal planning via exchange food list, purpose of diet, and importance of adherence to it

Instruct patient/family on hypoglycemic agent, including all aspects of sterilization, administration, drawing up correct dosage, as well as importance of testing urine regularly and maintaining activity levels

Instruct patient/family about safety measures and use of supportive devices, such as canes, walkers, and braces, as may be necessary

Instruct patient/family in measures to reduce discomforts and pain, as may be needed

Indicators for discharge
Adaptation to health status

Condition stable with blood sugar within acceptable range and urine free of sugar and acetone

Complications not evident
Health teaching completed
Referrals made
Pain controlled

Examples of community resources

Visiting Nurse Association or public health nurse
Pain clinics
Diabetic clinics
Social services

RETROSPECTIVE CRITERIA
Health

Condition stable with blood sugar within acceptable range and urine free of sugar and acetone
Complications not evident
Pain controlled

Activity

Ambulatory
Able to use canes, braces, or walker correctly
Able to plan diabetic meals, using exchange list correctly

Able to test urine correctly and to administer hypoglycemic agents

Knowledge

Understands importance of diet in control of diabetes; knows how to plan meals correctly; understands consequences of straying from diet
Understands therapeutic and restricted activities and can implement therapeutic ones
Understands and can implement proper administration of insulin with proper care of equipment
Understands and can implement pain-reducing measures
Understands and can implement safety measures

COMPLICATIONS

Acute or progressive renal failure
Amputation
Blindness
Degenerative vascular disease
Ocular disorders
Septicemia

Diabetes mellitus, osteomyelitis, chronic complications (Code: 250)

CONCURRENT CRITERIA
Identification of patient's physical and psychosocial needs and/or concerns

Relief from symptoms such as chills, fever, rapid pulse, profuse sweating, restlessness, nausea and vomiting, contractures, redness over infected area, pain, swelling, possible drainage, decubitus ulcers, weakness, and irritability
Understanding of disease process in terms of cause, course, treatment, nursing management, and prognosis, so that realistic plans for health maintenance after discharge can be made
Preventive measures for problems caused by immobility
Concern about loss of time from work or

school and possibility of having "leg cut off"
Reinforcement of diabetic control management teaching

Recommended nursing action consistent with diagnosis
Nursing services

Implement nursing measures to maintain adequate hydration, nutrition, and elimination consistent with diabetic control and osteomyelitis, including forcing fluids to 3,000 ml, if no contraindications, measuring all intake and output, administering parenteral fluids according to type, rate, and amount ordered

Implement measures to provide rest to the extremity and to promote healing, including elevation of affected extremity, application of warm, wet compresses, change of dressing as required; implement isolation if drainage present; apply splints properly as ordered; administer antibiotics as ordered

Implement measures to prevent problems from immobility, including maintaining correct position and alignment, using supportive devices, turning frequently, administering proper skin care, and initiating deep-breathing, coughing, and active range of motion exercises

Implement measures to assist patient in safe and proper crutchwalking

Closely observe vital signs, mental status, urinary output, and temperature; implement prompt nursing intervention should any signs of physical deterioration occur

Health education

Instruct on the name, purpose, dosage, frequency, side effects, action to take if side effects occur, and precautions of each discharge medication

Instruct as to proper wound care

Reinforce diabetic control management

Instruct regarding measures to prevent infection and reduce pain

Instruct as to therapeutic and restricted activities

Instruct as to when to return to clinic or physician's office for medical follow-up care

Indicators for discharge
Adaptation to health status

Condition stable with blood sugar within acceptable range and urine free of sugar and acetone

Complications not evident

Health teaching completed

Referrals made

Examples of community resources

Visiting Nurse Association or public health nurse

Diabetic clinic

Surgical clinic

Orthopedic clinic

RETROSPECTIVE CRITERIA
Health

Condition stable with blood sugar within acceptable range and urine free of sugar and acetone

Complications not evident

Wound healing

Activity

Ambulatory

Able to carry out wound care properly

Able to use canes, walker, or crutches properly

Able to carry out diabetic control regime properly

Knowledge

Knows name of each medication; understands purpose, dosage, frequency, side effects, action to take if side effects occur, and precautions for each

Understands and can implement measures to prevent infection and reduce pain

Understands therapeutic and restricted activities and can implement therapeutic ones

Understands when to return to physician's office or clinic for follow-up medical care

Understands importance of diet control

COMPLICATIONS

Acute or progressive renal failure

Amputation (may be necessary as the result of vascular insufficiency, gangrene, osteomyelitis, or possibly a chronically severe, nonhealing skin ulcer that resists grafting)

Blindness

Degenerative vascular disease

Ocular disorders

Septicemia

Diabetes mellitus, peripheral vascular disease, gangrene, nonhealing skin ulceration, chronic complications (Code: 250)

CONCURRENT CRITERIA
Identification of patient's physical and psychosocial needs and/or concerns

Anxiety over change in body image

Relief from symptoms of pain, intolerance to changes in temperature, pallor of extremity, "mottling" (sometimes), inability to perform duties because of pain

Understanding of condition in terms of relationship to diabetes, medical and surgical treatment, and nursing management, in order that realistic plans can be made for health maintenance after discharge

Preventive measures for problems from immobility

Understanding of community agencies available to assist patient after discharge

Recommended nursing action consistent with diagnosis
Nursing services

Implement measures to reduce pain

Implement measures to promote improved circulation and to stimulate healing of any skin ulcers, by elevating the leg, maintaining bed rest, cleansing the wound with hydrogen peroxide or other prescribed solution, administering appropriate antibiotics, and applying warm, sterile saline compresses

Implement measures to maintain adequate hydration, nutrition, and elimination in keeping with diabetic dietary regime

Implement measures consistent with surgical treatment of skin grafting or amputation—preoperatively including teaching through explanation of surgical procedure, recovery room, intravenous fluids, possible traction as appropriate to amputation, special dressings, estimated period of hospitalization, graduated steps to ambulation, exercises in preparation to ambulation, deep-breathing and coughing exercises, and physically preparing patient for surgery and postoperatively including reducing pain, assisting patient in dealing with grief over changes in body image, as in the case of amputation

Implement postoperative nursing measures, including close observations for shock, hemorrhage, infection of wound, pneumonia, urinary complications, circulatory impairment due to embolism or constriction of compression dressings, plaster dressings, or improper positioning, with prompt nursing intervention should any of the above occur; close monitoring of diabetic condition with appropriate administration of caloric needs in concurrence with dietary regime, administration of hypoglycemic agent, and monitoring spillage, with prompt intervention should signs of shock or diabetic coma occur; prevention of infection; rehabilitative exercises in preparation for proper use of cane, crutches, or walker; assisting patient in correct, safe use of cane, crutches, or walker; reinforcement of diabetic teaching and adherence to medical management of same; and prevention of problems from immobility

Health education

Teach wound care

Instruct patient to avoid activities that constrict circulation, such as crossing legs, sitting in one position for long periods, standing in one spot for long periods, wearing constrictive clothing, smoking, wearing inadequate clothing (cold temperatures cause vasoconstriction)

Reinforce diabetic control teaching, including diet, urine testing, administration of hypoglycemic agent, maintenance of activity level, skin care, measures to prevent infection

Teach drug name, purpose, dosage, frequency, side effects, action to take if side effects occur, and precautions as related to all discharge medications

Instruct as related to therapeutic and restricted activities

Instruct as to use of cane, crutches, or walker, application of prosthetic devices, and safety measures

Instruct as to when and why it is necessary to return to the clinic or the physician's office for follow-up medical care

Indicators for discharge
Adaptation to health status

Condition stable with blood sugar in acceptable range and urine free of sugar and acetone

Complications not evident

Health teaching completed

Referrals made

Examples of community resources

Visiting Nurse Association or public health nurse

Diabetic clinic

Social services

Physical and vocational rehabilitation centers

RETROSPECTIVE CRITERIA
Health

Condition stable with blood sugar in acceptable range and urine free of sugar and acetone

Complications not evident

Circulation improved to extremities

Activity

Ambulatory

Able to implement wound care correctly

Able to apply prosthesis correctly

Able to use crutches, canes, or walker correctly

Able to carry out diabetic regime correctly, including planning meals, administering insulin, and testing urine

Knowledge

Understands therapeutic and restricted activities and can implement therapeutic ones

Knows the name of each discharge medication and the purpose, dosage, frequency, side effects, action to take if side effects occur, and precautions for each

Understands and can implement safety measures

Understands the importance of preventing infections and can implement proper preventive measures

Understands the importance of avoiding activities that cause circulatory impairment and can implement same

Understands when to return for medical follow-up care

COMPLICATIONS

Acute or progressive renal failure

Amputation

Blindness

Degenerative vascular disease

Ocular disorders

Septicemia

Disability from miscellaneous causes (Codes: 135, 203, 342, 352)

CONCURRENT CRITERIA
Identification of patient's physical and psychosocial needs and/or concerns

Understanding of decreased mobility and motor ability

Assessment of sensory status

Fear of change in self-care ability, fear of dependency, and fear of loss of time from normal activities

Emotional reactions to disease process

Ability to negotiate in environment with safety and visual perception

Recommended nursing action consistent with diagnosis
Nursing services

Assess self-care ability and mobility; implement program to increase independence

Establish activities of daily living program with assistive devices as needed and an exercise program

Provide emotional assessment; intervene, if necessary

Reevaluate status every 2 hours

Establish safety program

Implement discharge planning for family and home assessment

Health education

Teach adaptations to activities of daily living

Explain disability, specific health maintenance program, and symptoms to report to physician

Instruct about medication, including the name, dosage, frequency, and side effects to report to physician

Indicators for discharge
Adaptation to health status

Goals in activities of daily living program attained

Health teaching completed

Symptoms resolved or controlled

Examples of community resources

Visiting Nurse Association or public health nurse

RETROSPECTIVE CRITERIA
Health

Symptoms resolved or controlled

Emotionally coping with disease process

Activity

Performs activities of daily living program independently or with minimal assistance

Completes exercise program independently or with minimum assistance

Knowledge

States disease process or disability limitations; knows what symptoms to report to physician

Knows activities of daily living program and exercise program

Understands medication instructions and side effects to report

COMPLICATIONS

Contractures

Decubitus ulcers

Pulmonary embolism

Thrombophlebitis

Disc, herniated cervical, osteophytosis, and cervical spondylosis
(Codes: 725, 756.5, 729.1)

CONCURRENT CRITERIA
Identification of patient's physical and psychosocial needs and/or concerns

Relief of symptoms, such as pain in cervical region, neurological deficits, muscle spasms

Assistance in dealing with long-term convalescence and increased dependence

Understanding of diagnostic and therapeutic medical and surgical procedures, including purpose, expected outcome, after-care, and possible alternatives

Understanding of measures in which recurrence of injury can be avoided

Understanding of community agencies available for assistance during convalescence

Recommended nursing action consistent with diagnosis
Nursing services

Implement nursing measures supportive of conservative therapy to include comfort measures, such as administration of muscle relaxants (carisoprodol), antiinflammatory medications (phenylbutazone), analgesics, and sedatives; apply moist hot compresses 10 to 20 minutes three or four times a day; assist patient in turning if medically permitted; use distractive techniques and waking-imagined analgesics; observe effects of drugs and other comfort measures; intervene if side effects from medication occur; apply collars and braces as needed; maintain cervical traction; implement measures to prevent problems from immobility while patient is bedridden; provide adequate hydration, nutrition, elimination, skin integrity, and muscle tone

Implement nursing measures supportive of surgical treatment, including assessment of preoperative status (by assessing motor and sensory function in arms, vital signs, respiratory status, possible injury to cord so severe that sensory and motor impairment is also present in trunk and lower extremities, signs of spinal shock) as related to establishment of a baseline, as well as observation for deterioration of patient's condition necessitating prompt intervention, physical and psychological preparation of patient for surgery by explaining typing and cross-matching of blood, surgical preparation, laboratory and x-ray diagnostic tests, explanation of procedure, purpose, expected outcome, special after-care units, and nursing management

Implement postoperative nursing care, including comfort measures, such as administration of analgesics, sedatives, muscle relaxants, and antiinflammatory drugs and positioning (keeping patient flat in bed with no pillow or very small pillow at the nape of neck and turning patient like a log, supporting head, arms, and legs, so that there is no twisting of the spine, neck, or head); provide adequate rest periods during and after nursing care; maintain skin integrity (massage of bony prominence); use protective devices, such as "specially rinsed linen," rubber sponge rings, air mattresses, lotions, and lambswool; give frequent skin cleansing as necessary; implement measures to ensure adequate hydration, nutrition, and elimination; apply collar and measures to ensure safety during ambulation

Health education

Instruct about medication, including the name, purpose, dosage, frequency, side effects, action to take should side effects occur, and precautions of each discharge medication

Implement activity, including gradual increase in activity as patient gains tolerance (convalescent period may extend 2 to 3 months); instruct to avoid prolonged traveling by car in early convalescence because of vibrations causing increased pain; instruct as to proper body mechanics, avoiding extreme flexion, extension, and rotation of cervical spine while working to help reduce or prevent future problems of cervical strain

Instruct patient to sleep on side or back, not prone, and to sleep with head in neutral position, avoiding use of several pillows (using one small, flat one, if necessary)

Instruct patient as to the importance of frequent regular medical checkups and possibly evaluation of physical requirements of job

Acquaint patient with community agencies available to assist with financial aid during convalescent period, to provide vocational guidance and rehabilitation in the event that return to previous employment is not possible and a different occupation or trade must be learned

Indicators for discharge
Adaptation to health status

Condition stable
Symptoms relieved or less severe
Complications not evident
Referrals made

Examples of community resources

Workmen's compensation or public assistance
Vocational guidance centers and social worker
Visiting Nurse Association or public health nurse

RETROSPECTIVE CRITERIA
Health

Pain and muscle spasms absent or controlled
Wound healing
Complications not evident
Sleeps with head in neutral position

Activity

Gradually increasing activity
Ambulatory with proper body mechanics
Able to carry out activities of daily living without extreme flexion, extension, or rotation of cervical spine

Knowledge

Understands and knows the name of each discharge medication and the dosage, purpose, frequency, side effects, action to take should side effects occur, and precautions for each drug
Understands therapeutic and restricted activities and can implement therapeutic ones
Understands recommendations for resting and sleeping positions
Understands importance of regular medical health surveillance and possibly job evaluation
Understands community agencies available for assistance after discharge

COMPLICATIONS

Atelectasis
Decubitus ulcers
Intractable pain
Paralysis
Pneumonia
Pulmonary embolism
Thrombophlebitis
Urinary tract infection
Wound infection

Disc, herniated lumbar (Code: 725.1)

Identification of patient's physical and psychosocial needs and/or concerns

Relief from symptoms, including low back pain, inability to bear weight, muscle spasms, sensory and motor impairment

Understanding of medical or surgical treatment and nursing management in order to make realistic plans for health maintenance after discharge

Concern over loss of time from work or school

Preventive measures for problems caused by decreased activity

Rehabilitation to maintain or promote maximum functioning with supportive medical and/or surgical treatment

Recommended nursing action consistent with diagnosis
Nursing services

Reduce pain by maintaining proper positioning and alignment (avoid hip and knee flexion) and pelvic traction, applying prescribed heat treatments, turning patient in log-like fashion, maintaining bed in flat position, administering analgesics, muscle relaxants, and tranquilizers, and implementing measures to promote rest

Provide adequate hydration, nutrition, and elimination

Prevent problems resulting from inactivity by implementing active or passive exercises, frequent turning, skin care, deep-breathing and coughing exercises, 3,000 ml daily fluid intake, adequate nutrition to prevent constipation, provide diversional activities

Observe for signs of physical deterioration, including motor and sensory deterioration, shock, urinary tract infections, hypostatic pneumonia, decubitus ulcers, or contractures; intervene if necessary

Implement preoperative nursing care and teaching; physically prepare patient for surgery

Postoperatively, reduce pain; monitor physiological responses; prevent complications; provide safety during ambulation; prevent wound infections; and provide cast care, if body cast used

Rehabilitate by muscle-strengthening exercises; passive or active exercises of lower extremities, avoiding twisting or jerking motions; gluteal and quadriceps setting, dorsiflexion of feet exercises, body mechanic exercises

Apply braces, corsets, or walker, as required

Health education

Instruct about discharge medications, including the name, purpose, dosage, frequency, side effects, action to take if side effects occur, and precautions for each

Explain therapeutic and restricted activities

Teach measures to reduce discomforts during convalescence, to avoid future injury to back, and to prevent complications from decreased activity

Explain wound care (if any indicated) and signs of wound infection

Instruct about application and use of brace or corset and when to wear

Emphasize importance of follow-up medical care and when to return to see physician

Indicators for discharge
Adaptation to health status

Low back pain and muscle spasms relieved

Able to bear weight

Muscle strength of lower extremities increased since admission

Complications not evident

Referrals made
Health teaching completed

Examples of community resources

Visiting Nurse Association
Physiotherapy clinic
Bureau of Vocational Rehabilitation
Orthopedic clinic
Social services

RETROSPECTIVE CRITERIA
Health

Low back pain and muscle spasms reduced
Wound healing
Weight bearing to lower extremities
Complications not evident

Activity

Ambulatory with proper body mechanics
Able to apply corset or brace correctly

Knowledge

Knows the name, and understands the purpose, dosage, frequency, side effects, action to take if side effects occur, and precautions for each discharge medication
Understands therapeutic and restricted activities and can implement therapeutic ones

Understands and can implement discomfort-reducing measures and measures to prevent future injury to back
Understands and can implement any necessary wound care
Understands and can implement measures to prevent problems from decreased activity
Understands how to apply and when to wear brace or corset
Understands when and why it is necessary to return to the clinic or physician's office for follow-up care

COMPLICATIONS

Arrhythmias
Atelectasis
Cauda equina syndrome
Drug reaction
Hemorrhage
Paralysis
Pneumonia
Pulmonary embolism
Temperature of 100° F or over at time of discharge
Thrombophlebitis
Urinary incontinence
Urinary infections
Urinary retention
Wound infection

Dislocation of patella, recurrent (Code: 724.6)

CONCURRENT CRITERIA
Identification of patient's physical and psychosocial needs and/or concerns

Relief from pain, muscle spasms, and impairment of function
Understanding of diagnostic and surgical procedures, nursing management
Concern over loss of time from work or school
Prevention of problems resulting from decreased activity and provision of diversional activity

Rehabilitation to regain ambulatory status

Recommended nursing action consistent with diagnosis
Nursing services

Provide preoperative nursing care and teaching including explanation of surgical procedure (repair may be accomplished by tendon transplant, osteotomy with wedging to deepen the femoral groove, or the bone block procedure), recovery room, pain-reducing measures used postoperatively, deep-breathing and coughing exercises, quadriceps exercises, and physical preparation of patient for surgery

Postoperatively observe for signs of shock, excessive bleeding, circulatory impairment from constriction of compression dressing, deterioration of cardiopulmonary functioning, or lack of mental alertness, with prompt nursing intervention should signs of deterioration occur

Maintain adequate hydration, nutrition, and elimination

Prevent problems from inactivity by frequent turning, implementing deep-breathing and coughing exercises, skin hygiene, use of protective devices to prevent skin breakdown, adequate hydration, and prevention of wound infections

Promote safety and joint stability and function by elevating extremity on pillow with knee in slight flexion; observe for effusion; encourage quadriceps and straight leg–raising exercises; apply Ace bandages; supervise crutch-walking; implement safety measures while patient is ambulatory

Health education

Explain medications, including the name, purpose, dosage, frequency, side effects, action to take if side effects occur, and precautions for each discharge medication

Teach proper application of Ace bandages, purpose and duration of use

Teach proper technique for crutchwalking

Explain therapeutic and restricted activities

Advise when and why it is necessary to return to clinic or physician's office for a follow-up visit

Indicators for discharge
Adaptation to health status

Pain and muscle spasms relieved
Leg muscle strength increased
Complications not evident
Health teaching completed
Referrals made

Examples of community resources

Orthopedic clinic
Social worker
Physiotherapist

RETROSPECTIVE CRITERIA
Health

Pain and muscle spasms controlled
Knee joint stable and functioning
Leg muscle strength increased
Complications not evident

Activity

Performs quadriceps and straight leg–raising exercises
Ambulatory with crutches
Applies Ace bandages

Knowledge

Knows the name, purpose, dosage, frequency, side effects, action to take if side effects occur, and precautions for each discharge medication

Understands therapeutic and restricted activities and can implement therapeutic ones

Understands when and why it is necessary to return to clinic or physician's office for a follow-up visit

COMPLICATIONS

Chondromalacia of patella
Circulatory impairment
Decubitus ulcers
Degenerative joint disease
Hemorrhage
Pneumonia
Recurring dislocation of patella
Shock
Wound infection

Dislocation of shoulder, recurrent (Code: 724.1)

CONCURRENT CRITERIA
Identification of patient's physical and psychosocial needs and/or concerns

Relief from pain and impairment of function

Understanding of diagnostic and surgical procedures and nursing management

Concern over loss of time from work or school

Rehabilitation to regain use of joint function

Prevention of complications resulting from immobility or inactivity

Recommended nursing action consistent with diagnosis
Nursing services

Provide preoperative nursing care and teaching, including explanation of surgical procedure (repair may be accomplished by placing tendon of long head of biceps through head of humerus or by suturing capsule and labium to anterior lip of glenoid fossa), recovery room, duration of hospitalization, pain-reducing measures to be used postoperatively, and importance of frequent change of position and deep-breathing exercises; administration of pain-reducing measures; and physical preparation of patient for surgery

Implement postoperative nursing care, including providing adequate hydration, nutrition, and elimination; preventing hypostatic pneumonia, skin breakdown, urinary tract infection, decubitus ulcers, and wound infection; and observing for signs of circulatory impairment if Velpeau's bandage or a compression dressing is used and for other complications

Implement pain-reducing measures

Health education

Instruct patient on pendulum exercises to start when medically feasible

Explain the name, purpose, dosage, frequency, side effects, action to take if side effects occur, and precautions for each discharge medication

Explain about therapeutic and restricted activities

Instruct about wound care

Advise when and why it is necessary to return to clinic or physician's office for a follow-up visit

Indicators for discharge
Adaptation to health status

Pain controlled
Shoulder function increased
Complications not evident
Health teaching completed
Referrals made

Examples of community resources

Orthopedic clinic
Physiotherapist
Social worker

RETROSPECTIVE CRITERIA
Health

Pain relieved
Shoulder function increased
Wound healing
Complications not evident

Activity

Ambulatory
Able to do prescribed exercises

Knowledge

Understands frequency and mechanics of therapeutic exercises

Knows the name, purpose, dosage, frequency, side effects, action to take if side effects occur, and precautions for each discharge medication

Understands therapeutic and restricted activities

Understands and can implement wound care, if any

Understands when and why it is necessary to return to clinic or physician's office for follow-up visit

COMPLICATIONS

Circulatory impairment
Decubitus ulcers
Hemorrhage
Pneumonia
Recurrent anterior dislocation
Shock
Tear of musculotendinous cuff
Traction injury of circumflex (axillary) nerve
Urinary tract infection
Wound infection

Diverticular disease of colon (Code: 562)

CONCURRENT CRITERIA
Identification of patient's physical and psychosocial needs and/or concerns

Relief from symptoms, including colicky pains and tenderness in the lower left quadrant, nausea, loss of appetite, fever, constipation or diarrhea, increased gas, dehydration, possibly bowel obstruction, peritonitis, fistula, or frank bleeding

Understanding of medical, surgical, and nursing management so realistic plans for health maintenance after discharge can be made

Maintenance of vital body functions

Concern over loss of time from work or school, change in body image, or fear of cancer

Prevention of problems from inactivity

Recommended nursing action consistent with diagnosis
Nursing services

Maintain vital body functions, including cardiovascular functions, fluid replacement, conservation of body heat, ventilation with oxygen administration, administration of vasopressors, if ordered

Implement nursing measures consistent with medical management, including observation for physical deterioration with intervention in case of complications

Maintain adequate hydration, nutrition, elimination, and activity, by adminis-
tering parenteral fluids for patient if nothing by mouth allowed and by implementing an oral hygiene program, a progressive diet, intake and output recording, measures to avoid constipation, relief from anxiety, and promotion of activity

Provide preoperative nursing care and teaching, including explanation of procedure, course in recovery room, postoperative intravenous solutions, duration of nothing by mouth order, nasogastric suction, monitoring of vital signs, chest physiology, pain relief or control measures, progressive ambulation, dressing care, and possibility of special care unit; physically prepare patient for surgery

Implement postoperative nursing care, including observation of physiological responses, postoperative care intervention, support to patient for dealing with fears of cancer, changes in body image, or financial problems; promote wound healing

Implement rehabilitation measures related to colostomy, including acceptance of colostomy, control of diet, skin care, application of appliance, irrigations, odor control, discharge care

Health education

Explain diet, including cooking methods to avoid, permitted foods and foods to be avoided (for medically managed patient, frequently a low residue diet, high in protein and calories, avoiding foods like clams, oysters, meat fibers—pureed meats are sometimes permitted—sweet potatoes, whole grains, corn, carrots, nuts, cabbage, and lettuce; for colostomy patient, a similar diet, avoiding gas-forming foods, but frequently graduating to a regular diet with only those foods restricted that cannot be tolerated by the individual

Teach the name, purpose, dosage, frequency, side effects, action to take if side effects occur, and precautions for all discharge medications

Instruct about therapeutic and restricted activities

Instruct colostomy patient on skin care, equipment needed for home care and where to purchase, appliance application, irrigation methods, techniques for controlling regularity and odor, and what to do about problems with leakage and accidents; stress the fact that a colostomy patient can live a normal life; stress the positive—that which can be done by the patient, not what cannot

Instruct medically managed patient on the importance of good skin care; instruct patient with a resection on wound care

Instruct patient when to return to the physician's office or clinic; stress the importance of continual medical follow-up care

Indicators for discharge
Adaptation to health status

Hydrated
Gastrointestinal symptoms controlled
Stools formed or colostomy functioning
Complications not evident
Health teaching completed
Referrals made

Examples of community resources

Visiting Nurse Association or public health nurse
Social services
Medical or surgical clinic
Ostomy club

RETROSPECTIVE CRITERIA
Health

Increased diet tolerance
Stools formed or colostomy functioning and wound healing
Coping with change in body image
Complications not evident

Activity

Ambulatory
Able to carry out activities of daily living
Able to apply colostomy appliance and administer colostomy irrigations correctly, if applicable
Able to carry out wound care correctly, if applicable
Able to implement skin hygiene

Knowledge

Understands and can implement diet correctly
Understands name, purpose, dosage, frequency, side effects, action to take if side effects occur, and precautions of all discharge medications
Understands importance and method of achieving good skin care and preventing excoriations; medical patient understands method of controlling diarrhea or constipation by diet; colostomy patient understands colostomy care, including application of appliance, irrigations, prevention of stricture, and diet control
Understands when and why it is necessary to return to physician's office or clinic for medical follow-up care

COMPLICATIONS

Abscess
Complete intestinal obstruction
Constipation

Dehydration	Nausea
Diarrhea	Perforation
Fistula	Peritonitis
Hemorrhage	Skin excoriation
Infection	Shock
Mental depression	

Drug abuse (Code: DSM II 304)

CONCURRENT CRITERIA
Identification of patient's physical and psychosocial needs and/or concerns

Evaluation of health status

Documentation of need for protective environment

Expression of concerns, such as hospitalization and treatment

Identification of concerns, such as for significant others and job

Determination of mental status

Recommended nursing action consistent with diagnosis
Nursing services

Observe for symptoms of drug withdrawal

Provide for improvement and/or maintenance of health status, such as skin care and nutrition

Provide for a safe physical environment

Administer medication as required to control symptoms

Make recommendations for treatment plan

Health education

Inform patient and significant others of treatment plan and realistic expectations of the plan

Teach patient and significant others about physical effects of drug abuse

Indicators for discharge
Adaptation to health status

Achievement of inpatient treatment goals

Follow-up treatment plan established; plan understood by patient and significant others

Dependency on drugs absent

Examples of community resources

Community halfway house

RETROSPECTIVE CRITERIA
Health

Regular sleep pattern
Improved nutritional status
Withdrawn from drugs
Complications not evident

Activity

Able to perform activities of daily living
Interacting in personal and group relationships

Knowledge

Understands how to set goals and make plans

Patient verbalizes understanding that nonverbal behavior should confirm verbal expression of feelings

Patient verbalizes a positive attitude toward abstinence from drug

COMPLICATIONS

Acute anxiety
Acute psychedelic reaction
Acute respiratory distress
Cardiac arrhythmia or arrest
Coma
Drug reaction
Gastric distress
Hepatitis
Hyperpyrexia
Hypertensive crisis
Hypotension
Malnutrition
Psychiatric problems
Psychosis
Skin problems
Withdrawal seizures

Dysrhythmias (Code: 781.7)

CONCURRENT CRITERIA
Identification of patient's physical and psychosocial needs and/or concerns

Relief of symptoms, including fast or slow heart rate, chest pain, dyspnea, syncope, weakness, nausea and/or vomiting

Explanation of hyper- or hypotension

Fear and concern about heart palpitations, interrupted life-style, and/or impending death

Adaptation to coronary care unit environment

Understanding of nature of condition, course, management, and prognosis

Recommended nursing action consistent with diagnosis
Nursing services

Begin cardiac monitoring and vital signs within 5 minutes of admission to coronary care unit

Initiate delegated medical directions immediately such as intravenous solutions, medications, and oxygen

Record and document rhythm strips (electrocardiogram)

Reassure patient that environment is safe; provide emotional support to patient and family

Physically assess patient for signs of embolization

Health education

Explain purpose of techniques and procedures, including drugs, pacemaker, if indicated, and cardioversion, if indicated

Cooperate with plan of care contributing to recovery

Explain activity limitations (physical and sexual)

Explain diet, drugs, restrictions, and importance of medical follow-up

Explain contributory risk factors

Indicators for discharge
Adaptation to health status

Syncope and dyspnea absent

Heart rate and vital signs controlled within normal range

Activity tolerated without signs and symptoms of cardiac stress

Acceptance of diagnosis verbalized

Knowledge of restrictions or limitations of activities verbalized

Embolization not evident (pulses in extremities palpable)

Examples of community resources

Visiting Nurse Association or public health nurse

American Heart Association

RETROSPECTIVE CRITERIA
Health

Diet controlled
Chest pain absent
Heart rate within normal range
Complications not evident

Activity

Ambulatory without symptoms of cardiac stress
Self-care

Knowledge

Patient and/or significant other verbalizes understanding of diagnosis, risk factors (according to the American Heart Association), diet, drugs, and importance of follow-up medical care

COMPLICATIONS

Cardiac arrest
Ventricular fibrillation
Ventricular tachycardia

Encephalitis (Code: 323)

CONCURRENT CRITERIA

Identification of patient's physical and psychosocial needs and/or concerns

Relief of symptoms, including high fever, severe headache, disorientation, diplopia, sleepiness, lethargy, insomnia, coma

Family/patient understanding of cause, identifiable as related to insect bites or to related systemic infections such as measles, chickenpox, mumps, herpes simplex, mononucleosis; prognosis; outcome; and medical and nursing management

Concern about possible infection of other members of the family

Family protection, such as through immunization against previously mentioned viral infections and, when possible, community protection through insect (particularly mosquitoes) eradication

Recommended nursing action consistent with diagnosis
Nursing services

Implement safety measures during restlessness, seizures, or coma

Maintain vital body functions, including hydration, nutrition, adequate ventilation, elimination, and cardiovascular functions

Closely observe for desired effects and side effects of medications and therapeutic procedures, such as lumbar punctures, with prompt nursing intervention should untoward reactions occur; prevent deterioration of patient's condition and complications, including problems from immobility such as circulatory stasis; observe for increased intracranial pressure

Reduce anxiety within patient/family about the nature of the disease and about possible contagion to others

Health education

Explain to patient/family purpose and duration of initial isolation and method for maintaining it

Explain to patient/family means of preventing contagion to other members of the family, if source of encephalitis is identifiable

Explain to patient/family medical and nursing management, including purpose, expected outcome, preparation, and duration of medical and nursing regime, special care units, medications, intravenous solutions, nasogastric tubes, lumbar punctures, suctioning, positioning, artificial airways, ventilatory devices, seizure care, and isolation units

Identify community agencies that may appropriately assist patient once discharged

Indicators for discharge
Adaptation to health status

Afebrile

Maximum improvement after medical and/or surgical therapy

Family/patient understanding of what is necessary for home care or convalescence

Referral agencies contacted for follow-up care

Examples of community resources

Visiting Nurse Association or public health nurse

Department of Public Health

Social services and other appropriate referrals for financial assistance

Speech, physical, and vocational rehabilitation centers

School nurse to survey health status of child; teacher for guidance where learning disability may be present or where referral to exceptional child center would be appropriate

Health

Afebrile

Maximum improvement achieved for neurological deficits

Activity

Independent in activities of daily living with minimal assistance

Knowledge

Patient/family understands importance of prompt medical attention to viral infections

Patient/family understands rehabilitative care necessary for home management of patient with residual neurological deficits and is capable of implementing that care

Patient/family understands care as related to medications for epileptic individual, safety precautions, measures for decreasing occurrence, and legal implications

Patient/family understands the importance of follow-up medical surveillance

Patient/family aware of and understands the function of community agencies that can appropriately help after discharge

COMPLICATIONS

Bronchial pneumonia
Decubitus ulcers
Epilepsy
Infection
Mental deterioration
Parkinsonism
Urinary retention

Encephalocele, cranium bifidum (Code: 743.9)*

CONCURRENT CRITERIA
Identification of patient's physical and psychosocial needs and/or concerns

Correction of defect and control or relief from symptoms that vary with location of encephalocele and location of incomplete closure of bones in skull

Assistance to parents in coping with having a deformed child

Understanding by parents of cause (if identifiable), course, treatment, nursing management, and prognosis, so that realistic plans for child's care can be made

Understanding by parents of the importance of continuous regular medical checkups and evaluation as child matures

Acquaintance by parents with community agencies available for assistance after discharge

Recommended nursing action consistent with diagnosis
Nursing services

Implement preoperative and supportive nursing measures, including protection from infection and trauma and avoidance of exposure to drafts, personnel with infections, and trauma to sac and head; observe child's behavior and reactions to care daily for signs of deterioration (by checking color, temperature, quality and rate of respirations and pulse, increased drowsiness, apathy, vomiting, convulsions, and daily measurement of the head—hydrocephalus is frequently associated with encephalocele and cranium bifidum); ensure adequate hydration and nutrition; physically prepare child for surgery

---

*Criteria are for child through 16 months. Criteria must be modified for child having surgery subsequent to the initial repair or for older child being hospitalized for other problems relating to encephalocele or cranium bifidum.

Implement postoperative nursing measures, including close observation for signs of shock, meningitis, pneumonia, fever, decubitus ulcers, impairment of motor function, spasticity, and contractures by checking color, temperature, quality and rate of respiration and pulse and by watching for increased drowsiness, apathy, vomiting, or convulsions; ensure adequate hydration and nutrition; prevent increased intracranial pressure by elevating the head 20 to 30 degrees and restricting fluids, as ordered; prevent decubitus ulcers by frequent repositioning with proper support and "props"; prevent wound infection; consult with parents about a plan to provide emotional support for child

Initiate appropriate referrals

Implement measures to aid parents in adjusting to having a deformed child

Health education

Instruct parents in physical care of child, including skin care and measures to ensure adequate hydration and nutrition, to provide for emotional security, and to prevent infection

Instruct parents in ego-supportive measures and necessity of imposing limits on child as child grows older

Instruct parents as to importance of regular medical checkups and psychological testing at prescribed intervals in order to determine realistic long-range and short-term goals

Instruct parents about possible outcome of surgery, intensive care or special care units, visiting hours, and possibility of residual permanent neurological defects or death

Indicators for discharge
Adaptation to health status

Condition stable

Complications not evident

Necessary health teaching completed

Referrals made

Parents coping with having a deformed child

Examples of community resources*

National Cerebral Palsy Association or social services

Visiting Nurse Association, public health nurse, or school nurse

Rehabilitation centers (depending on age of child) or exceptional child centers

RETROSPECTIVE CRITERIA
Health

Condition stable

Afebrile

Wound infection or breakdown of sac not evident

Increased intracranial pressure not evident

Activity

Parents coping with having a deformed child

Activity according to medical expectations and appropriate for age

Parents take measurement of child's head daily

Knowledge

Parents understand and can implement necessary physical care of child, such as skin care, adequate hydration and nutrition, measures to promote emotional security, and measures to prevent infection

Parents understand and can implement ego-supportive measures and necessary limits on child as child grows older

Parents understand importance of frequent regular medical checkups and psychological testing of child; parents have means by which to secure this type of health surveillance

Parents understand and know the name, dosage, frequency, purpose, side effects, action to take if side effects occur, and precautions for each discharge medication

Parents understand and are able to imple-

---

*Parents should be made aware of services available for later period, if not appropriate at this time

ment care as related to residual permanent neurological deficits

COMPLICATIONS

Convulsions
Decubitus ulcers
Developmental defects in brain
Hydrocephalus
Increased intracranial pressure
Infections
Joint contractures
Meningitis
Nausea and/or vomiting
Pneumonia
Shock
Spasticity
Thromboembolism
Wound infection

Encephalopathy (toxic-metabolic) (Code: 781.7)

CONCURRENT CRITERIA
Identification of patient's physical and psychosocial needs and/or concerns

Relief from symptoms, including changes in consciousness level, convulsions, withdrawal symptoms such as delirium, tremors, and hallucination from toxic agents, polyneuritis, loss of positional sense, ataxia, parkinsonian tremors

Explanation of cause of encephalopathy, if known, prognosis, and medical and nursing management

Family genetic counseling as related to encephalopathies caused by hereditary conditions, such as porphyria, phenylketonuria, galactosemia, lipoidosis, or Tay-Sachs disease or following lateral sclerosis

Protection from injury possibly resulting from changes in mental ability, disorientation, impairment of sensory and motor function, and generalized weakness resulting from metabolic disturbance

Maintenance of vital body functions, including hydration, nutrition, elimination, respiration, and cardiovascular functioning

Recommended nursing action consistent with diagnosis
Nursing services

Closely observe for signs of physical deterioration; implement immediate nursing intervention if signs occur

Implement safety measures to protect patient from injury possibly resulting from impaired judgment, sensory or motor loss, and/or weakness

Initiate referrals

Implement measures to maintain or improve hydration, nutrition, elimination, respiration, and cardiovascular functioning

Implement measures to improve impaired motor function in the presence of residual neurological deficits

Health education

Teach the name, dosage, frequency, purpose, side effects, action to take should side effects occur, and precautions of each discharge medication

Teach safety measures related to impaired judgment, sensory or motor loss, and/or weakness

Explain special diet and restrictions related to alcohol and drugs (barbiturates and narcotics)

Teach proper storage of toxic agents, correction of health hazards related to occupation and toxic agents; provide genetic counseling related to hereditary metabolic disorders

Teach measures to maintain optimal functioning within limits of neurological deficits or mental changes

Indicators for discharge
Adaptation to health status

Condition stable

Symptoms relieved or reduced in severity

Referrals made

Examples of community resources

Visiting Nurse Association or public health nurse

Social services

Department of Public Health (industrial health hazards as related to toxic agents and drug abuse)

Drug abuse treatment centers

Medical clinics as related to metabolic disorders

Genetic counseling centers

Exceptional child centers and physical, speech, and vocational rehabilitation centers

RETROSPECTIVE CRITERIA
Health

Special diet and dietary restrictions tolerated

Hydration improved

Condition stable

Symptoms relieved or less severe

Complications not evident

Activity

Ambulatory

Able to perform activities of daily living

Knowledge

Patient/family understands name, dosage, frequency, purpose, side effects, action

to take if side effects occur, and precautions for each medication

Patient/family understands special diet and restrictions related to foods and alcohol

Patient/family understands necessary safety measures and is capable of implementing them

Patient/family understands proper storage of toxic agents and has acceptable plan for avoiding or correcting health hazards related to toxic agents in occupation; when appropriate, patient/family understands significance of hereditary factors related to metabolic-induced encephalopathy and has means of obtaining genetic counseling

Patient/family understands and is capable of implementing measures to maintain optimal functioning level within limits of neurological deficits and/or mental changes

COMPLICATIONS

Bronchial pneumonia

Convulsions

Decubitus ulcers

Dehydration

Epilepsy

Hallucinations

Infection

Mental deterioration

Parkinsonism

Urinary retention

Enteritis, chronic, in children (Code: 563.9)

CONCURRENT REVIEW CRITERIA
Identification of patient's physical and psychosocial needs and/or concerns

Maintenance of hydration and electrolyte balance

Cessation of diarrhea and/or vomiting

Understanding of basic nutrition

Understanding by patient/family of purpose of restricting fluids and food intake

Oral stimulation if nothing by mouth allowed

Recommended nursing action consistent with diagnosis
Nursing services

Carefully regulate intravenous fluids

Control amount of oral intake

Keep accurate account and description of any vomiting and/or diarrhea

Record daily weights
Give emotional support

Health education

Teach patient/family about diet ordered by physician and importance of restricted diet

Explain to patient/family importance of seeing each stool and/or vomitus

Stress importance of a happy environment

Indicators for discharge
Adaptation to health status

Diarrhea and/or vomiting controlled
Proper dietary instructions received and understood
Ambulatory
Afebrile

Examples of community resources

Referral usually not indicated

RETROSPECTIVE REVIEW CRITERIA
Health

Diarrhea and/or vomiting controlled
Diet tolerated
Afebrile

Activity

Ambulatory

Knowledge

Patient/family understand diet ordered by physician
Patient/family understand causes of chronic enteritis and ways to prevent and/or manage condition

COMPLICATIONS

Cerebral edema
Fluid and electrolyte imbalance
Metabolic acidosis or alkalosis
Pulmonary or peripheral edema
Skin irritation

Epilepsy (Code: 353.1)

CONCURRENT REVIEW CRITERIA
Identification of patient's physical and psychosocial needs and/or concerns

Control of seizures
Acceptance of disorder by self and others
Understanding of disorder, cause, chronicity, restrictions, and legal aspects
Understanding of medical, surgical, and nursing management
Support of family and community

Recommended nursing actions consistent with diagosis
Nursing services

Observe and record seizure characteristics
Protect patient from bodily harm during and after seizure
Protect patient from psychological trauma

Observe for desired and toxic effects of drug therapy
Explain purpose, preparation, and outcome of diagnostic or therapeutic procedures

Health education

Teach the name, purpose, dosage, frequency, desired effect, and side effects of each medication; explain necessity of good oral hygiene while using anticonvulsant drugs and continual maintenance of therapeutic blood levels of anticonvulsant drugs; emphasize importance of regular medical follow-up supervision
Give instructions about incision care, diet, and activities for home care consistent with surgery
Help devise plan for regulating activities and avoiding emotional stress, physical

excitement, excessive fatigue, and alcohol to decrease occurrence of convulsions

Stress importance of wearing a medical tag or carrying identification signifying medications being taken as an epileptic

Teach signs and symptoms of aura, if present, and appropriate action to take should aura occur; teach emergency care during seizures

Indicators for discharge
Adaptation to health status

Toxic effects from medication not evident

Convulsions absent for 3 to 5 consecutive days prior to discharge

Discharge environment suitable

Referral initiated for follow-up care

Examples of community resources

Visiting Nurse Association

Alcoholics Anonymous (if appropriate)

Bureau of Vocational Rehabilitation

National Association to Control Epilepsy

Mental health agencies

RETROSPECTIVE REVIEW CRITERIA
Health

Alcohol avoided (if appropriate)

Seizures controlled or suppressed by adherence to drug regimes

Complications not evident

Activity

Avoids hazardous occupations and driving

Independent in activities of daily living

Avoids excessive fatigue

Knowledge*

Demonstrates knowledge of symptoms and of aura, when present, and appropriate action to take; understands emergency care during seizures

Understands relationship of stress, fatigue, inactivity, and alcohol to precipitation of convulsions

Understands importance of continuing drug therapy; knows name, purpose, dosage, frequency, desired effect, side effects, and action to take if side effects occur for each medication; understands importance of regular medical follow-up supervision

Has knowledge of appropriate referral agencies and means of contacting them, if further aid after discharge is necessary

Understands legal implications of convulsive state

COMPLICATIONS

Automatisms

Disorientation

Drug reaction

Erratic behavior

Excitement

Fractures or soft tissue injuries

Hallucinations

Incoherent speech

Irritability

Mental and emotional changes

Mental dullness

---

*In all cases where there is a physical and/or mental disability preventing learning, the family or a responsible party must demonstrate required knowledge, and this must be indicated in the nurse's notes.

Esophageal atresia and tracheoesophageal fistula in children
(Codes: 750.2, 750.3)

CONCURRENT CRITERIA
Identification of patient's physical and psychosocial needs and/or concerns

Relief from excessive salivation and thick mucus

Evaluation of cyanosis that improves with oxygen and suctioning but recurs as secretions build up again

Prevention of infection

Reduction of reflux of gastric juices into the trachea and lungs by proper positioning—keeping head and chest elevated

Provision of psychological needs of sucking, warmth, and comfort

Recommended nursing action consistent with diagnosis
Nursing services

Maintain a constant, low suction on the indwelling replogle tube of upper pouch to prevent overflow of secretions into the lungs preoperatively

Keep infant in an upright position to avoid reflux of gastric juices into trachea and lungs

Postoperatively, suction only to depth indicated by physician

Postoperatively, prevent hyperextension of head and neck

Allow sucking on a nipple as soon as the physician will permit; make infant as comfortable as possible

Health education

Explain to parents all the necessary equipment being used

Stress importance of preventing infection

Explain diet

Upon discharge, explain possibility of a stricture and that vomiting should be reported to physician immediately

Indicators for discharge
Adaptation to health status

Afebrile
Diet tolerated
Weight gained
Wound healed; sutures removed

Examples of community resources

Public health nurse or Visiting Nurse Association for follow-up

RETROSPECTIVE CRITERIA
Health

Afebrile
Weight gained
Wound healed; sutures removed

Activity

Active
Alert

Knowledge

Responsible party understands measures to take to prevent infection

Responsible party understands diet

Responsible party understands importance of calling the physician if repeated vomiting occurs

COMPLICATIONS

Anastomotic leak
Pneumonia
Sepsis
Stricture
Vomiting
Wound infection

Facelift, surgical (Code: 94.3)

CONCURRENT REVIEW CRITERIA
Identification of patient's physical and psychosocial needs and/or concerns

Correction of scars, deformities, facial palsy, or aging marks that create poor body image or socioeconomic disadvantages or impair muscular functions

Full understanding of surgical procedure and anticipated outcome as well as adjunctive therapy to be used, so that realistic plans for health maintenance can be made

Preventive measures for complications of surgery and inactivity

Maintenance of adequate nutrition and hydration

Rehabilitiative measures supportive of surgical procedure

Recommended nursing action consistent with diagnosis
Nursing services

Provide preoperative care and teaching, including explanation of surgical procedure, recovery room, appearance of wound immediately after surgery, use of pressure dressings and possible drains, duration of hospitalization, possible limitations of surgical procedure, use of adjunctive therapy (such as makeup consultations, contact lenses, and dental correction); explain when patient may resume social or business activities; prepare patient regarding comments well-meaning friends may make during convalescent period; physically prepare patient for surgery

Implement postoperative nursing care, including pain-reducing measures, proper hydration, nutrition, and elimination, prevention of wound infection, scarring, or deterioration of cosmetic or functional effect

Assess for impairment of circulation every 4 hours; observe for hemorrhage or development of a hematoma every 4 hours; implement prompt interventive measures should any of the above occur; provide adequate ventilation and a patent airway; prevent complications from decreased activity

Implement measures to assist patient in using adjunctive therapy to maximize the effects of surgical therapy

Implement measures to assist patient in coping with changing body image postoperatively; initiate discharge planning and referrals

Health education

Instruct on medications, including name, purpose, dosage, frequency, side effects, action to take if side effects occur, and precautions of all discharge medications

Teach wound care

Instruct patient on use of adjunctive therapy according to instructions of cosmetology consultant, or, if no contact with consultant prior to discharge, instruct patient on measures to reduce discomforts from wound healing and embarrassment of scars during convalescence

Instruction restricted and therapeutic activities

Instruct patient when and why it is necessary to return to office or clinic for follow-up medical care

Indications for discharge
Adaptation to health status

Condition stable
Complications not evident
Health teaching completed
Referrals made
Wound healing

Examples of community resources

Cosmetologist
Social services
Surgical clinic

RETROSPECTIVE REVIEW CRITERIA
Health

Condition stable
Wound healing
Complications not evident

Activity

Ambulatory
Independent in activities of daily living
Performs wound care correctly

Knowledge

Knows the name, purpose, dosage, frequency, side effects, action to take if side effects occur, and precautions of each discharge medication
Understands how to give wound care correctly
Understands and can implement the use of adjunctive therapy

Understands and can implement restricted and therapeutic activities
Knows when to return to clinic or physician's office and understands the importance of follow-up medical care

COMPLICATIONS

Arrhythmias
Atelectasis
Drug reaction
Hematoma
Hemorrhage
Pneumonia
Pulmonary embolism
Scarring
Temperature of 100° F or over at time of discharge
Thrombophlebitis
Urinary infections
Wound infection

Failure to thrive in children (Code: 269.9)

CONCURRENT REVIEW CRITERIA
Identification of patient's physical and psychosocial needs and/or concerns

Relief of failure to grow
Resolution of malnutrition
Understanding by parents about condition, prognosis, treatment, and delay in motor and social development
Relief of dehydration (resulting from vomiting, diarrhea, anorexia, and apathy)
Increase in expression of affection toward child and in sensory stimulation

Recommended nursing action consistent with diagnosis
Nursing services

Carefully observe for determination of cause of failure to thrive
Chart each feeding, noting child's manner of eating, amount eaten, and presence of vomiting and/or diarrhea
Provide understanding and praise for parents during feeding of child

Help establish positive self-images in parents and appropriate parent-child identification
Create an environment of understanding; be available to listen to parents/child

Health education

Discuss proper methods of child care with parents; reinforce learning about the child
Teach parents the importance of cuddling and loving their child
Foster feelings of worth in parents as to their ability to care for the child

Indicators for discharge
Adaptation to health status

Afebrile
Eating well; gaining weight
Parents able to feed child
Parents able to meet physical and emotional needs of child

Examples of community resources

Social worker
Public health nurse or Visiting Nurse Association

RETROSPECTIVE REVIEW CRITERIA
Health

Afebrile
Eating well; gaining weight
Physical and emotional needs met

Activity

Alert and responsive

Knowledge

Parents able to feed child
Parents know when to bring child in for medical follow-up
Parents able to identify child's nonverbal cues and provide appropriate physical and/or emotional support

COMPLICATIONS

Congenital heart disease
Dehydration
Malnutrition
Mental retardation
Renal insufficiency
Sensory deprivation
Urinary tract infection

Fluid and electrolyte imbalance in children (Codes: 790, 790.2, 790.3)

CONCURRENT CRITERIA
Identification of patient's physical and psychosocial needs and/or concerns

Correction of dehydration and electrolyte imbalance
Maintenance of basic nutrition
Monitoring of acid-base imbalance
Patient/parent understanding of the importance of intravenous fluids
Resolution of vomiting and/or diarrhea

Recommended nursing action consistent with diagnosis
Nursing services

Regulate and carefully record administration of intravenous fluids
Regulate oral intake; record properly
Keep accurate account of urine output
Keep accurate record of any vomiting and/or diarrhea
Maintain proper positioning to protect intravenous equipment; prevent aspiration of fluids, if vomiting occurs
Administer prompt, thorough cleansing of skin after each episode of vomiting and/or diarrhea

Health education

Explain importance of intravenous solutions to family and patient

Explain diet limitations
Implement a teaching program based on the parents' knowledge and understanding of causative factors

Indicators for discharge
Adaptation to health status

Progressive improvement in hydration and electrolyte balance, as evidenced by adequate skin turgor and urine output
Control of vomiting and/or diarrhea
Ambulatory
Tolerating usual diet for 48 to 72 hours

Examples of community resources

Visiting Nurse Association or public health nurse (to evaluate home situation and possible precipitous causes)

RETROSPECTIVE CRITERIA
Health

Afebrile
Control of vomiting and/or diarrhea
Tolerating diet

Activity

Ambulatory

152

Knowledge

Parents understand and can implement diet ordered by physician

Parents understand methods to correct causative factors

COMPLICATIONS

Cardiac arrhythmias

Circulatory overload

Dehydration

Hypovolemic shock

Metabolic acidosis and alkalosis

Skin breakdown

Thrombophlebitis

Fracture of ankle—trimalleolus, medial malleolus, lateral malleolus, or bimalleolus

Closed reduction (Code: 824)

Open reduction (Code: 824.7)

CONCURRENT CRITERIA

Identification of patient's physical and psychosocial needs and/or concerns

Relief from symptoms and disabilities, including pain, swelling, muscle spasms, deformity, impaired function, and false motion

Explanation of diagnostic and surgical procedures and nursing management

Reassurance about increased dependence during convalescence

Assistance in protection against injury and problems caused by immobility

Rehabilitative measures to regain ambulatory status

Recommended nursing action consistent with diagnosis

Nursing services

Provide preoperative nursing measures, including reduction of swelling and pain by elevation, positioning, sand bags, ice, pillows, and medication; maintain proper position of bone segments and alignment prior to reduction; explain reduction procedure, recovery room, estimated healing time, length of hospitalization, postoperative patient participation, deep breathing, coughing, and pain reduction; promote circulation; physically prepare patient for procedure; maintain adequate hydration; closely observe patient for signs of complications prior to reduction procedure, including disturbances in sensory or motor function, fat embolism, shock, or infection, with prompt nursing intervention in event of abnormality

Implement postoperative nursing measures, including observation and monitoring for abnormalities in vital signs, presence and quality of peripheral pulses, skin color, skin temperature, motor and sensory function (particularly in affected foot), urinary output, mental alertness, degree of swelling in foot, or severe pain or bleeding with prompt nursing intervention in event of abnormality; implement pain reduction via elevation, positioning, medication, and ice; maintain adequate nutrition, hydration, and elimination; provide cast care, including drying, protecting, petaling, and care of surrounding skin, and assistance and instruction in proper use of crutches in successive stages of ambulation

Implement rehabilitative measures, including cast care, progressive ambulation, range-of-motion exercises, methods to reduce dependent edema, and complete health education program

Health education

Control pain through appropriate positioning and comfort measures, and medication

Provide cast care, including cleaning and protecting; observe for danger signs such as extreme pain, swelling, discoloration or numbness of skin; implement steps to remediate such symptoms

Instruct in safe crutchwalking with return demonstration

Teach discharge medications, including the name, purpose, dosage, frequency, and precautions for each

Explain the purpose, frequency, and importance of orthopedic clinic follow-up

Explain measures to reduce dependent edema and discomfort

Indicators for discharge
Adaptation to health status

Condition stable, including stable vital signs, no abnormal pain, swelling, or circulatory problems, and no complications evident

Pain controlled through nursing measures and oral medication

Bones properly aligned, as confirmed by postoperative x-rays

Patient knowledgeable regarding cast care and crutchwalking; understands limitations of activities

Referrals completed

Examples of community resources

Orthopedic clinic

RETROSPECTIVE CRITERIA
Health

Peripheral pulses strong
Pain and swelling controlled

Condition stable
Complications not evident
Fractured bones properly aligned

Activity

Ambulatory
Able to use crutches appropriately
Provides own cast care

Knowledge

Patient has knowledge and demonstrates ability to implement measures regarding cast care, including recognizing danger signs and symptoms and maintaining cleanliness, protection, and prevention of infection

Patient understands and is able to use discharge medications; knows the name, purpose, dosage, frequency, effects, side effects, and precautions for each

Patient understands safety procedures regarding crutchwalking

Patient understands and can implement pain-reduction measures other than medication

Patient understands purpose and time of orthopedic clinic follow-up appointment

COMPLICATIONS

Ankle joint stiffness
Degenerative joint disease
Fat embolism
Hemorrhage
Impaired peripheral circulation
Muscle spasms
Nonunion or malunion
Shock
Swelling
Tear of tibiofibular ligament
Wound infection

Fracture of cervical, dorsal, or lumbar vertebrae (Codes: 806, 806.2, 806.4)

CONCURRENT CRITERIA
Identification of patient's physical and psychosocial needs and/or concerns

Relief of symptoms and disability, including severe pain and inability to bear weight

Reassurance about increased dependence during convalescence or about time away from work or school

Close observation for deterioration of condition and injuries to spinal cord, including severe pain, (especially on movement), sensory and motor function impairment below level of injury, or spinal shock

Explanation of diagnostic, medical, and/or surgical procedures as well as nursing management

Rehabilitative measures to regain ambulatory status

Recommended nursing action consistent with diagnosis
Nursing services

Closely observe for physical deterioration or cord damage by frequently monitoring vital signs, sensory and motor function, urinary output, skin color and temperature and watching for signs of paralytic ileus (such as distention and vomiting), with prompt nursing intervention should signs of deterioration occur

For uncomplicated fracture of the lumbar dorsal spine

Implement pain-reducing measures; maintain skin integrity and circulation, by turning patient frequently in log-like fashion, massaging skin gently to promote circulation, providing protective devices such as sheepskin to prevent skin breakdown, keeping skin clean and dry, and encouraging patient to do isometric exercises; maintain adequate hydration, nutrition, and elimination; prevent problems from immobility (such as thrombophlebitis, decubitus ulcers, urinary tract infections, and hypostatic pneumonia) by encouraging patient to do isometric, deep-breathing, and coughing exercises, frequently turning via "log-rolling technique," and maintaining high fluid intake

Apply full-length brace to back when patient becomes ambulatory; implement safety measures during ambulation; provide diversional activity

For moderate or severe fracture of the lumbar and dorsal spine

Implement pain-reducing measures; maintain hyperextension of back by gradual increasing angle of Gatch bed to specified degree of hyperextension until reduction is accomplished or by implementing measures prior to manual hyeprextension and casting, explain procedure, which is done under anesthesia, including where patient will be casted (from neck to hips), recovery room, and duration of cast; physically prepare patient for hyperextension and casting

Teach cast care, including proper handling (with palms) while wet to prevent indentations, proper support of curves with small pillows so that cast does not crack while drying, need for frequent turning (using sufficient personnel to properly support cast) to facilitate drying, and petaling rough edges when cast is dry; implement measures to protect cast from deterioration as the result of dampness or soiling

Maintain skin integrity and promote circulation by massaging accessible skin, turning patient frequently, avoiding positioning patient, when turning, so that pressure is produced on shoulders, chest, or abdomen; encourage patient to do isomettric and active and passive exercises; maintain adequate hydration, nutrition, and elimination by avoiding gas-forming foods that could cause abdominal distention and discomfort, providing foods with high residue content, if no contraindications, and providing large amounts of fruit or fruit juices; prevent problems related to immobility, such as thrombophlebitis, urinary tract infections, and hypostatic pneumonia, by encouraging the patient to do isometric, active and passive (when possible), deep-breathing and coughing exercises frequently turning patient, and ensuring adequate intake of fluids; observe patient for circulatory or respiratory distress resulting from constriction of cast, for acute duodenal obstruction, or for infection from decubitus ulcers inside cast; implement prompt nursing intervention should signs of complications occur

After cast is removed and patient begins ambulation, apply Taylor's apparatus during ambulation; implement safety measures while patient is ambulating

For cervical fracture

Implement pain-reducing measures; maintain proper traction on Crutchfield or Vinke tongs, by keeping head of bed at the proper elevation and by keeping the prescribed weights on tongs; keep weights hanging free; implement measures to maintain proper alignment, by using a footboard to prevent footdrop and proper space to allow suspension of heels and by using trochanter rolls to maintain alignment of extremities

Implement measures to maintain skin integrity and to promote circulation by frequently turning patient on Stryker frame or Circ-O-lectric bed, gently massaging skin over sacrum, hips, knees, heels, and shoulders each time, keeping skin clean and dry, encouraging the patient to do isometric exercises, if not contraindicated, and passive range-of-motion exercises to extremities; implement measures to maintain adequate hydration, nutrition, and elimination and to prevent infection of tong sites, hypostatic pneumonia, and urinary tract infection; observe for neurological damage or spinal shock; implement prompt nursing action if signs of complications occur

Implement safety measures once tongs are removed and patient becomes ambulatory (patient may have body cast applied once tongs are removed or may only need to wear a brace when ambulatory); provide diversional activities

For cord compression associated with fractured vertebrae

Provide preoperative nursing care with pain-reducing measures; explain surgical procedure, recovery room, measures to reduce postoperative discomfort, and deep-breathing and coughing exercises; physically prepare patient for surgery

Implement postoperative measures to maintain adequate hydration, nutrition, and elimination; prevent wound infection; maintain skin integrity and promote circulation by turning patient in log-like fashion, avoiding extreme knee flexion while patient is on side, gently massaging bony prominences of back, keeping skin clean and dry, and using protective devices such as lambswool or lotion; encourage exercise of the extremities, avoiding extreme flexion of knees; implement measures to prevent complications from decreased activity, such as hypostatic pneumonia, urinary tract infections, thrombophlebitis

Implement safety measures when patient becomes ambulatory

Health education

Teach the name, purpose, dosage, frequency, side effects, action to take if side effects occur, and precautions for each discharge medication

Explain proper body mechanics, therapeutic activities, and avoidance of activities that produce flexion strain on spine, including safety considerations

Teach measures to reduce discomfort

Teach proper application of braces, or use of crutches or walkers

Indicators for discharge
Adaptation to health status

Pain controlled

Able to bear weight

Therapeutic and restricted activities applied

Fractured vertebrae properly aligned

Complications not evident

Health teaching completed

Referrals made

Examples of community resources

Vocational rehabilitation center, in the event the patient cannot go back to previous type of employment

Visiting Nurse Association or public health nurse

Orthopedic clinic

RETROSPECTIVE CRITERIA
Health

Pain controlled

Condition stable

Complications not evident

Activity

Ambulatory with weight bearing

Able to use crutches or apply brace properly

Applies techniques of proper body mechanics

Knowledge

Knows the name and understands the purpose, dosage, frequency, side effects, action to take if side effects occur, and precautions of each discharge medication

Understands therapeutic and restricted activities

Understands proper body mechanics

Understands safety measures

Understands and can implement measures to reduce discomfort

Understands when and why it is necessary to return to clinic or physician's office for follow-up visit

COMPLICATIONS

Circulatory distress

Decubitus ulcers

Malunion and nonunion

Paralysis—paraplegia or quadriplegia

Paralytic ileus

Pneumonia

Pulmonary embolism

Sensory or motor impairment

Shock

Thrombophlebitis

Urinary tract infections

Fracture of femoral neck of hip

Closed reduction (Code: 820)

Open reduction (Code: 820.1)

CONCURRENT CRITERIA
Identification of patient's physical and psychosocial needs and/or concerns

Relief of symptoms, including pain, swelling, deformity, muscular spasms, impairment of function, and possibly crepitus

Explanation of diagnostic and surgical procedures as well as nursing management, including preoperative teaching, explanation of special care unit, and postoperative teaching

Concern over time lost from work, long-term convalescence, and/or loss of independence

Protection against injury and problems caused by immobility and instability

Rehabilitative measures to regain use of hip

Recommended nursing action consistent with diagnosis
Nursing services

Implement preoperative nursing measures, including pain reducing through positioning, sand bags, ice bags, and medication; maintain proper traction and correct alignment; teach need, purpose, and method of turning with patient participation and deep-breathing and coughing exercise used to reduce postoperative discomfort; explain surgical procedure, recovery room, bed rest, progressive steps to ambulation, active and passive exercises and range-of-motion exercises to assist in prevention of complications; maintain adequate nutrition, hydration, and elimination; physically prepare patient for surgery

Implement postoperative nursing measures, including close observation for abnormalities by monitoring vital signs, quality and presence of peripheral pulses, skin color, motor and sensory functions, urinary output, and mental alertness, with prompt nursing intervention if necessary; maintain adequate hydration, nutrition, elimination, intravenous therapy, and catheterization as ordered; provide reduction of pain through positioning and maintenance of proper alignment by use of trapeze, pillows, sand bags, traction, ice bags as ordered, analgesics, and antispasmodics; prevent problems resulting from immobility through active and passive exercises, frequent turning, use of supportive devices to maintain proper body alignment (in relation to decubitus ulcers, hypostatic pneumonia, urinary tract infection, and contractures); implement supportive measures

to promote early ambulation through transfer techniques, muscle-strengthening exercises (qudriceps setting exercises), and use of prosthetic devices (canes, walkers, and crutches)

Control coexistent medical problems via close observation and prompt intervention

Implement cast care and safety measures related to fracture and disabilities of age

Initiate appropriate referrals

Health education

Teach name, dosage, purpose, side effects, precautions, and measures to counteract side effects for each medication

Teach measures to reduce discomfort, such as pacing techniques and positioning

Teach prevention of immobility problems, including decubitus ulcers, contractures, constipation, urinary tract infections, pneumonia, and thrombophlebitis

Teach proper use of prosthetic or assistive devices (crutches, walker, and cane) by muscle strengthening and graduated activity

Explain safety measures to prevent falling in home

Indicators for discharge
Adaptation to health status

Vital signs stable and within normal limits

Fracture healing in proper position

Complications not evident

Health teaching completed with reasonable response

Referrals made

Examples of community resources

Visiting Nurse Association or public health nurse

Orthopedic clinic

Social services

Physical therapist (in outpatient clinic or home, dependent on patient's needs)

RETROSPECTIVE CRITERIA
Health

Condition stable; coexisting medical problems under control
Complications not evident
Fracture healing and stable

Activity

Ambulatory with crutches, walker, or cane
Performs activities of daily living with limited assistance
Performs muscle-strengthening exercises

Knowledge

Patient understands and can implement methods to reduce discomfort, including pacing techniques and regular rest periods, prevention of problems from restricted activity, safe and appropriate use of prosthetic and assistive devices, such as walker, crutches, or cane; and correct performance of muscle-strengthening exercises
Knows name, purpose, dosage, frequency, mode, side effects, and remediation of side effects for each discharge medication

COMPLICATIONS

Avascular necrosis of femoral head
Constipation
Decubitus ulcers
Degenerative joint disease of hip
Hemorrhage
Joint contractures
Joint stiffness
Motor impairment
Nonunion or malunion
Pneumonia
Sciatic nerve lesion
Shock
Thrombophlebitis
Urinary tract infection
Wound infection

Fracture of femur, proximal (Codes: 820-820.5, 820.9)

CONCURRENT CRITERIA
Identification of patient's physical and psychosocial needs and/or concerns

Control of pain
Immobilization of affected part and proper alignment of bone
Understanding of disease process procedures, medical and nursing management, rehabilitation measures, expected duration of immobilization
Concern about immobility, loss of time from normal activities, and dependency
Diversionary activities to help adjustment to hospitalization

Recommended nursing action consistent with diagnosis
Nursing services

Implement pain control measures
Provide preoperative nursing care and teaching, including adequate nutrition, hydration, elimination, and explanation about surgical procedure, recovery room, postoperative pain control, chest physiology exercises, and wound care; maintain proper bone alignment at all times; observe patient for fat embolism
Maintain mobility of unaffected joints; implement muscle-strengthening exercises pre- and postoperatively
Maintain skin integrity by changing patient's position and massaging bony prominences every 2 hours, pre- and postoperatively
Provide postoperative nursing care, including assessing physiological response parameters; providing adequate nutrition, hydration, and elimination; preventing infections, impaired circulation, decubitus ulcers, or hemorrhage; providing wound care and

pain control; permitting expression of feelings by patient

Provide diversionary activities

Health education

Teach about condition, treatment, medical and nursing management, pre- and postoperative care, symptoms to report to physician, and cast care, if indicated

Explain rehabilitation measures for range of motion and muscle-strengthening exercises and assistive devices for ambulation

Teach skin inspection and skin care

Instruct about medications, including the name, dosage, frequency, duration, and side effects to report to physician for each

Indicators for discharge
Adaptation to health status

Fracture site stabilized or healed

Ambulatory (with or without assistive devices)

Wound healing (if surgery performed)

Health teaching completed

Examples of community resources

Physical rehabilitation center

Visiting Nurse Association or public health nurse

RETROSPECTIVE CRITERIA
Health

Wound healing (if surgery performed)

Fracture site stabilized or healed

Muscle strength of affected leg increasing

Activity

Ambulatory (with or without assistive devices)

Independent in activities of daily living

Performs muscle-strengthening exercises

Knowledge

Understands and can verbalize rehabilitation measures of range of motion and muscle-strengthening exercises; skin, wound, or cast care; symptoms to report to physician; and medication instructions

COMPLICATIONS

Avascular necrosis of femoral head

Decubitus ulcers

Degenerative joint disease of hip

Fat embolism

Hemorrhage

Joint contractures

Nonunion, delayed union, or malunion

Painful, swollen calf

Persistent knee joint stiffness

Pulmonary embolism

Shock

Thrombophlebitis

Urinary tract infection

Wound infection

Fracture of hip, intertrochanteric, open reduction (Code: 820.2)

CONCURRENT CRITERIA
Identification of patient's physical and psychosocial needs and/or concerns

Relief of symptoms and disability, including pain, swelling, false motion, deformity, and/or impairment of function

Explanation of diagnostic and surgical procedures and nursing management

Concern over increased dependence, long-term convalescence, and implications of time away from normal responsibilities

Prevention of secondary injuries and complications from instability and immobility

Rehabilitative measures, including cost, methodology, and length of time involved in order to regain ambulatory status

Recommended nursing action consistent with diagnosis
Nursing services

Provide pre-operative nursing measures, including pain-reducing measures and traction and correct alignment (usually Russell traction, which maintains the knee in a neutral plane and the hip in flexion)

Provide preoperative teaching, including the necessity of frequent turning; methods for patient participation in turning; means of reducing discomfort during the turning process; the purpose and method of deep breathing and coughing; measures to reduce discomfort postoperatively; explanation of the surgical procedure regarding the use of Neufeld nail, Jewett nail, Smith-Petersen nail, Austin Moore pin, or a Thornton plate; explanation of recovery room, and duration of bed rest status, progressive steps to ambulation, and active and passive exercises used to aid in the prevention of complications

Maintain adequate nutrition, hydration, and elimination

Physically prepare patient for surgery

Implement postoperative nursing measures, including closely observing for signs of physical deterioration by monitoring vital signs, quality and presence of peripheral pulses, skin color, motor and sensory functions, urinary output, mental alertness, and excessive drainage from wound, with prompt nursing intervention if necessary; providing adequate hydration, nutrition, and elimination; maintaining correct alignment; preventing problems from immobility or infection through passive and active exercises, frequently turning patient and using supportive devices for proper alignment; and providing wound care, chest physiology, and catheter care

Implement supportive measures to promote early ambulation, including hourly quadriceps-setting exercises, arm strenthening with flexion and extension exercises, nonweight-bearing techniques for ambulation, and related safety measures

Control coexistent medical problems of elderly patient via close observation and prompt intervention if necessary

Provide discharge planning with initiation of appropriate referrals

Health education

Explain medication, including the name, purpose, dosage, frequency, side effects, action to take if side effects occur, and precautions for each

Teach safety measures to prevent falling

Explain measures to prevent problems from restricted activity during convalescence

Demonstrate proper use of prosthetic devices, such as crutches, walkers, and canes

Instruct about muscle-strengthening exercises, graduated increased levels in activity, measures to reduce discomfort, pacing techniques, and the need for regular rest periods

Indicators for discharge
Adaptation to health status

Fracture site stabilized; wound healing
Ambulatory without weight bearing
Coexisting medical problems controlled
Complications not evident
Referrals made
Health teaching completed

Examples of community resources

Visiting Nurse Association or public health nurse
Orthopedic clinic
Social services
Physical therapy clinic

RETROSPECTIVE CRITERIA
Health

Wound healing
Peripheral pulses strong

Afebrile
Coexisting medical problems controlled
Complications not evident

Activity

Ambulatory without weight bearing, using prosthetic devices such as canes, walker, or crutches

Independent in activities of daily living or requiring minimal assistance

Performs muscle-strengthening exercises

Knowledge

Knows the name of each discharge medication; understands the dosage, frequency, purpose, side effects, action to take if side effects occur, and precautions for each

Understands and can implement safety measures

Understands and can implement measures to prevent problems related to restricted activity during convalescence

Understands and can use prosthetic devices correctly

Understands and can implement pain-reducing measures, pacing techniques, and rest periods

Understands and can implement muscle-strengthening exercises

Understands and can implement non-weight-bearing techniques for ambulation

COMPLICATIONS

Avascular necrosis of femoral head
Constipation
Decubitus ulcers
Degenerative joint disease of hip
Hemorrhage
Joint contractures
Joint stiffness
Motor impairment
Nonunion, malunion, or delayed union
Pneumonia
Shock
Thrombophlebitis
Urinary tract infection
Wound infection

Fracture of pelvis (Code: 808.6)

CONCURRENT REVIEW CRITERIA
Identification of patient's physical and psychosocial needs and/or concerns

Relief from symptoms and disability, including pain on bearing weight, swelling, and tenderness at fracture site

Concern over increased dependence during convalescence or over loss of time from school or work

Explanation of diagnostic and surgical procedures and nursing management

Protection against further injury and deterioration resulting from complications of immobility

Close observation for internal injuries, such as intra-abdominal hemorrhage and urethral, bladder, and rectal injuries

Recommended nursing action consistent with diagnosis
Nursing services

Closely observe for deterioration in physical condition, by frequently monitoring vital signs, sensory and motor functions, mental alertness, skin color, urinary output, presence or absence of peripheral pulses, and skin temperature and checking for bleeding or nausea (as related to fat embolism, thromboembolism shock, laceration of iliac artery, or nerve injury), with prompt nursing intervention should any signs occur

Maintain proper alignment of bone segments, either by use of traction (Buck's extension or skeletal traction on the leg of the fractured side may be used to reduce overriding segments) or by proper positioning of compression sling

For patient with hip spica cast (used when hip joint is involved)

Implement cast care, including supporting curves of cast with small pillows to prevent cracking while it is still wet, keeping patient's head and chest flat while cast is drying, handling wet cast with palms to avoid indenting the cast, turning patient frequently to facilitate cast drying on posterior, and petaling rough edges when cast is dry

Maintain skin integrity and promote circulation, by turning patient frequently with adequate personnel to ensure safety, massaging pressure areas, avoiding twisting cast or positioning patient with pressure on the groin, back, chest, or abdominal areas, providing good skin hygiene around cast edges and perineal area, and supervising isometric exercises

Maintain adequate hydration, nutrition, and elimination, including avoiding foods that cause gas and abdominal distention, forcing fluids to at least 2,800 ml daily, and encouraging intake of fruits and foods with residue and bulk

Prevent complications of thrombophlebitis, urinary tract infection, and pneumonia

Observe for circulatory impairment (numbness, sensory and motor disturbances, severe pain, odor from cast, discoloration of cast which comes from within it, absence of pedal pulse, temperature change in the skin), respiratory impairment, or cast syndrome (acute duodenal obstruction occurring after cast application), with prompt nursing intervention should any signs occur

Maintain cleanliness and prevent deterioration of cast

Reduce discomfort

For patient in a pelvic sling

Reduce discomfort

Maintain adequate hydration, nutrition, elimination, and skin integrity; promote circulation by *not turning* patient, but massaging skin on buttocks and back by reaching under the sling

Maintain skin cleanliness

Line sling with sheepskin to prevent decubitus ulcers; *caution: do not loosen sling unless specifically ordered to do so*

Encourage isometric exercises

Prevent thrombophlebitis, urinary tract infection, and pneumonia by encouraging deep-breathing and isometric exercises and by forcing fluids

Provide diversional therapy

For patient on bedrest with or without a pelvic girdle or Buck's extension

Reduce discomfort

Maintain adequate hydration, nutrition, and elimination

Maintain skin integrity and promote circulation by *not turning patient unless specifically ordered to do so,* but rather by elevating patient via overhead trapeze or another nurse's assistance to give back care; use protective devices such as sheepskin to protect back from decubitus ulcers; when a girdle is used, line girdle with flannel or some other soft material to prevent pressure areas; encourage patient to do isometric exercises; maintain proper position of extremities to avoid deformities and pressure on heels; keep skin clean and dry

Prevent thrombophlebitis, pneumonia, and urinary tract infections by encouraging deep-breathing and isometric exercises and exercising of uninvolved extremities, and by forcing fluids

Maintain proper positioning of girdle with adequate degree of support, remembering the binder or girdle should be applied without snugness when the iliac bone is fractured, with snugness when the ischium or pubic bones are involved, and very tightly when the symphysis pubis is separated

Provide diversional therapy

Health education

Explain the name, purpose, frequency, dosage, side effects, action to take if side effects occur, and precautions for each discharge medication

Explain activities, including mobilization within therapeutic limits and restrictions

Teach crutchwalking without bearing weight on the affected side

Apply pelvic girdle when weight bearing is started; explain type of girdle, application, and duration of usage

Teach proper body mechanics to avoid trauma to back and pelvis in the future

Implement measures to reduce discomfort, including usage of a firm mattress, use of bed boards, supportive shoes, and rest periods

Advise when and why it is necessary to return for follow-up medical surveillance

Indicators for discharge
Adaptation to health status

Fracture stabilized

Pain controlled

Complications not evident

Health teaching completed

Referrals made

Examples of community resources

Visiting Nurse Association or public health nurse

Social services

Orthopedic clinic

RETROSPECTIVE REVIEW CRITERIA
Health

Fracture stabilized

Pain controlled

Complications not evident

Activity

Ambulatory

Able to use crutches or apply pelvic girdle properly

Implements proper body mechanics

Knowledge*

Knows the name of each discharge medication; understands the purpose, dosage, frequency, side effects, action to take if side effects occur, and precautions for each

Understands therapeutic and restricted activities and can implement therapeutic ones

Understands and can implement proper body mechanics

Understands and can implement measures to reduce discomfort

Understands when and why it is important to return to clinic or physician's office for follow-up visit and the importance of same.

COMPLICATIONS

Acute duodenal obstruction

Bladder injury

Circulatory impairment

Decubitus ulcers

Extravasation of urine

Fat embolism

Hemorrhagic shock

Injuries to sacral plexus of nerves

Internal hemorrhage

Laceration of iliac artery

Motor impairment

Pneumonia

Thromboembolism

Thrombophlebitis

Urethra injury

Urinary tract infection

---

*If the patient is unteachable and there is no family, the responsible party assuming health care supervision is required to be knowledgeable in these areas, and this must be documented on the nurse's notes.

Fracture of shaft of tibia and/or fibula

Closed reduction (Code: 823.4)
Open reduction (Code: 823.5)

CONCURRENT CRITERIA
Identification of patient's physical and psychosocial needs and/or concerns

Relief from symptoms and disability, including pain, swelling, deformity, impaired function, false motion, or muscle spasms

Explanation of diagnostic and surgical procedures and nursing management

Concern about loss of time from normal activities such as work, school, or homemaking and about increased dependence during convalescence

Provision of rehabilitative measures to regain ambulatory status

Protection against injury and/or complications resulting from instability and immobility

Recommended nursing action consistent with diagnosis
Nursing services

Implement preoperative nursing measures, including reduction of pain and swelling via positioning, ice bags, and medication; maintenance of adequate nutrition, hydration, and elimination; and traction and alignment to prevent further bone displacement

Provide preoperative teaching regarding operative procedure, casting, recovery room, duration of bed status and hospitalization, progressive steps to ambulation; deep-breathing and coughing exercises, and patient participation in reduction of postoperative pain; explain and prepare patient for all diagnostic procedures; give patient information concerning cast drying, positioning, and care

Physically prepare patient for surgery

Implement postoperative nursing measures, including reduction of pain and swelling by positioning, alignment, and medication or ice bags; closely observe patient for signs of significant abnormalities regarding vital signs, quality and presence of peripheral pulses, skin color, blanching, and skin temperature, sensory and motor function, urinary output, unusual or severe pain, mental alertness, or bleeding, with prompt nursing intervention in response to abnormalities

Prevent problems from immobility, such as thrombophlebitis, contractures, urinary tract dysfunction or infection, pneumonia, pulmonary embolism, decubitus ulcers, or constipation or complications of the surgery itself, like shock, infection, or fat embolism

Maintain adequate hydration, nutrition, and elimination

Implement cast care as related to drying, petaling, protection, cleanliness, and safe transfer techniques (because casts are frequently used for immobilization in addition to internal fixation by intramedullary nailing, plating, or screws in open reduction procedures)

Health education

Teach measures to control pain and prevent dependent edema

Teach wound care if no cast, otherwise teach cast care including protection, cleanliness, danger signs, such as extreme pain or swelling, discoloration from within, numbness, or blueness of toes and action to initiate if signs and symptoms occur

Teach proper use of crutches dependent on instructions regarding weight bearing, including nonweight-bearing techniques and safety measures

Teach prevention of problems resulting from immobility if discharged on wheelchair status, including change of position, isometric exercises, active and passive exercise of unaffected limbs, and daily inspection of skin

Instruct about name, purpose, dosage, frequency, side effects, and precautions of each discharge medication

Indicators for discharge
Adaptation to health status

Condition stable, including vital signs, and abnormal pain, swelling or circulatory problems absent

Pain controlled with oral medication and usual nursing measures

Bones in proper alignment; cast in correct position as confirmed by postoperative x-rays

Patient knowledgeable about cast care or wound care, if open dressing; able to demonstrate safe transfer techniques; understands limitations or physical mobility

Complications not evident

Referrals made

Examples of community resources

Orthopedic clinic

Visiting Nurse Association or public health nurse

Social services

RETROSPECTIVE CRITERIA
Health

Fracture site stabilized

Pain controlled

Wound healing

Complications not evident

Tibia and fibula in proper alignment

Activity

Ambulatory with or without assistive devices such as crutches or walker

Independent in activities of daily living

Knowledge

Understands causes, prevention, and treatment of swelling and dependent edema, muscle spasms, and pain and can implement care accordingly

Understands and can implement wound and/or cast care, including cleaning, protecting, recognizing danger signs and symptoms, carrying out remediation measures, and can implement modes of safe transfer with cast

Knows name, dosage, frequency, side effects, and precautions of each discharge medication

Uses crutches (with nonweight-bearing techniques, when necessary) and/or other assistive devices in appropriate and safe manner

Understands and can implement prevention of problems of immobility through exercise

COMPLICATIONS

Ankle joint stiffness

Arterial injury

Constipation

Decubitus ulcers

Delayed union, nonunion, or malunion

Dependent edema

Fat embolism

Hemorrhage

Joint contractures

Lateral popliteal nerve injury

Muscle spasms

Persistent swelling

Pneumonia

Pulmonary embolism

Shock

Thrombophlebitis

Urinary tract infection

Wound infection

Fracture of skull (Codes: 803-803.9, 804-804.9)

CONCURRENT REVIEW CRITERIA
Identification of patient's physical and psychosocial needs and/or concerns

Relief from symptoms, including unconsciousness, headache, focal neurological deficits, drainage from ear or nose, or from shock

Assistance in regaining orientation and adjusting to alteration in body image or life-style

Explanation of diagnostic and therapeutic medical and/or surgical and nursing procedures, including purpose, preparation, outcome, prognosis, special discharge care, and rehabilitation measures

Recommended nursing action consistent with diagnosis
Nursing services

Observe for changes in condition by monitoring level of consciousness, vital signs, motor functions, and pupillary signs and by checking for convulsions, nuchal rigidity, otorrhagia, personality changes related to tissue damage associated with depressed fragments or bone, cerebral hematoma, or hemorrhage, with immediate intervention should signs of deterioration occur

Protect patient from injury and prevent complications by using side rails, avoiding restraints, implementing eye care to prevent corneal ulcerations (as related to unconsciousness), reducing cerebral edema, avoiding oversedation, and preventing contractures, decubitus ulcers, urinary tract infections, pneumonia, and problems related to stasis

Maintain vital body functions, as related to cerebral tissue damage associated with fractured skull by providing adequate airway, ventilation, nutrition, hydration, and elimination; controlling body temperature; and maintaining cardiovascular function; provide cardiopulmonary resuscitation in case of respiratory or cardiac arrest

Implement rehabilitative measures designed to minimize residual neurological deficits resulting from original trauma or surgery

Implement nursing measures to enhance medical treatment, which may include observation of patient, analgesics, steroid therapy, use of antibiotics, osmotic diuretics, parenteral or tube feedings, mechanical respiration, bur holes, craniotomy, subdural taps, or physical, occupational, or speech therapy, depending on extent of damage

Health education

Explain surgical treatment, including purpose, pre- and postoperative teaching, nursing management, the surgical procedure itself, and special care units

Explain medical management, including the purpose, preparation, outcome, and special aftercare, if any, of each diagnostic test; the name, purpose, dosage, frequency, side effects, action to take if side effects occur, and precautions for each medications; therapeutic and restricted activities; diet; and the purpose and duration of special care units

Explain specific nursing management, including rehabilitative measures as related to improvement of sensory and motor functions, bowel and bladder control programs, activities of daily living programs, speech and visual improvement, and prevention of complications from inactivity

Advise about community agencies available for assistance after discharge

Instruct about methods of dealing with possible posttrauma aftereffects, such as headaches, dizziness, emotional instability, and epilepsy

Indicators for discharge
Adaptation to health status

Neurological deficits improved
Mental status improved
Complications not evident
Health teaching completed
Referrals made

Examples of community resources

Medical or surgical clinic
Social services
Visiting Nurse Association or public health nurse
Physical, occupational, or speech rehabilitation centers, when appropriate
Mental health agencies

RETROSPECTIVE REVIEW CRITERIA
Health

Conscious
Neurological deficits improved
Mental status improved
Complications not evident

Activity

Ambulatory
Independent in activities of daily living

Knowledge

Understands the name, dosage, frequency, purpose, side effects, actions to take if side effects occur, and precautions for each discharge
Understands medication and can implement appropriate care for posttrauma after effects, such as headaches, dizziness, convulsions, and emotional instability
Understands rehabilitative measures as related to sensory and motor functions, bowel and bladder control measures, activities of daily living measures, speech and visual improvements, and prevention of complications caused by inactivity
Understands community agencies available for assistance after discharge

COMPLICATIONS

Aneurysm
Cerebral edema
Cerebrospinal fluid rhinorrhea
Contractures
Contusion of brain surface
Convulsions
Corneal ulcerations
Decubitus ulcers
Emotional instability
Extradural hemorrhage
Herniation of lower brainstem
Intracranial infection
Laceration of meningeal blood vessels
Otorrhea
Pneumonia
Shock
Subdural hematoma
Transtentorial herniation
Trauma to cranial nerves
Urinary tract infection

Fractures of upper extremity, group

Fracture of elbow, humerus lower end (Code: 812.5)
Fracture of elbow, humerus, lower end radius (Code: 812.4)
Fracture of elbow, radius, and ulna, upper end, closed reduction (Code: 813)
Fracture of elbow, radius, and ulna, upper end, open reduction (Code: 813.1)
Fracture of shaft of humerus, closed reduction (Code: 812.3)
Fracture of shaft of humerus, open reduction (Code: 812.4)

CONCURRENT REVIEW CRITERIA
Identification of patient's physical and psychosocial needs and/or concerns

Relief of symptoms, including pain, swelling, muscle spasms, false motion, and impairment of function

Relief of malposition and functional disability

Attention to mental and emotional concerns, including modification of activities; about loss of time from work, school, or homemaking for adult; and about fear of separation from parent and/or fear of permanence of condition for child

Explanation and understanding of diagnostic, surgical, and follow-up procedures

Knowledge of rehabilitation measures for regaining strength and function

Recommended nursing action consistent with diagnosis
Nursing services

Reassure about notification of significant persons; give reasonable explanation of possible functional ability and potential for return to usual life-style

Implement preoperative nursing measures, including reduction of pain by positioning, maintenance of proper body alignment by traction and/or pillows, sandbags, splint prior to surgery, and icebags and/or elevation of limbs to reduce swelling, and/or administration of analgesics and antispasmodics as ordered

Educate patient preoperatively regarding diagnostic, surgical, and rehabilitation procedures, bodily responses to surgery, need for deep breathing, recovery process, and aids in maintaining balance and mobility in bed, including use of trapeze when appropriate

Implement other preoperative measures, including x-ray and laboratory procedures; maintenance of ventilation, nutrition, hydration, elimination, and normal body temperature; administration of preoperative medication; and monitoring of vital signs with observation for shock and disturbance of sensory-motor functions, with prompt nursing intervention if necessary; physically prepare patient's limb for surgical procedure or casting

For open reduction of compound fracture, use sterile dressing technique to prevent infection; control bleeding (via pressure); implement and monitor traction, as appropriate

Provide postoperative nursing measures, including close monitoring of vital signs, peripheral pulses, limbs for skin color, temperature, sensory-motor functions, swelling, urinary output, mental alertness, bleeding, and pain, with prompt nursing intervention if abnormalities are noted; ensure adequate nutrition, hydration, and elimination

Control pain through appropriate positioning and body and limb alignment, utilizing preoperative measures plus traction and/or other support

Provide stimulation for mobility, as appropriate, including turning, sitting, walking, and performance of isometric exercises to prevent postoperative complications; promote independence in activities of daily living

Health education

Teach dressing care, when no cast, precautions to prevent infection, and instruction in dressing change, if no visiting nurse is available

Instruction cast care, including protection from moisture, padding to prevent pressure and irritation, causes of discoloration, sling support and on observing for danger signs regarding circulatory impairment, abnormal discoloration, and action to initiate in response to complications

Explain medications, including the purpose, side effects, precautions, administration, dosage, frequency, and mode for each

Instruction exercises, including pendulum and isometric exercises and permitted and restricted activities within lifestyle

Explain the purpose, frequency, and mode of intermittent medical supervision, including the role of the visiting nurse, when referral is made, and the importance of orthopedic clinic follow-up

Indicators for discharge
Adaptation to health status

Condition stable, including vital signs, sensorium, affect within normal limits

Bleeding, pain, discoloration, need for traction or *abnormal* swelling absent

Complications not evident

Health education completed, with evidence of patient knowledge and understanding of condition and future therapeutic regime

Examples of community resources

Orthopedic clinic referral for all patients

Social services referral as indicated by mode of injury, economic, and psychological status

Visiting Nurse Association or public health nurse referral for open reductions requiring frequent dressing changes and observation

Physical rehabilitation center

RETROSPECTIVE REVIEW CRITERIA
Health

Afebrile

Vital signs stable

Primary wound healing

Bone alignment appropriate with cast in proper position and fitting correctly

Complications of respiration, circulation, elimination, ambulation, or infection not evident

Pain controlled with usual comfort measures and oral medication

Activity

Patient independent in performance of activities of daily living

Patient able to complete therapeutic exercise program

Patient/family member able to correctly apply sling

Patient ambulatory

Knowledge

Patient/family understands and can demonstrate and/or describe areas of wound care and adverse symptoms; cast care and adverse symptoms or response; modes of maintaining comfort and preventing edema, pressure, or pain, and correct use of assistive devices

Knows medications, including the name, purpose, mode, precautions, and side effects for each

Understands role of referral agencies in treatment and follow-up

COMPLICATIONS

Decubitus ulcers

Degenerative joint disease

Delayed union, nonunion, malunion, or crossunion

Dependent edema

Elbow joint stiffness

Injury to branchial artery

Injury to circumflex (axillary) nerve
Median nerve injury
Persistent shoulder joint stiffness
Radial nerve injury
Sensory-motor function disturbance

Shock
Skin breakdown
Volkmann's contracture
Wound infection

Fracture-subluxation or subluxation of cervical spine
(Codes: 805, 887)

CONCURRENT CRITERIA
Identification of patient's physical and psychosocial needs and/or concerns

Relief from symptoms, including pain and loss of or impairment of cervical flexion, extension, and rotation with or without sensory and/or motor impairment below the nipple line

Reassurance about concern over increased dependence, changes in body image, and life-style

Explanation of extent of injury, surgical treatment, outcome, possible neurological deficits, and rehabilitative medical and nursing management

Assistance in dealing with possible long-term convalescence, paralysis, change in body image, and life-style

Knowledge of community agencies available for assistance after discharge

Recommended nursing action consistent with diagnosis
Nursing services

Maintain proper traction as established via Crutchfield or Vinke tongs

Implement measures to prevent infection of tong sites, hypostatic pneumonia, or urinary tract infection

Closely observe for deterioration, such as changes in rate and character of respiration, cyanosis, or dyspnea as related to cord damage; respiratory distress from pressure on the diaphragm caused by a paralytic ileus; changes in blood pressure, pulse, and temperature as related to infection and cord damages; or changes in motor and sensory function

Maintain adequate circulation, hydration, nutrition, elimination, and skin integrity

Implement measures to assist patient in coping with long-term convalescence, change in independent status either temporarily or permanently as related to cord damage, and changes in body image and/or life-style

Health education

Teach name, purpose, dosage, frequency, side effects, action to take if side effects occur, and precautions of each discharge medication

Teach safety measures for ambulation during convalescent period

Explain restricted and therapeutic activities, including duration away from work, evaluation of job prior to hospitalization in terms of patient's ability to return to same occupation, and body mechanics

Teach application and use of neck brace or collar

Refer to community agencies available for assistance after discharge

Indicators for discharge
Adaptation to health status

Fracture site stabilized
Ambulatory with neck brace
Complications not evident
Health teaching completed
Symptoms relieved or reduced in severity
Referrals made

Examples of community resources

Social services

Visiting Nurse Association or public health nurse

Physical rehabilitation center (in the case of paralysis)

Vocational guidance center for job reevaluation and vocational training center (in the event occupation must be changed)

RETROSPECTIVE CRITERIA
Health

Fracture site stabilized

Complications not evident

Symptoms relieved or reduced in severity

Activity

Ambulatory

Able to apply brace or collar correctly

Independent in activities of daily living

Knowledge

Understands name, dosage, purpose, frequency, side effects, action to take if side effects occur, and precautions of each discharge medication

Understands and can implement safety measures

Understands restriction on activities and therapeutic activities and can implement therapeutic ones

Understands function of community agency that can best be of assistance after discharge

COMPLICATIONS

Decubitus ulcers

Motor impairment

Paralysis

Paralytic ileus

Pneumonia

Respiratory distress

Rheumatoid arthritis

Shock

Spinal cord compression

Spinal cord transection

Thrombophlebitis

Urinary tract infection

Wound infection

Gastroenteritis in children (Codes: 003, 004, 005, 008, 009)

CONCURRENT CRITERIA
Identification of patient's physical and psychosocial needs and/or concerns

Maintenance of hydration and electrolyte balance

Resolution of vomiting and/or diarrhea

Maintenance of basic nutrition

Understanding by patient/parents of purpose of restricting fluid and food intake

Emotional support for adjustment to hospitalization

Recommended nursing action consistent with diagnosis
Nursing services

Carefully regulate intravenous fluids

Regulate oral intake with proper recording

Accurately record any vomiting and/or diarrhea with description

Record daily weight

Properly position patient to prevent aspiration of food or fluids if vomiting occurs

Administer prompt, thorough skin cleansing after vomiting or diarrhea occurs

Health education

Explain to patient/parents importance of restricted diet to decrease irratibility of gastrointestinal tract

Stress importance of notifying nurse to see any vomitus and/or diarrheic stools

Teach proper feeding methods and importance of restricted amounts of food; explain diet ordered by physician

Stress good hand washing
Explain importance of restricted activity to keep intravenous tubing in place

Indicators for discharge
Adaptation to health status

Afebrile
Vomiting and/or diarrhea controlled
Ambulatory
Proper dietary information received and understood

Examples of community resources

Referral usually not indicated

RETROSPECTIVE CRITERIA
Health

Hydrated
Gaining weight
Vomiting and/or diarrhea controlled

Diet tolerated for 48 hours prior to discharge
Afebrile
Complications not evident

Activity

Ambulatory or activity appropriate for age

Knowledge

Parents understand diet ordered by physician
Parents understand possible causes of gastroenteritis, such as poor hand washing or inappropriate dietary management

COMPLICATIONS

Dehydration
Fluid and electrolyte imbalance
Metabolic acidosis or alkalosis
Skin breakdown

Gastrointestinal tract surgeries, group

Diverticular disease, with surgical intervention (Codes: 562, 562.1, 562.3)
Esophageal disease, with esophageal surgery (Code: 530)
Fissure-in-ano (Code: 455)
Fistula-in-ano (Code: 465)
Gastric or duodenal ulcer, with surgical intervention (Code: 533)
Hemorrhoids (Code: 565.1)
Hiatal hernia (Codes: 551.5, 553.5)
Neoplasm, stomach, malignant, with surgical intervention (Code: 151)
Peptic ulcer (Code: 533)
Ventral hernia (Codes: 551.3, 551.4)

CONCURRENT CRITERIA
Identification of patient's physical and psychosocial needs and/or concerns

Control of pain
Adjustment to surgical invasion of body and change in life style, role, or dependency during hospitalization
Fear of death or presence of malignancy
Explanation and understanding of surgical procedures, expected pre- and postoperative courses, prognosis, treatment, nursing management, and realistic plans for care after discharge

Relief of symptoms
   Peptic ulcer: relief of epigastric distress (40 to 60 minutes after meals), nocturnal pain, epigastric tenderness and guarding, anemia, or occult blood in stool
   Diverticular disease: relief of left lower quadrant pain, constipation, fever, bloody stools, dysuria
   Fissure-in-ano: relief of acute pain during and after defecation, spotting of bright red blood at stool, constipa-

tion through fear of pain, and spasm of anal canal

Fistula-in-ano: relief of purulent discharge, local itching, tenderness or pain aggravated by bowel movements, and recurrent anal abscesses

Hemorrhoids: relief of straining at stool, constipation, discomfort from prolonged sitting, anal infection, and local pain and/or itching

Hiatal hernia: relief of pressure sensation, severe pain, burning behind lower sternum, pain aggravated by recumbency or increase of abdominal pressure, cough, dyspnea, palpitation, or tachycardia

Esophageal disease: relief of dysphagia progressing as more is eaten, bad breath, foul taste in mouth, regurgitation of undigested or partially digested food from first portion of a meal, irritating cough, swelling in neck with eating, increased salivation, or gurgling

Malignant neoplasm of stomach: relief of weight loss, anemia, occult blood in stools, nausea, sensations of pressure, belching, heartburn, decline in general health and strength, diarrhea, hematemesis, or melena

Recommended nursing action consistent with diagnosis

Nursing services

Relieve pain through medication, positioning, and comfort measures

Give preoperative nursing care, including rest, nutrition, hydration, and elimination, and teaching, including explanation of surgical procedures, expected outcomes, recovery room, estimated period of hospitalization, progressive ambulation, chest physiology exercises, and possible use of chest tubes for esophageal surgery

Physically prepare patient for surgery

Implement postoperative nursing care, including pain control, rest, nutrition, hydration, elimination, wound care, and fluid and electrolyte balance

Monitor chest tube and observe for signs of physical deterioration, such as shock, excessive bleeding, respiratory difficulty, or changes in mental status, with prompt nursing intervention should any signs occur

Provide emotional support

Health education

Teach importance of avoiding constipation through diet, adequate fluid intake, stool softeners, and mild laxatives

Explain discharge medications, including the name, purpose, dosage, frequency, side effects, and action to take if side effects occur for each

Give diet instructions; explain restrictions

Give wound care instruction

Advise when and why it is necessary to return to physician for follow-up medical care

Advise about community agencies available to assist with discharge care, if patient has posthospitalization care needs

Indicators of discharge

Adaptation to health status

Normal physiological responses reestablished, including tolerating discharge diet for 2 to 3 days prior to discharge

Independent in activities of daily living

Wound healing

Complications not evident

Examples of community resources

Referral usually not indicated, except for malignant neoplasm of stomach (referred to Visiting Nurse Association or public health nurse and American Cancer Society)

RETROSPECTIVE CRITERIA

Health

Normal physiological parameters reestablished

Wound healed satisfactorily

Pain controlled

Diet tolerated for 2 to 3 days prior to discharge

Activity

Independent in activities of daily living
Ambulatory

Knowledge

Understands wound care
Understands activity level permissible
Has some understanding of surgery performed and prognosis
Understands discharge diet
Understands name, dosage, purpose, frequency, side effects, action to take if side effects occur, and precautions of each discharge medication

COMPLICATIONS

Atelectasis
Constipation
Esophageal rupture and/or perforation (with esophageal disease)
Gastrointestinal obstruction
Hemorrhage
Intraperitoneal abscess
Peritonitis
Pneumonia
Postoperative pancreatitis (with peptic ulcer)
Shock
Thrombosis (with hemorrhoids)
Wound infection

Guillain-Barré syndrome (Code: 354)

CONCURRENT REVIEW CRITERIA
Identification of patient's physical and psychosocial needs and/or concerns

Relief of symptoms, including pain, palatal weakness, hoarseness, flaccid paralysis, and paresthesia of fingers, toes, extremities, trunk, and face
Understanding of pathology, cause, course, prognosis, outcome, and medical and nursing management
Anxiety over helplessness and absence from work or school
Protection from injury and physical deterioration; maintenance of vital body functions during acute and convalescing stages
Rehabilitative measures to restore muscle function

Recommended nursing action consistent with diagnosis
Nursing services

Closely monitor temperature, pulse, respiration, circulatory status, blood pressure, level of consciousness, hourly urinary output, fluid intake, and central venous pressure for circulatory failure

Prevent deterioration and injury; immediately notify physician of any changes in respiratory pattern; implement nasopharyngeal or tracheal suctioning, hot packs for pain; avoid central nervous system depressing analgesics and sedatives; encourage deep-breathing and coughing exercises and turning to prevent pneumonia and decubitus ulcers, passive range-of-motion alignment and supportive devices to prevent atrophy of muscles, and small, frequent feedings to prevent inanition
Initiate rehabilitation measures, including gradually increased muscle-strengthening and active exercises and activities self-care in feeding and performing light hygiene as condition of shoulder girdle, arms, and hands permit; sitting, when no tenderness in back extensors, gluteus maximus, or hamstrings; standing and ambulation, when no tenderness in gastrocnemius or weakness in gluteus medius; and bowel and bladder control program, as warranted by degree of muscle weakness
Decrease emotional distress within pa-

tient/family resulting from dependency, image and role changes, and long-term illness

Maintain vital body functions, such as nutrition, respiration, elimination, hydration, and cardiovascular function

Health education

Explain cause, course, prognosis, and possible residual effects of disorder to family/patient

Explain medical diagnostic and therapeutic procedures, including purpose, preparation, outcome, and special care units, to family/patient

Explain nursing management, such as eye care, suction, passive exercises, turning, and skin care, to family/patient

Educate family/patient about community agencies to assist them postdischarge

Teach family/patient about restrictions during home convalescing period

Indicators for discharge
Adaptation to health status

Accepts diagnosis

Muscle strength improved

Daily living activities assumed with minimal assistance

Complications not evident

Community agencies contacted for follow-up assistance postdischarge

Health teaching completed

Examples of community resources

School district for tutoring

Visiting Nurse Association or public health nurse

Social services for financial aid

Physiotherapy clinic

RETROSPECTIVE REVIEW CRITERIA
Health

Muscle strength improved

Complications not evident

Activity

Able to carry out activities of daily living with minimal assistance

Ambulatory

Knowledge

Patient/family understands nursing management (such as prevention of decubitus ulcers and urinary tract infection, if Foley catheter present, maintenance of bowel and bladder care, and continuation of exercises), if full recovery of all muscle function has not occurred by time of discharge

Patient/family understands need for gradual increase in activities and avoidance of fatigue

Patient/family understands purpose and has the means of contacting appropriate community agencies should the need arise postdischarge

COMPLICATIONS

Atelectasis

Decrease in muscle function

Decubitus ulcers

Emotional distress

Muscle atrophy

Pneumonia

Pulmonary embolism

Thrombophlebitis

Urinary incontinence

Urinary retention

Urinary tract infection

Head trauma (cerebral trauma, including subdural hematoma)
(Code: 850)

CONCURRENT CRITERIA
Identification of patient's physical and psychosocial needs and/or concerns

Close observation for changes in condition, with immediate intervention should signs of deterioration in level of consciousness, vital signs, motor function, or pupillary signs occur or if convulsions, nuchal rigidity, otorrhagia, or neurological deficits (that is, sensation or personality changes occur)

Maintenance of vital body functions, including adequate airway and ventilatory action, nutrition and hydration for fluid and electrolyte balance, temperature, elimination, and cardiovascular function

Protection from injury and prevention from complications, by side rails, avoidance of restraints, eye care to prevent corneal ulcerations, measures to reduce cerebral edema, avoidance of oversedation and improper sedation, and prevention of contractures, decubitus ulcers, urinary tract infections, pneumonia, and problems from stasis

Understanding by family/patient of diagnostic and therapeutic medical and/or surgical procedures, including purpose, preparation, outcome, prognosis, and special after-care, if any

Awareness of aftereffects of a head injury, including headaches, dizziness, emotional instability, possible convulsions (posttraumatic epilepsy), and personality changes, as related to posttraumatic neuroses and psychoses

Recommended nursing action consistent with diagnosis
Nursing services

Maintain vital body functions, including adequate airway, ventilation, fluid and electrolyte balance, temperature control, elimination, hydration, and cardiovascular functioning; maintain environmental control

Protect from injury and prevent complications by side rails; eye care; turning, coughing, and deep-breathing exercises; graded range-of-motion exercises; skin care; positioning; alignment; and supportive devices; explain nursing procedures and medical, surgical, and nursing management

Implement rehabilitation to minimize neurological deficits resulting from orginal trauma or postsurgery, trauma including speech rehabilitation, vision corrective measures, physical therapy, and bowel and bladder regimes

Assist patient in regaining orientation and adjusting to alterations in body image or life-style

Health education

Explain surgical treatment, such as evacuation of subdural hematoma, including the purpose, the surgical procedure, nursing management, and special care units

Explain medical management, such as diagnostic tests, including the purpose, preparation, outcome, and special care, if any

Teach the name, purpose, frequency, dosage, side effects, and precautions, if any (such as not to drive if on any medication that induces drowsiness) of each discharge medication; explain the amount of activity and "exercises" that are therapeutic and specific activity restrictions, if any, as a result of the condition; explain diet, including graduating from nothing by mouth allowed to solid foods as condition becomes more stable postinjury or postsurgery;

explain purpose, duration, and restrictions of diet; explain special care units, including the purpose and duration posttrauma or postsurgery

Instruct about specific nursing management, including rehabilitation measures, range-of-motion exercises, speech therapy, measures to minimize visual problems, skin care, and bowel and bladder regime, as may be necessary to relieve anxiety and appropriate for home care should the patient have residual neurological deficits

Identify posttrauma aftereffects and methods of dealing with them, including ice packs, mild analgesics, and avoiding emotional or physical stress for headaches; methods of moving to minimize severity of dizziness; mental hygiene guidance for emotional instability; avoiding fatigue, alcohol, and emotional stress and continuing therapeutic blood levels of anticonvulsant for epilepsy

Indicators for discharge
Adaptation to health status

Neurological deficits improved
Mental status improved
Complications not evident
Afebrile
Necessary knowledge acquired by family/ patient to manage home care properly
Proper referrals made for necessary follow-up care

Examples of community resources

Surgical or medical clinic for epileptic
Social services
Visiting Nurse Association or public health nurse
Speech, physical, or vocational rehabilitation centers, if appropriate
Mental health agencies

RETROSPECTIVE CRITERIA
Health

Neurological deficits improved
Mental status improved
Complications not evident

Activity

Able to carry out activities of daily living with minimal or no assistance
Ambulatory

Knowledge

Family/patient understands name, purpose, dosage, frequency, side effects, and precautions of each medication

Family/patient understands rehabilitation measures appropriate to any residual neurological deficits; that is, bowel and bladder program, speech therapy exercises, measures to minimize visual deficits, range-of-motion and quadriceps-and triceps-strengthening exercises, and transfer techniques

If patient is semiinvalid, family understands measures by which complications can be prevented, such as skin care to prevent decubitus ulcers, frequent turning to prevent pneumonia, and positioning and alignment to prevent contractures; family also can demonstrate correct use of supportive devices

Family/patient understands posttrauma aftereffects (headaches, dizziness, emotional instability, and epilepsy), and measures of dealing with them

COMPLICATIONS

Brain stem compression
Coma
Contractures
Contralateral hemiparesis
Convulsions
Decubitus ulcers
Dizziness
Emotional instability
Headaches
Increased intracranial pressure
Ipsilateral hemiparesis
Paralysis
Persistent headaches
Personality changes
Pneumonia
Uncal herniation
Wound infection (posttrauma or postsurgery)

Head trauma in children (Codes: 850, 851, 854)

CONCURRENT CRITERIA
Identification of patient's physical and psychosocial needs and/or concerns

Close observation for neurological signs indicative of brain injury, including level of consciousness, vital signs, motor function, pupillary signs, convulsions, nuchal rigidity, otorrhagia, neurological deficits, or personality changes

Maintenance of airway and ventilatory function

Limitation of fluids to prevent cerebral edema

Provision of quiet environment and protection from injury or complications, by using side rails, avoiding restraints, providing eye care to prevent corneal ulcerations, avoiding oversedation, and preventing contractures, decubitus ulcers, urinary tract infections, and pneumonia

Understanding of aftereffects of head injury, including headaches, dizziness, emotional instability, and possible convulsions or personality changes, as related to posttraumatic neuroses and psychoses

Recommended nursing action consistent with diagnosis
Nursing services

Monitor neurological vital signs carefully, including level of consciousness, temperature, blood pressure, and pupillary size and reaction; check response to pain every 15 to 30 minutes; check and monitor weakness

Limit fluids to prevent cerebral edema

Observe for bleeding from ears, nose, or mouth

Turn patient frequently from side to side

Decrease environmental stimuli

Health education

Teach parents symptoms of increased intracranial pressure and to report them to physician

Instruct parents in posttrauma aftereffects and methods to relieve them, including ice packs and mild analgesics; prevent headaches by avoiding emotional stress; prevent seizures by avoiding fatigue and emotional stress and by administering anticonvulsant medication

Teach parents the name, dosage, frequency, side effects, and precautions of discharge medications

Indicators for discharge
Adaptation to health status

Neurological vital signs within normal limits

Sensorium normal

Symptoms absent

Examples of community resources

Referral usually not indicated

RETROSPECTIVE CRITERIA
Health

Normal neurological signs

Normal sensorium

Activity

Alert

Ambulatory or activity appropriate for age

Knowledge

Parent recognizes symptoms of increased intracranial pressure (vomiting, headache, bulging fontanelle in infant, lethargy, irritability); knows to report these to physician

Parents know name, dosage, frequency, side effects of discharge medications

COMPLICATIONS

Cerebral edema
Coma
Contractures
Convulsions
Decubitus ulcers
Difficulties with gait
Dysarthria
Dysphasia
Headaches
Hydrocephalus
Hyperthermia
Impaired consciousness
Incoordination
Increased intracranial pressure
Intracranial hematoma
Papilledema
Pressure necrosis from endotracheal tube
Pulmonary infection
Urinary tract infection

Headache, including migraine (Codes: 346, 791)

CONCURRENT CRITERIA
Identification of patient's physical and psychosocial needs and/or concerns

Relief from symptoms, including sweating, chilling, pain, nasal stuffiness, edema, pallor, visual disturbances, nausea, vomiting, chills, photophobia, and tremors

Understanding of cause, if identifiable, course, and prognosis of disorder

Understanding of diagnostic, and therapeutic medical and surgical procedures, including the purpose, preparation, outcome, and specific after-care, if any, of each

Assistance for patient/family in identifying and dealing with the psychosocial aspects of patient's life as related to occurrence, frequency, and severity of headaches

Understanding of appropriate community agencies available for assistance

Recommended nursing action consistent with diagnosis
Nursing services

Implement and evaluate plans for dealing with pain and associated symptoms, including physical comfort measures, positive feedback measures, awake-imagined analgesic techniques; distraction techniques; analgesic and/or other medication; relaxation and rest-promoting measures, cutaneous stimulation, behavioral therapy, environmental control, and adaptive or coping mechanisms

Implement and evaluate plan for identifying psychosocial aspects of patient's life as related to occurrence, frequency, and severity of headaches; symptoms in terms of personality traits, cultural conditioning, work habits, aspirations, family relationships, reaction to stress; assess calendar or daily diary of headaches, activities, drinking, somatic changes, and sleep habits, as related to headache

Implement and evaluate plan for assisting patient to change life-style, as appropriate and possible

Observe for desired and side effects of medications as related to frequency of headaches

Health education

Teach desired effects, side effects, name, dosage, frequency, precautions, and restrictions for each medication and when to take medications for optimal relief of symptoms

Teach pain-reducing measures and methods of utilizing physical comfort measures, positive feedback methods, awake-imagined analgesic techniques, distraction techniques, relaxation and

180

rest-promoting measures, and cutaneous stimulation

Teach approaches to reduce emotional tension and to modify or correct inadequate adaptive measures

Explain need to avoid upper respiratory infection or allergen, if associated with sinusitis or allergic response

Indicators for discharge
Adaptation to health status

Headaches decreased in severity, duration, frequency, and occurrence

Patient understands measures for reducing or alleviating symptoms

Patient understands medical management and is able to follow through with its implementation

Appropriate community agencies have been contacted for referral

Examples of community resources

Pain, allergy, or hypertension clinics

Mental health agencies

Environmental and industrial health agencies

Visiting Nurse Association or public health nurse

Social services

RETROSPECTIVE CRITERIA
Health

Afebrile

Headaches decreased in severity, frequency, and occurrence

Associated symptoms absent

Drug toxicity not evident

Activity

Ambulatory

Able to perform activities of daily living

Knowledge

Understands pain-reducing measures

Knows the name of each medication; understands desired and side effects, precautions, dosage, and frequency for each

Understands psychosocial aspects affecting occurrence, frequency, and severity of headaches

COMPLICATIONS

Adverse drug reaction

Status migrainus

Heart disease, arteriosclerotic (Code: 412.9)

CONCURRENT CRITERIA
Identification of patient's physical and psychosocial needs and/or concerns

Relief from prolonged angina and/or heart palpitations

Explanation of abnormal electrocardiogram, elevated blood pressure, cyanosis, dyspnea, edema, distended neck veins, pulsus alternans, weakness, or fatigue

Fear of pain and/or threat of death

Recommended nursing action consistent with diagnosis
Nursing services

Maintain physical and emotional rest with serene environment

Restrict sodium and fluid intake; keep accurate record of intake and output

Observe cardiac rhythm, vital signs, and emotional reactions

Initiate medical orders to alleviate chest pain or pressure

Maintain good skin care and passive leg exercises

Health education

Teach about disease process, signs and symptoms, and complications

Explain relationship of normal heart function and anatomy to patient's diseased heart

Explain risk factors and the importance of

avoiding emotional stress, fatigue, and lifting

Instruct about diet, medications, self-management during pain episodes, and plan of care

Reinforce explanation of physician's diagnosis in simple terminology to patient and/or family

Indicators for discharge
Adaptation to health status

Symptoms, such as pain and dyspnea, controlled or stabilized

Activity tolerated without signs and symptoms of cardiac stress

Acceptance of diagnosis verbalized

Knowledge about restrictions and limitations of activities verbalized

Heart rate controlled within normal range

Examples of community resources

Cardiac rehabilitation (depending on local offerings)

American Heart Association

RETROSPECTIVE CRITERIA
Health

Chest pain absent

Heart rate within normal range

Restricted diet tolerated

Complications not evident

Activity

Ambulatory

Self-care without angina

Knowledge

Patient/family verbalizes understanding of diagnosis, risk factors, diet, drugs, and medical follow-up

Knows to avoid fatigue, emotional stress, and lifting

COMPLICATIONS

Acute myocardial infarction

Angina pectoris

Arrhythmias

Heart failure

Preinfarction angina

Heart disease, congenital, in children (Codes: 744-747.2)

CONCURRENT REVIEW CRITERIA
Identification of patient's physical and psychosocial needs and/or concerns

Identification of primary disease signs, including cyanosis, acyanosis, or polycythemia

Evaluation of cardiopulmonary function; individualized treatment of potential complications, including cardiac arrhythmias or congestive heart failure

Adjustment of parents/child to life-style consistent with congenital cardiac anomalies and abnormalities

Acceptance of diagnostic tests and intrusion of body by surgical procedures (if surgery indicated); diversionary activities; and continuation of schoolwork for school-aged patients

Recommended nursing action consistent with diagnosis
Nursing services

Observe for physiological responses, including heart rate, cyanosis, blood pressure, dyspnea, pulse, respiration, weight, and exercise tolerance

Promote adequate body functioning, including nutrition, hydration, elimination (sufficient intake to ensure output of 800 to 1,000 ml every 24 hours), respiration, electrolyte balance, and activity tolerance

If surgery indicated, implement preoperative nursing care (physical and psychological); provide postoperative nursing care, including close observation of cardiac monitoring, prevention of complications, promotion of wound healing, increase in activity tolerances, encouragement of parent/child interactions

Initiate cardiac rehabilitation program for adjustment to appropriate levels of dependence and independence

Isolate patient from those with infections, especially upper respiratory infections

Health education

Explain to parents/child about cardiac anomaly, treatment plan, medical and nursing management expectations, family participation in care, diet restrictions, and activity limitations

Instruct in procedures to prevent infections, including upper respiratory infections, and signs and symptoms to report to physician

Instruct child in specific methods of treatment; encourage independence according to age and activity tolerance

Reinforce physician's explanation of surgery and pre- and postoperative course; familiarize parents/child with equipment to be used, such as cardiac monitors and intravenous equipment

Teach parents to assess signs and symptoms of potential complications, including change in pusle rate, increase in cyanosis, increase in fatigue with minimal exercise

Educate parents about available community resources for discharge care

Indicators for discharge
Adaptation to health status

Oxygen therapy discontinued; dyspnea or other complications not evident for 24 hours prior to discharge

Afebrile and vital signs stable

Activity tolerance increasing and normal activities resuming

Weight gained or stabilized; food and fluids tolerated

Deficit, corrections, and restrictions accepted; patient/parent education about home care completed

If problem surgically corrected, cyanosis not evident for 24 hours prior to discharge and wound healing

Examples of community resources

Visiting Nurse Association or public health nurse

American Heart Association

RETROSPECTIVE REVIEW CRITERIA
Health

Afebrile

Dyspnea controlled, if not absent; edema and heart failure symptoms absent

Oxygen not needed; vital signs stable

If surgery, wound healing

If surgery, pain and cyanosis absent

Weight gained; food and fluids tolerated

Complications not evident

Activity

Activities consistent with age resumed and tolerated

Knowledge

Parents/child understand activity restrictions but are not overprotective

Parents/child understand to avoid respiratory and dental infections if possible

Parents/child understand need for prophylactic antibiotics; know name, dosage, frequency, action to take if side effects occur, and precautions of each discharge medication

Parents understand possible complications; know when and to whom to report them

COMPLICATIONS

Arrhythmias
Atelectasis
Bacterial endocarditis
Brain abscess
Congestive heart failure
Dental infections
Drug reaction

Dyspnea	Polycythemia
Hypertension	Pulmonary embolism
Hypoxemia	Shock
Pneumonia	Wound infection

Heart disease, valvular (Code: 424.9)

CONCURRENT CRITERIA
Identification of patient's physical and psychosocial needs and/or concerns

Relief and/or control of anxiety and apprehension

Adjustment to reduced tolerance for physical activity

Relief of symptoms, including dyspnea, weakness, diaphoresis, palpitation, and chest pain

Explanation of disease process, course, prognosis, treatment alternatives, medical and nursing management, duration of hospitalization, and expected outcomes

Fear of death or change in life-style

Recommended nursing action consistent with diagnosis
Nursing services

Monitor body functions, including vital signs, heart rate, heart rhythm, respiration, tolerance for activity, nutrition, hydration, and elimination

Relieve discomfort

Prepare patient for diagnostic testing, including comprehensive explanation to patient/family

Provide psychological support for expression of feelings and fears

Maintain nutrition to reach normal weight

Health education

Explain disease process, course, treatment, medical and nursing management, and symptoms to report to physician

Teach measures to avoid recurrences, such as avoiding exposure to streptococcal infections, completing antibiotic therapies, receiving prompt and adequate treatment of infections caused by hemolytic streptococci

Instruct about name, dosage, purpose, frequency, and side effects to report to physician of each medication

Teach measures to prevent fatigue, promote rest, and continue productive life even with reduced exercise tolerance

Instruct about nutrition, including maintaining a balanced diet and normal weight to avoid obesity

Indicators for discharge
Adaptations to health status

Symptoms resolved or controlled
Afebrile
Heart rate within normal range
Health teaching completed
Referrals made

Examples of community resources

Vocational rehabilitation center
Visiting Nurse Association or public health nurse

RETROSPECTIVE CRITERIA
Health

Heart rate within normal limits
Weight within or approaching normal limits
Chest pain absent
Complications not evident

Activity

Ambulatory without chest pain or dyspnea
Performs activities of daily living with minimal assistance
Uses rest periods to avoid fatigue

Knowledge

Understands and can verbalize medication instructions, disease process, preventive measures, measures to adapt to reduced exercise tolerance, and symptoms to report to physician

COMPLICATIONS

Anemia
Aortic stenosis
Cardiac arrhythmias
Congestive heart failure
Obesity

Heart failure, congestive (Code: 420)

CONCURRENT CRITERIA
Identification of patient's physical and psychosocial needs and/or concerns

Relief of dyspnea, edema, cyanosis, rales, and distended neck veins

Fear of death

Reduction of physical and emotional stress and anxiety

Understanding of auscultatory gallop rhythm

Recommended nursing action consistent with diagnosis
Nursing services

Maintain physical and emotional rest with serene environment

Restrict sodium and fluid intake; keep accurate intake and output records

Monitor cardiac rhythm and vital signs

Initiate medical directions

Maintain good skin care and passive leg exercises

Health education

Explain disease process (signs and symptoms of congestive heart failure) and risk factors

Explain diet restrictions and medication

Maintain special care unit environment

Initiate plan of care (ability to cooperate)

Indicators for discharge
Adaptation to health status

Improved and free of dyspnea, edema, cyanosis, rales, distended neck veins, irregular pulse

Verbalizes understanding of disease

Verbalizes understanding of diet restrictions and drug therapy

Verbalizes understanding of medical follow-up

Examples of community resources

Visiting Nurse Association or public health nurse

American Heart Association

RETROSPECTIVE CRITERIA
Health

Sodium restricted diet tolerated

Chest pain absent

Respiration normal

Weight stable

Complications not evident

Activity

Ambulatory without chest pain or dyspnea

Self-care

Knowledge

Patient and/or significant other verbalizes understanding of diagnosis, risk factors (of the American Heart Association), diet, medication, and medical follow-up

COMPLICATIONS

Cardiac cirrhosis

Electrolyte disturbance

Peripheral arterial embolism

Pulmonary edema

Pulmonary embolism

Pulmonary infections

Refractory cardiac failure

Renal failure

Hematoma, hypertensive intracerebral, spontaneous (Codes: 400, 438.3)

CONCURRENT REVIEW CRITERIA
Identification of patient's physical and psychosocial needs and/or concerns

Correction of change in condition, including level of consciousness, behavior, vital signs, temperature, urinary output, cardiovascular functioning

Maintenance of vital body functions, including adequate ventilation and elimination, normal body temperature, cardiovascular functioning, and adequate hydration and nutrition

Minimization of functional loss from initial accident; prevention of physical trauma and physical deterioration as related to nutrition, hydration, contractures, fractures, circulatory problems from stasis, infections, sensory disturbances, corneal ulcers, and aspiration

Restoration of motor function to optimal level possible, including mobility, bowel and bladder control, communication, visual correction, and activities of daily living

Assistance in adjusting to changes in body image; protection from mental trauma; prevention of intellectual regression; maintenance of interpersonal relationships

Recommended nursing action consistent with diagnosis
Nursing services

Promote mobility and improvement of motor functions; prevent complications

Provide adequate nutrition, hydration, elimination and prevent aspiration

Implement rehabilitation including bowel and bladder control program, communication improvement, circumvention of visual disturbances, modification of patient's life-style to fit needs for activities of daily living and restrictions imposed by condition

Provide preoperative and postoperative nursing measures including physical preparation and psychological preparation of patient/family, explanation of special care units, procedure, and aftercare

Assist patient/family to cope with alterations in body image and life-style

Health education

Explain medical and surgical management of patient

Teach nursing management of patient including rehabilitative and preventative measures

Provide family education concerning patient's emotional needs and behavior

Explain health agencies available for assistance after discharge

Indicators for discharge
Adaptation to health status

Condition stable

Motor, sensory, and mental status improved

Complications not evident

Health teaching completed

Examples of community resources

Visiting Nurse Association or public health nurse

Physical rehabilitation center

Speech therapist

RETROSPECTIVE REVIEW CRITERIA
Health

Conscious

Condition stable

Motor, sensory, and mental status improved

Complications not evident

Wound healing

Activity

Ambulatory, unless residual neurological deficit prevents

Independent in activities of daily living

unless residual neurological deficit prevents independence

Implements rehabilitative measures

Knowledge*

Understands and can implement safety measures necessary in case of residual neurological deficits, such as sensory and motor weakness, impaired judgment, and convulsions

Understands and can implement rehabilitative care, such as bowel and bladder control program, exercises, and application and use of adaptive and prosthetic devices

Knows the name, purpose, dosage, frequency, side effects, action to take if side effects are present, and precautions of all discharge medications

Understands and can implement care required to prevent problems resulting from immobility

---

*In all cases where the patient is unteachable and there is no family, the responsible party assuming health care supervision is required to be knowledgeable about discharge care, and this must be documented on the nurse's notes.

Understands and can implement special diet

Understands function of community agency available for assistance after discharge

COMPLICATIONS

Aspiration
Congestive heart failure
Convulsions
Corneal ulcers
Decubitus ulcers
Dehydration
Injury from falling
Intractable seizures
Joint contractures
Malnutrition
Neurological deficits
Peptic ulcer
Pneumonia
Recurrent bleeding and shock
Sensory disturbances
Thrombophlebitis
Wound infection

Hepatitis, viral, group

Infectious hepatitis (short incubation period) (Code: 070)
Serum hepatitis (long incubation period) (Code: 999.2)

CONCURRENT CRITERIA
Identification of patient's physical and psychosocial needs and/or concerns

Relief of symptoms, including anorexia, nausea, vomiting, malaise, symptoms of upper respiratory infection, aversion to smoking, fever, enlarged, tender liver, and jaundice

Understanding of disease process, transmission of disease, duration of hospitalization, and medical and nursing management

Isolation

Concern and fears about infectious process, possible contagion to others, and loss of time from normal activities

Recommended nursing action consistent with diagnosis
Nursing services

Place in isolation; explain procedure; give patient an opportunity to express feelings

Provide bed rest during acute initial phase, followed by gradual return to activities during convalescent period

Observe vital signs, skin and sclera for increasing jaundice, tolerance of fatty foods, urine output, and hydration; watch for presence of signs of hepatic coma, pruritus, change in serum glutamic-oxaloacetic transaminase (SGOT) and serum bilirubin, and bleeding into tissues; weigh patient daily

Provide emotional support for expression of fears and effects of isolation

Health education

Teach about personal hygiene, including perineal care after urination or defecation and skin care for pruritus

Explain disease process, mode of transmission, treatment regime, avoidance of alcohol, not donating blood, avoidance of upper respiratory infections; immediate reporting to physician of recurrence of signs and symptoms, and importance of medical follow-up

Instruct on the name, dosage, frequency, purpose, side effects, and adverse effects to report to physician of each medication

Teach methods to reduce tiring and prevent fatigue during convalescent period; reiterate restrictions and/or limitations

Indicators for discharge
Adaptation to health status

Laboratory reports of SGOT and serum bilirubin decreasing

Presenting symptoms relieved and/or controlled

High protein, high carbohydrate diet tolerated

Prohibition against donating blood understood

Examples of community resources

Infectious disease report to health department

Visiting Nurse Association or public health nurse

RETROSPECTIVE CRITERIA
Health

Presenting symptoms resolved or controlled

Laboratory results of SGOT and serum bilirubin decreasing

Diet tolerated

Activity

Increasing activities without fatigue

Independent in activities of daily living

Completes personal hygiene, including perianeal care after urination or defecation

Knowledge

Understands and can verbalize diet, medication, and avoidance of alcohol instructions; rationale for not donating blood, symptoms to report to physician, and necessity for continued medical supervision

COMPLICATIONS

Bleeding into tissue
Cirrhosis
Dehydration
Hepatic coma
Hypoprothrombinemia

Hernia, inguinal, and/or hydrocele in children (Codes: 550-550.2, 551, 551.1)

CONCURRENT CRITERIA
Identification of patient's physical and psychosocial needs and/or concerns

Prevention of straining of abdominal muscles preoperatively

Expression of fear of surgical invasion of body

Prevention of postoperative complications, including respiratory, wound, and intestinal complications and infections

Emotional support for child/parents

Explanation of condition, cause, treatment, prognosis, aspects of discharge care, and wound care

Recommended nursing action consistent with diagnosis
Nursing services

Gear child's diet to foods that will prevent constipation preoperatively; use simple diversions preoperatively, especially while child is allowed nothing by mouth

Give child fluids up to 2 hours prior to surgery, if possible

Use sterile technique when changing dressing or working with the incision

Use pediatric urine collector to keep urine off incision area

Use therapeutic communication to relieve anxiety of child/parents

Health education

Preoperatively, explain to child/parents surgical procedures to be undertaken

Instruct parents about care of incision

Indicators for discharge
Adaptation to health status

Vital signs stable and afebrile 24 hours prior to discharge

Inflammation or drainage at incision site not evident

Teaching about care of incision completed

Normal activity for age being resumed

Food and fluids being tolerated

Examples of community resources

Referral usually not indicated

RETROSPECTIVE CRITERIA
Health

Vital signs stable and afebrile 24 hours prior to discharge

Food and fluids being tolerated

Drainage or inflammation in incisional area not evident

Activity

Moderate activity for age

Knowledge

Parents understand and can implement protection and cleansing of incisional area

COMPLICATIONS

Constipation

Damage to testicle by compression of the pampiniform plexus in the cord

Hemorrhage

Incarceration

Intestinal obstruction

Respiratory infection

Wound infection

Hernia, umbilical, in children (Code: 551.2)

CONCURRENT CRITERIA
Identification of patient's physical and psychosocial needs and/or concerns

Prevention of straining of abdominal area

Prevention of infection, postoperatively

Provision of emotional support for child/parents

Provision of teaching about care of incision

Expression of fear of surgical invasion of body

Recommended nursing action consistent with diagnosis
Nursing services

Reinforce pressure dressing as needed

Give child fluids up to 2 hours prior to surgery, if possible, and as soon as nausea abates following surgery

Use pediatric urine collector to keep incisional area dry

Use sterile technique when changing dressing or cleaning incision

Use therapeutic communication to relieve anxiety of parents and develop a trusting relationship with child

Health education

Teach family about diet and other measures to prevent straining of abdominal area

Preoperatively, explain to child/parents surgical procedures to be undertaken

Instruct parents about care of incision

Indicators for discharge
Adaptation to health status

Vital signs stable and afebrile for 24 hours prior to discharge

Inflammation or infection at operative site not evident

Wound care teaching completed

Normal activity for age being resumed

Food and fluids being tolerated

Examples of community resources

Referral usually not indicated

RETROSPECTIVE CRITERIA
Health

Vital signs stable and afebrile for 24 hours prior to discharge

Food and fluids being tolerated

Drainage or inflammation in incisional area not evident

Activity

Moderate activity for age

Knowledge

Parents understand and can implement protection and cleansing of incisional area

COMPLICATIONS

Anxiety

Hemorrhage

Postoperative intestinal obstruction

Wound complications such as hematoma, infection, and dehiscence

Herpes zoster (Code: 053.9)

CONCURRENT CRITERIA
Identification of patient's physical and psychosocial needs and/or concerns

Relief of symptoms, including pain, blisters, fever, or itching

Adjustment to changes in body image during acute phase

Fear of possible scarring during convalescence

Concern over contagion to others

Understanding of medical and nursing management

Recommended nursing action consistent with diagnosis
Nursing services

Reduce pain and itching

Prevent secondary infection and debilitation, especially if patient is elderly

Maintain good hydration and nutrition

Aid in adjustment to changes in body image during acute phase

Health education

Teach methods by which to avoid secondary infection

Teach avoidance of viral infections

Explain cause, course, and prognosis of disorder

Explain diet

Indicators for discharge
Adaptation to health status

Afebrile

Pain absent

Complications not evident

Examples of community resources

Referrals usually not indicated

RETROSPECTIVE CRITERIA
Health

Afebrile

Symptoms controlled

Complications not evident

Diet tolerated

Activity

Ambulatory

Independent in activities of daily living

Knowledge

Understands importance of avoiding viral infections

Understands and can implement maintenance of adequate diet

COMPLICATIONS

Ocular involvement that may lead to blindness

Adverse drug reactions

Malnutrition

Postzoster neuralgia

Temporary palsy

Hodgkin's disease (Code: 201)

CONCURRENT REVIEW CRITERIA
Identification of patient's physical and psychosocial needs and/or concerns

Understanding of systemic symptoms, including fever, night sweats, weight loss, fatigue, or pruritus

Relief of pain or discomfort

Feelings about disease, treatment, and prognosis

Adjustment to change in body image, including enlargement of nodes or organs (superior or inferior vena cava syndrome), dyspnea, or intractable itching

Understanding of irradiation or chemotherapy techniques, including desired results, possible side effects, frequency, and duration

Recommended nursing action consistent with diagnosis
Nursing services

Check temperature every 6 hours and weight daily

Treat pain and pruritus

Allow frequent rest periods

Provide emotional support for patient/family; allow ventilation of feelings

Observe and report side effects of irradiation or chemotherapy

Health education

Instruct about chemotherapy sequence, potential complications, measures to decrease nausea and/or vomiting, and possible alopecia

Explain importance of taking food with steroids

Explain rationale of treatments and medications

Prevent infections

Explain need for medical follow-up evaluation

Indicators for discharge
Adaptation to health status

Resolution of admitting problems

Verbalization of information about medication regime

Knowledge of disease and specific treatment goals

Completion of plans for appropriate care and follow up after discharge

Adjustment to change in body image

Examples of community resources

Public health nurse or Visiting Nurse Association

Social services

American Cancer Society

RETROSPECTIVE REVIEW CRITERIA
Health

Afebrile

Relief of admission symptoms

Control of pain

Activity

Maximum level of mobility reached

Initiates frequent rest periods

Knowledge

Patient/family can verbalize knowledge of medications, disease, and treatment goals

Patient/family knows when to return for continuation of irradiation or chemotherapy

COMPLICATIONS

Alopecia

Bone marrow depression

Diarrhea and/or constipation

Drug reaction

Gastrointestinal disturbances

Mucositis

Nausea and vomiting

Progressive deterioration

Pulmonary embolism

Septicemia

Tissue breakdown

Toxicity beyond therapeutic limits

Unsuitable discharge environment

Huntington's chorea (Code: 331)

CONCURRENT REVIEW CRITERIA
Identification of patient's physical and psychosocial needs and/or concerns

Coping with choreiform movements, mental deterioration, and chronic progressiveness of disease

Understanding by family/patient of disease ramifications for making realistic plans following discharge

Concern over change in body image and increased dependency role

Assistance in coping with changes in body image and role and increased dependency

Assistance in maintaining independence by use of adaptative measures and alterations in life-style

Maintenance of good hydration, nutrition, elimination, and muscle tone

Recommended nursing action consistent with medical diagnosis
Nursing services

Implement safety measures to prevent injury resulting from motor impairment, suicidal intentions, or impairment of judgment

Implement measures to ensure adequate nutrition, hydration, and elimination, including adaptative devices for self-feeding, easily managed foods, such as "finger foods," and small, frequent feedings; feed patient as necessary; measure intake and output; force fluids; insert catheter for elimination; encourage activity

Observe for desired effects and side effects of medications, with prompt nursing intervention should side effects occur

Implement measures to promote activity within limitations, including frequent turning in bed if bedridden, range-of-motion exercises, positioning, aligning, transfer techniques if wheelchair is used, and use of canes or walkers, to encourage ambulation, when possible

Control physical environment to facilitate patient remaining independent; have items for self-care within reach

Health education

Provide genetic counseling about hereditary disease

Explain ramifications of disease, regarding present disabilities in light of realistic plans for care after discharge, course, prognosis, and treatment plan

Educate family about measures by which to modify patient's life-style to promote independence for a longer period of time with assistance, including trips to grocery stores and advanced preparation of foods to minimize the need to cook

Educate family about community agencies available to assist with care after discharge and about possibility of custodial care as related to mental changes or physical impairments

Teach measures to maintain adequate hydration, nutrition, elimination, and maximum mobility within limitations of disease

Indicators for discharge
Adaptation to health status

Mental state more manageable
Motor disorder more manageable
Complications not evident
Referrals made

Examples of community resources

Meals on Wheels
Social services
Mental health centers or clinics
Physical or occupational rehabilitation centers (if appropriate)
Visiting Nurse Association or public health nurse
Genetic counseling center

Health

Mental state more manageable

Motor disorder more manageable

Complications not evident

Coping with choreiform movements, mental deterioration, progressiveness of disease, and increased dependency

Activity

Able to carry out activities of daily living with minimal assistance

Ambulatory either with assistance of individuals or with use of adaptive equipment

Knowledge*

Knows the name of each discharge medication, understands the dosage, frequency, desired effects, side effects, and precautions for each

---

*In all cases where the patient is unteachable and there is no family, the responsible party assuming health care or health supervision is required to be knowledgeable about discharge care, and this must be noted on the nurse's notes.

Understands the ramifications of the disease and has made appropriate plans for care after discharge

Understands and can implement measures to promote activities within limitations and to maintain adequate hydration, nutrition, elimination, and muscle tone

Understands and can implement safety measures

Understands purposes of referral agencies that have been contacted for assistance after discharge

COMPLICATIONS

Adverse drug reaction

Aspiration of food and fluids

Decubitus ulcers

Inanition

Mental depression

Persistent fever

Respiratory arrest

Urinary tract infection

Hyaline membrane disease (Code: 776.1)

CONCURRENT REVIEW CRITERIA
Identification of patient's physical and psychosocial needs and/or concerns

Relief of symptoms, including cyanosis, decreased peripheral circulation, tachypnea, labored rapid breathing, grunting, retractions of intercostal or xiphoid area, irregular breathing, edema, fatigue, changes in heart rate

Emotional support for parents, including ongoing information regarding child's condition; tactile stimulation for infant

Control of temperature instability

Reiteration of physician's explanations of physiology of respiratory distress syndrome, expectations of treatment, duration of hospitalization, and medical and nursing management

Maintenance of body function by use of umbilical arterial and/or venous catheters

Recommended nursing action consistent with diagnosis
Nursing services

Maintain neutral thermal environment that permits observation and treatment of unclothed infant

Monitor oxygen therapy constantly to maintain appropriate arterial blood gases, which are monitored every 4 hours while oxygen concentration is high

Observe for physical deterioration, including changes in respiratory pattern, increased cyanosis, apnea, variations in cardiopulmonary functions, with appropriate nursing intervention

Promote ventilation through patent airway, frequent suctioning, humidified oxygen, turning, and chest percussion every 2 to 4 hours

Maintain electrolyte and fluid balance by careful regulation of intravenous fluids

Implement respirator care, if indicated

Provide emotional support to parents, who may feel emotionally unprepared for parenting role—especially with high risk infant

Health education

Explain equipment, care, procedures, and expectations of hospitalization to parents

Teach parents about preventing infections after discharge

Instruct and encourage parents to participate in care of infant while hospitalized, including bathing, feeding, providing tactile stimulation, changing diaper, providing cord care, monitoring rectal temperature

Teach formula preparation and sterilization procedures

Instruct parents to use discharge day from hospital instead of birthdate for anticipating growth and development patterns

Advise when to return to physician; stress the importance of continued medical care

Indicators for discharge
Adaptation to health status

Afebrile
No apnea or cyanosis
Weaned from oxygen
Good appetite; gaining weight
Parents demonstrated ability to care for infant

Examples of community resources

Visiting Nurse Association or public health nurse
Parent groups

RETROSPECTIVE REVIEW CRITERIA
Health

Afebrile
No further apnea or cyanosis
Weaned from oxygen

Activity

Good appetite with weight gain
Alert and active

Knowledge

Parents understand the importance of avoiding crowds for the first few months to avoid any respiratory infections

Parents understand importance of continued medical supervision and know symptoms to report to physician

Parents familiar with community agencies and parent groups available for assistance after discharge

Parents know methods of bathing, feeding, tactiley stimulating, diaper changing, cord care, and monitoring rectal thermometer

COMPLICATIONS

Acidosis
Bronchopulmonary dysplasia
Cerebral hemorrhage
Electrolyte imbalance
Hyperbilirubinemia
Pneumonia
Pneumothorax
Retrolental fibroplasia
Sepsis

Hydrocephalus (Code: 743.9)

Identification of patient's physical and psychosocial needs and/or concerns

Relief of symptoms, including deterioration of memory and intellectual abilities, inability to concentrate, bizarre or antisocial behavior, labile emotional responses, incontinence of bowel and bladder, inability to feed self, unsteady gait, or total motor impairment; correction of cause, if possible

Understanding by family/patient of the purpose, preparation, and after-care of diagnostic and therapeutic procedures

Understanding by family/patient of the purpose, preparation, and after-care of surgical intervention (atrioventricular shunt), prognosis, course, anticipated outcome of surgery, and possibility of residual neurological deficits, so that realistic plans and goals can be made

Rehabilitation measures and assistance during long-term convalescence

Understanding by family/patient of community agencies available for assistance during convalescence

Recommended nursing action consistent with diagnosis
Nursing services

Implement safety measures to protect patient from injury resulting from poor judgment, sensory or motor impairment, emotional disturbances, or convulsions

Implement measures to ensure adequate nutrition and hydration, with special considerations for the hyperactive patient as well as for the underactive patient

Implement measures to maintain adequate elimination

Observe patient for signs and symptoms of deterioration or complications, by monitoring pupillary size, reaction to light, level of consciousness, extremity movement, and vital signs and by watching for excessive bleeding from head and neck dressing and complications from immobility; implement prompt nursing intervention should any occur

Assist family/patient in coping with knowledge that adult hydrocephalus may be caused by degenerative brain disease that has progressed to brain atrophy

Initiate rehabilitation measures, such as range-of-motion exercises, use of adaptive devices, and referrals

Health education

Instruct family/patient as related to name, purpose, dosage, frequency, side effects, action to take if side effects occur, and precautions of each medication

Instruct family/patient as to safety measures as related to impaired judgment and sensory or motor functions and to convulsions

Instruct family/patient as related to maintenance and improvement of motor functions as well as to application of prosthetic and adaptive devices

Instruct family/patient as related to community agencies available for assistance after discharge

Instruct family/patient as related to anticipated surgery, special care units, anticipated outcome of surgery, and medical and nursing care after surgery

Indicators for discharge
Adaptation to health status

Condition stable

Complications not evident

Maximum benefits from inhospital care achieved

Referrals made

Bowel and bladder program established to relieve incontinence

Examples of community resources

Visiting Nurse Association or public health nurse
National Association for Epilepsy
Visual, physical, speech, and vocational rehabilitation centers
Social services
Long term care facility

RETROSPECTIVE CRITERIA
Health

Symptoms more manageable
Wound healing; shunt functioning
Complications not evident

Activity

Able to carry out exercise program
Able to carry out activities of daily living with or without individual assistance or with the use of prosthetic and adaptive devices
Ambulatory

Knowledge

Family/patient knows the name of each discharge medication; understands the dosage, purpose, frequency, side effects, action to take if side effects occur, and precautions for each
Family/patient understands and can implement safety measures as related to judgment, sensory or motor functions, and convulsions

Family/patient understands and can implement methods of maintaining and/or improving motor functions by range-of-motion, active, passive, and resistive exercises
Family/patient able to apply and use adaptive and/or prosthetic devices
Family/patient understands and can implement techniques used to perform activities of daily living
Family/patient understands function of community agencies available for assistance after discharge

COMPLICATIONS

Bowel incontinence
Cardiac arrhythmias
Contractures
Decubitus ulcers
Dehydration
Inanition
Increased intracranial pressure
Persistent fever
Pneumonia
Sepsis
Shunt malfunction
Urinary incontinence
Urinary retention
Urinary tract infections
Thromboembolism
Wound infection

Hydrocephalus in children (Code: 743.9)

CONCURRENT CRITERIA
Identification of patient's physical and psychosocial needs and/or concerns

Relief of symptoms, including macrocephaly, abnormal rate of head growth, signs and symptoms of increased intracranial pressure (such as headache, retardation, vomiting, lethargy, scalp vein distention, full fontanelle, and sunsetting eyes)
Understanding by parents of cause, course, treatment, prognosis, nursing management, possible outcomes as related to residual neurological deficits, and possible repeat shunting procedures as the child grows older, so that realistic plans for the child's care can be made
Understanding by parents of purpose, preparation, and after-care of diagnostic studies and surgical procedures; with ventriculogram, parents should be aware, so as not to be alarmed of shaving head and use of restraints;

parents should be aware of type of surgery, such as atrioventricular shunt, ventriculoperitoneal or ventriculoureteral shunt, lumboureteral or lumboperitoneal shunt

Understanding by parents of the importance of ego-supporting measures for child, frequent and regular medical check-ups, including psychological testing, and imposing limits as the child grows older

Understanding by parents of community agencies available for assistance in care of child after discharge

Emotional support for parents to assist them in coping with infant's congential deformity

Recommended nursing action consistent with diagnosis
Nursing services

Implement preoperative, supportive nursing care, including frequent turning and use of protective devices, such as sponge rubber pad or lambswool, to prevent decubitus ulcers of the skull and earlobes; frequent turning to prevent hypostatic pneumonia; observation for signs of increasing intracranial pressure, degree of irritability, and changes in vital signs, with prompt reporting to physician should they occur; measures to maintain skin integrity and prevent infection; measures to prevent vomiting and to maintain adequate hydration and nutrition and to prevent aspiration of food and fluids; physical preparation of child for surgery; and psychological and emotional preparation of parents for child's surgery, by explaining all procedures, nursing measures, equipment, and special care units

Implement postoperative nursing care, including observation for increased intracranial pressure or excessive bleeding, with prompt nursing intervention should either occur; frequently check vital signs; observe for increased irritability, restlessness, bulging of the fontanelles, fever, lethargy, vomiting, elevated systolic blood pressure, widened pulse pressure, slowing or changing pulse and respiratory rates, changes in body temperature, excessive bleeding from incision site, swelling and tenderness along shunt tract, odor and purulent drainage from wound site; implement measures to ensure proper hydration and nutrition, with preventive measures against circulatory overload, cardiac failure, and aspiration of food and fluids, with close observation of electrolyte studies for electrolyte imbalance; maintain proper positioning to help decrease cerebral edema and to facilitate shunt functioning (recommended positioning varies with type of shunt and coexisting problems); implement measures to prevent infection and shunt malfunctioning; observe for signs of increased intracranial pressure if shunt fails; ensure avoidance of personnel with any type of infection; implement proper techniques in carrying out care of child and pumping of shunt

Initiate proper referrals

Provide supportive measures to assist parents in coping with a defective child requiring long-term care

Health education

Instruct parents as to physical care of child, including skin care, hydration, proper handling of child, turning, methods to assist child in strengthening muscles and improving motor function, prevention of decubitus ulcers and hypostatic pneumonia, measures to stimulate normal growth and development such as play therapy, convulsive care should the child be subject to seizures, and pumping of shunt

Instruct as to the danger of too rapid pumping of shunt, signs and symptoms of shunt failure or infection, and appropriate actions to take

Instruct as to the name, purpose, dosage, frequency, side effects, action to take if side effects occur, and precautions of discharge medications

Explain the need for continuous, regular medical surveillance with psychological testing

Explain appropriate community agencies available for assistance after discharge and for aid that may become necessary as the child grows

Indicators for discharge
Adaptations to health status

Wound healing; shunt functioning
Complications not evident
Referrals made
Parents demonstrated ablility to care for infant and to cope with infant's congenital abnormality

Examples of community resources

Visiting Nurse Association or public health nurse
Social worker
Exceptional children's center

RETROSPECTIVE CRITERIA
Health

Tolerating diet; gaining weight
Absence of signs of increased intracranial pressure
Shunt wound healing and generally good skin integrity
Shunt pump functioning
No evidence of complications
Parents can care for infant

Activity

Activity appropriate for age

Knowledge

Parents understand and can implement physical care of child, including skin care, diet, hydration, proper handling of child, turning, methods of assisting the child in strengthening muscles and improving motor functioning, and prevention of pressure sores and hypostatic pneumonia

Parents understand the dangers of pumping shunt too rapidly and the signs and symptoms of infection and shunt failure; parents know proper action to take

Parents understand and know the name, dosage, frequency, side effects, action to take if side effects occur, and precautions of each discharge medication

Parents understand need for regular medical check-ups and psychological testing

Parents understand function of community agencies available to assist after discharge

COMPLICATIONS

Aspiration of food and fluids
Bowel incontinence
Cardiac failure
Cerebral edema
Contractures
Decubitus ulcers
Dehydration
Electrolyte imbalance
Hemorrhage
Inanition
Increasing intracranial pressure
Persistent fever
Pneumonia
Sepsis
Shunt malfunction or failure
Spina bifida
Thromboembolism
Urinary incontinence
Urinary retention
Urinary tract infection
Wound infection

Hypertension (Code: 401)

CONCURRENT CRITERIA
Identification of patient's physical and psychosocial needs and/or concerns

Relief from headache, chest pain, impaired vision, and decreased urine output

Prevention of complications, such as cerebrovascular accident, heart failure, angina pectoris, cerebral hemorrhage, cerebral thrombosis, renal failure, myocardial infarction, or cardiac arrhythmia

Evaluation of elevated blood pressure over 150 systolic and 115 diastolic

Fear of hospital environment, death, and incapacitation

Explanation of nature of disease, cause, prognosis, management, and plan for care

Recommended nursing action consistent with diagnosis
Nursing services

Monitor heart rate, heart rhythm, and vital signs

Observe for changes in behavioral characteristics, symptoms of stroke, decreased urine output, and chest pain

Maintain restful and serene environment

Initiate medical directions

Restrict sodium intake and monitor output in accordance with drug therapy (diuretics)

Health education

Teach risk factors (obesity, smoking, activity, and stress)

Explain diet (restriction of sodium intake)

Explain disease process (the problem and what it does to the heart and other organs)

Explain relationship of normal cardiac tension to hypertension

Help patient develop plan of care to be self-administered

Indicators for discharge
Adaptation to health status

Diastolic blood pressure below 100 mm Hg

Pain absent

Mentally alert

Activity tolerated without dyspnea or shortness of breath

Understanding of diet restrictions verbalized

Understanding of diagnosis and prescribed drugs verbalized

Antismoking program implemented, if appropriate

Examples of community resources

Local chapter of the American Heart Association

Visiting Nurse Association or public health nurse

Hypertension clinic

RETROSPECTIVE CRITERIA
Health

Diastolic blood pressure below 100 mm Hg

Urine output approaching normal range

Complications not evident

Diet restrictions tolerated

Mentally alert

Activity

Ambulatory

Self-care

Knowledge

Patient-family verbalizes an understanding of diagnosis, diet, drugs, activity limitations, and importance of medical follow-up

COMPLICATIONS

Acute hypertensive crises

Angina pectoris

Cardiac arrhythmia

Cerebral hemorrhage

Cerebral thrombosis
Cerebrovascular accident
Congestive heart failure
Headache
Myocardial infarction
Renal failure

Hypertension in children (Codes: 400, 438.3)

CONCURRENT CRITERIA
Identification of patient's physical and psychosocial needs and/or concerns

Observation for and report of signs and symptoms of hypertension, such as elevated blood pressure and oliguria
Relief from irritability and poor appetite
Emotional support and entertainment to help accomplish bed rest
Concern about increased dependency, diet restrictions, limited activities, and surgical invasion of body
Understanding of nature of disease, surgical procedures, prognosis, management, and plan of care

Recommended nursing action consistent with diagnosis
Nursing services

Weigh twice daily (same time every day)
Check blood pressure at least every 4 hours around the clock
Monitor intake and output, limiting oral intake to amount ordered by physician
Provide quiet entertainment to make bed rest less confining
Prepare patient for surgical intervention, if indicated; implement appropriate pre- and postoperative nursing care

Health education

Explain low-salt diet and its importance to patient/parents
Explain meaning and importance of bed rest to both patient/family
Instruct parents on taking blood pressure at home, if indicated
Emphasize to parents the importance of continuous medical follow-up

Indicators for discharge
Adaptation to health status

Hypertension under control
Urine output sufficient
Required surgery completed
Afebrile
Salt intake restricted

Examples of community resources

School nurse

RETROSPECTIVE CRITERIA
Health

Afebrile
Weight stabilized
Diastolic pressure below 100 mm Hg
Wound healing, if surgical patient

Activity

Ambulatory

Knowledge

Parents understand and can implement restricted low-salt diet
Parents can take child's blood pressure at home, if indicated
Parents understand importance of continuous medical follow-up
Parents know the name, dosage, frequency, side effects, action to take if side effects occur, and precautions of each discharge medication

COMPLICATIONS

Acute hypertensive crisis
Cerebrovascular accident
Congestive heart failure
Renal failure
Wound infection

Hyperthyroidism with surgical intervention (Code: 242.9)

CONCURRENT CRITERIA
Identification of patient's physical and psychosocial needs and/or concerns

Relief of symptoms, including weakness; sweating; weight loss; nervousness; loose bowel movements; heat intolerance; tachycardia; warm, thin, soft, moist skin; exophthalmos; tremors; irritability; fatigue; ravenous appetite; goiter; and/or rapid speech

Nonstimulating, cool, restful, and quiet physical and emotional environment

Diet with large meals, high in calories, protein, and vitamins, offered frequently; avoidance of stimulating drinks like tea or coffee

Protection of eyes when exophthalmos is present by use of dark glasses, eye shield, and nonglaring light and by protection from dust

Explanation to patient/family about patient's altered anatomy and physiology, which accounts for patient's extreme sensitivity and irritability

Understanding by patient/family about disease process, surgical treatment, medical and nursing management, duration of hospitalization, and expected outcome

Fears of surgery, presence of noticeable scar tissue on neck, change in body image, and/or death

Recommended nursing action consistent with diagnosis
Nursing services

Provide great quantities of food to counter patient's negative nitrogen and calcium balance and increased metabolic needs

Provide stable environment for bed rest, including anticipating patient's needs, avoiding discrepancies in performing nursing care, and restricting emotionally upsetting visitors

Monitor physiological response parameters postoperatively, including vital signs every 4 hours; fluid intake to 4,000 ml per day; frequency and amount of urine and stool output; level of fatigue, restlessness, or nervousness; weight loss; heart rate and rhythm; respiratory status; elevation in temperature, indicating possible thyroid crisis or storm; changes in voice or speech pattern; presence of edema in lower extremities; observe for incision for pain, swelling, redness, drainage, or complaints of tight dressing; signs of tetany; and presence of bleeding at side and back of neck

Provide psychological support and understanding to help patient cope with disease process, change in body image, presence of scar tissue, and fear of surgery and/or death

Health education

Explain disease process, surgical treatment, medical and nursing management, and discharge care

Instruct about the name, dosage, frequency, and side effects of medication; stress importance of continuous thyroid replacement therapy

Implement rehabilitation measures, including flexion, lateral movement, and hyperextension of head and neck exercises; wound care; scar care, stressing stroking neck upward with moisturizing cream; progressive ambulation; rest and relaxation techniques; and avoidance of emotionally disturbing situations

Give diet instruction, stressing good nutrition and returning to normal weight

Teach patient/family to identify symptoms of recurrent hyperthyroidism, hypothyroidism, or infection of incision that should be reported to physician

Indicators for discharge
Adaptation to health status

Protein-bound iodine (PBI), thyroxine, and triiodothyronine maintained at above normal levels
Presenting symptoms relieved or controlled
Wound healing
Health teaching completed
Complications not evident

Examples of community resources

Referral usually not indicated

RETROSPECTIVE CRITERIA
Health

Symptoms relieved or controlled
Normal physiological responses reestablished
Wound healing
Nutritional state improving, with decrease in food consumption and increase in weight
Metabolic needs returning to normal
Complications not evident

Activity

Independent in ambulation and activities of daily living

Self-administration of daily thyroid medication
Supports head to prevent tension on incision

Knowledge

Understands and can verbalize medication and diet instructions, rehabilitation measures, disease process, and potential discharge complications and symptoms to report to physician

COMPLICATIONS

Cardiac complications (tachycardia, congestive heart failure, or atrial fibrillation)
Edema of trachea
Exophthalmos
Hemorrhage
Hypercalcemia
Hypoparathyroidism, leading to tetany
Laryngeal nerve damage
Myxedema
Nephrocalcinosis
Persistent fever
Posttreatment hypothyroidism
Thyroid crisis or storm
Thyrotoxicosis

Hypoglycemia in diabetes (Code: 251)

CONCURRENT REVIEW CRITERIA
Identification of patient's physical and psychosocial needs and/or concerns

Relief of symptoms, including nausea, feelings of shakiness, hunger pains, lethargy, frequent yawning, weakness, distorted vision, pale, moist skin, slow pulse, low blood glucose, excitement, dizziness, sweating; as condition progresses, there may be palpitations, tachycardia, high blood pressure, convulsions, and/or coma
Fear of death or invalidism
Understanding of disease, course, prognosis, and medical and nursing management, so that realistic plans for

health maintenance can be made for after discharge
Dietary control teaching

Recommended nursing action consistent with diagnosis
Nursing services

Determine precipitating causes of hypoglycemia, by assessing food intake in terms of "skipping" meals, retention of food, excessive activity, an error in insulin dosage, or possibly the presence of infection; implement corrective action, including calling for "weighback" from the dietician when part of a meal is not eaten, reinforcement of diet teaching, reinforcement of teaching concerning insulin administration and activity, and reporting findings to physician so appropriate measures can be taken for insulin dosage reevaluation or for treatment of infection

Administer oral glucose or inject glucagon, according to orders; repeat as necessary until patient responds, then follow rapid-acting carbohydrate or glucose with a feeding of protein or fat

Alleviate fears of invalidism or death

Implement hypoglycemia prevention measures, including preventing prolonged fasting periods that could interfere with dietary control and/or insulin administration, administering prescribed snacks, and monitoring sugar and acetone urine spillage

Health education

Provide diabetic teaching, including diet, recognition of signs and symptoms of hypoglycemia, use of candy or sugar lump, carrying medical alert information, need to prevent infections, skin care, activity level, and insulin and glucagon administration

Instruct about the name, purpose, dosage, techniques of administration, frequency, side effects, and precautions of each discharge medication, including insulin

Instruct about importance of follow-up medical care

Indicators for discharge
Adaptation to health status

Blood glucose level above 40 mg per 100 ml and less than 130 mg per 100 ml before meals

Complications not evident

Health teaching completed

Referrals made

Examples of community resources

Visiting Nurse Association or public health nurse

Diabetic clinic

Social services

RETROSPECTIVE REVIEW CRITERIA
Health

Blood glucose level stabilized

Glucosuria controlled

Urine free of ketone bodies

Weight approaching accepted limits

Precipitating cause controlled

Complications not evident

Activity

Able to administer hypoglycemic agent using correct dosage and technique; when insulin is the drug, can rotate sites properly, sterilize equipment properly, and use correct technique

Able to test urine correctly

Able to plan meals correctly, using exchange food system of diabetic diet

Ambulatory

Knowledge*

Understands importance and measures of preventing infections

Understands activity level and importance of adherence to it

Understands diet and importance of adherence to it

Knows the name, purpose, dosage, frequency, side effects, action to take if side effects occur, and precautions of each discharge medication

Family understands administration of oral glucose or injection of glucagon according to order; repeat as necessary until patient responds, then provide feeding of protein or fat

Understands and can implement convulsive care

Knows when and why it is necessary to return to physicians's office or clinic for follow-up medical care

COMPLICATIONS

Cerebrovascular hemorrhages

Coma

Convulsions

Paroxysmal tachycardia

Prolonged hypoglycemia

*If the patient is unteachable and there is no family, the responsible party assuming health care supervision must know the above and this must be documented on the nurse's notes.

Hypospadias in children (Code: 752.2)

CONCURRENT CRITERIA
Identification of patient's physical and psychosocial needs and/or concerns

Correction of deformity according to the degree in which it interferes with normal urination, future procreation, and normal psychological development

Maintenance of patency of urinary drainage system; decrease of bladder spasm; protection from wound infection

Assistance to parents in coping with feelings of guilt or anxieties regarding possible sterility, homosexuality, or defectiveness of child

Expression by child of fears of mutilation

Play therapy or diversionary activities to help child adjust to hospitalization

Recommended nursing action consistent with diagnosis
Nursing services

Implement nursing measures to aid parents and child in dealing with feelings of guilt or defectiveness

Provide preoperative care, including adequate hydration and nutrition and prevention or correction of infection of urinary tract or skin; preoperatively, explain surgical procedure, recovery room, intravenous equipment, if any, dressings, estimated time of hospitalization to parents and to child, as appropriate for age

Physically prepare child for surgery

Implement postoperative nursing care, including those to reduce discomforts to maintain adequate hydration, nutrition, and elimination; and to prevent wound infection, skin breakdown, hypostatic pneumonia, or urinary tract infection; closely observe for hemorrhage, hematoma, edema, or shock, with prompt nursing intervention, if necessary; prevent trauma to operative site by restraining or applying mittens to child's hands, if necessary

Administer medications, especially to decrease bladder spasms

Provide emotional support to child and parents; initiate play therapy to aid child in expression of fears

Health education

Teach the name, purpose, dosage, frequency, side effects, action to take if side effects occur, and precautions of each discharge medication

Teach wound care

Explain signs and symptoms of wound or urinary tract infection and action to take if either should appear

Discuss with parents the effect that surgery will have on child's body image and that child may have to relearn method of voiding

Instruct parents on need for medical follow-up to ensure urinary patency and anatomical functioning of penis

Indicators for discharge
Adaptation to health status

Condition stable
Voiding adequate if catheter removed
Blood in urine absent
Afebrile with wound healing
Health teaching completed
Child's and parents' fears expressed and being handled

Examples of community resources

Visiting Nurse Association or public health nurse

RETROSPECTIVE CRITERIA
Health

Afebrile
Wound healing
Adequate voiding
Absence of blood in urine

Activity

Ambulatory

Activity consistent with age of child and normal health

Knowledge

Parents know the name, dosage, frequency, purpose, side effects, action to take if side effects occur, and precautions of each discharge medication

Parents understand and can implement correct wound care

Parents understand the signs and symptoms of wound or urinary tract infection and can implement appropriate action should either occur

Parents can implement catheter care, if child discharged with catheter

Parents understand need for medical follow-up to ensure urinary patency and anatomical functioning of penis

Parents and child understand the basis of fears and can cope

COMPLICATIONS

Arrhythmias
Edema
Fistula formation
Hematoma
Hemorrhage
Pneumonia
Pulmonary embolism
Shock
Temperature of 100° F or over
Thrombophlebitis
Urinary incontinence
Urinary infection
Urinary retention
Wound infection

Internal derangement of knee (Code: 724.4)

CONCURRENT CRITERIA
Identification of patient's physical and psychosocial needs and/or concerns

Relief from pain or disability in terms of knee locking or giving away at unexpected times

Concern over time away from school or work

Understanding of injury in terms of prognosis and medical and nursing management

Rehabilitative measures to regain function of knee

Recommended nursing action consistent with diagnosis
Nursing services

Implement comfort measures

Provide preoperative explanation of procedure, recovery room, use of casts or splints, deep breathing and coughing, measures to reduce pain postoperatively, use of crutches, and estimated period of hospitalization

Physically prepare patient for surgery

Implement postoperative nursing measures, including close observation of patient for signs of physical deterioration, such as shock, bleeding, respiratory distress, infection, circulatory impairment; measures to facilitate cast drying and to maintain cleanliness (cast not always used); and safety measures for ambulation with crutches or splint

Control pain

Supervise prescribed quadriceps-setting and straight leg–raising exercises

Ensure adequate hydration, elimination, and nutrition

Health education

Explain medications, including the name, purpose, dosage, frequency, side effects, action to take if side effects occur, and precautions of each discharge medication

Teach cast care

Instruct about crutchwalking, applying

splints, using supportive knee devices, and duration of knee support usage

Instruct on therapeutic activities as well as on duration of restricting activities

Instruct patient when to return to physician's office or clinic

Indicators for discharge
Adaptation to health status

Condition stable
Complications not evident
Health teaching completed
Referrals made
Cast care implemented

Examples of community resources

Visiting Nurse Association or public health nurse
Social worker
Orthopedic clinic

RETROSPECTIVE CRITERIA
Health

Pain controlled
Wound healing
Knee stabilized
Complications not evident

Activity

Ambulatory with crutches or knee support
Initiates prescribed exercises

Knowledge

Knows the name of each discharge medication; understands the purpose, dosage, frequency, side effects, action to take if side effects occur, and precautions for each

Understands therapeutic and restricted activities and can implement therapeutic ones

Understands signs of circulatory impairment as related to the cast; can implement proper action should signs occur

Understands and can implement cast care

Understands when and why it is necessary to return to physician's office or clinic for follow-up medical supervision

COMPLICATIONS

Circulatory impairment
Hemorrhage
Infection
Joint contractures
Pneumonia
Respiratory distress
Shock

Intestinal obstruction, acute organic (Code: 560.9)

CONCURRENT CRITERIA
Identification of patient's physical and psychosocial needs and/or concerns

Relief of symptoms, including colicky abdominal pain, fecal vomiting, constipation, progressive shock, tender distended abdomen without peritoneal irritation, weakness, perspiration, anxiety, restlessness, dehydration, or tachycardia

Understanding of disease process, course, medical and nursing management, surgical procedures, and prognosis

Fear of death, surgical invasion of body, change of body image, change in role, and loss of time from normal activities

Correction of fluid and electrolyte imbalance

Recommended nursing action consistent with diagnosis
Nursing services

Maintain fluid balance; record intake and output

Implement measures to relieve colicky

abdominal pain, vomiting, and other presenting symptoms

Provide preoperative nursing care, including adequate nutrition, hydration, and elimination; explain about surgical procedure, recovery room, postoperative pain control, turning, coughing, deep breathing, bowel function expectations, and equipment

Physically prepare patient for surgery

Implement postoperative nursing care, including assessing physiological response parameters; maintaining nutrition, hydration, and elimination; preventing wound or respiratory infections; observing for complications and providing emotional support

Assist in early self-care and progressive ambulation

Health education

Instruct on the name, dosage, frequency, duration, and side effects to report to physician of each medication

Instruct on diet restrictions and methods to avoid constipation

Teach postoperative turning, coughing, and deep breathing rationale; infection prevention; wound care; and self-care

Instruct about disease process, surgical procedure, and symptoms to report to physician

Advise when and why it is necessary to return for follow-up medical care

Indicators for discharge
Adaptation to health status

Pain absent
Gas and feces passed via rectum

Normal physiological responses reestablished, including tolerating diet for 2 to 3 days prior to discharge

Wound healing
Complications not evident
Health teaching completed

Examples of community resources

Referral usually not indicated

RETROSPECTIVE CRITERIA
Health

Normal physiological responses reestablished

Wound healing
Pain controlled
Gas and feces passed via rectum

Activity

Independent in ambulation and activities of daily living

Knowledge

Understands wound care, activity level, medication instructions, disease process, and symptoms to report to physician

COMPLICATIONS

Anastomotic leak or obstruction
Constipation
Fluid and electrolyte imbalance
Gangrenous bowel
Hemorrhage
Pneumonia
Sepsis
Thrombophlebitis
Wound infection

Intestinal obstruction in children (Code: 560)

CONCURRENT CRITERIA
Identification of patient's physical and psychosocial needs and/or concerns

Fear of mutilation and increased dependency

Implementation of play therapy or diversional activities to help child adjust to hospitalization

Explanation to parents/child about condition, prognosis, medical and nursing management, and discharge care

Observation and report of signs of obstruction, such as nausea, vomiting, abdominal distention, absence of stools, severe abdominal cramps, and dehydration

Provision of adequate nutritional intake

Recommended nursing action consistent with diagnosis
Nursing services

Position patient on right side or stomach; elevate head to prevent aspiration with vomiting

Maintain patency of nasogastric tube; measure and record amount of gastric output

Keep accurate intake and output records

Maintain fluid and electrolyte balance by administering ordered intravenous fluids and by replacing gastric loss

Provide for routine postoperative care for intestinal surgery, if applicable

Health education

Explain procedures and equipment to child/parents to help alleviate some of their fears

Explain to child/parents importance of turning, coughing, and deep breathing

Explain condition, prognosis, medical and nursing management, and discharge care

Indicators for discharge
Adaptation to health status

Afebrile
Tolerating diet
Wound healing
Complications not evident
Health teaching completed

Examples of community resources

Referral usually not indicated

RETROSPECTIVE CRITERIA
Health

Fear alleviated
Afebrile
Tolerating diet
Wound healing
Normal bowel habits reestablished
Complications not evident

Activity

Ambulatory
Alert and active

Knowledge

Parents understand and can implement feeding techniques and dietary needs

Parents can implement home incisional care, if applicable

Parents understand condition, prognosis, and necessity of continued medical supervision

COMPLICATIONS

Anastomotic leak or obstruction
Constipation
Fluid and electrolyte imbalance
Gangrenous bowel
Hemorrhage
Pneumonia
Sepsis
Wound infection

Intussusception in children (Code: 560)

Identification of patient's physical and psychosocial needs and/or concerns

Relief from repeated reflux vomiting, paroxysmal, colicky, intermittent abdominal pain or tumor-like mass at site of intussusception, "current jelly," bloody, and mucoid stools; shock; and dehydration

Fear of mutilation from surgery, fear of increased dependency and change in body function

Parent/child understanding of condition, prognosis, medical and nursing management, and discharge care

Play therapy or diversional activities to help child adjust to hospitalization

Recommended nursing action consistent with diagnosis
Nursing services

Evaluate child's reaction to the pain (cries loudly, becomes pale, draws legs up sharply on abdomen)

Implement preoperative supportive nursing care, including measures to prevent vomiting and aspiration; maintain adequate hydration and nutrition via intravenous therapy; keep accurate and descriptive intake and output records; observe for signs of bowel necrosis; monitor vital signs at least every 4 hours; maintain patent and working gastric suction; physically and emotionally prepare patient/family, as appropriate; explain all procedures, nursing measures, and equipment

Provide postoperative nursing care, including implementing turning, coughing and, deep breathing every 1 to 2 hours postoperatively, ambulating as soon as physician permits, and proper hydration and nutrition with measures to prevent intestinal overload; observe for signs of recurrent intestinal obstruction, shock, abdominal distention, or

odor from the incision and report if present

Health education

Instruct parents on possibility of recurrence and possible causative factors, such as diarrhea, constipation, or any overstimulation of the bowel

Explain procedures and equipment to child/parents, to help alleviate some of their fears

Instruct on signs of intestinal obstruction and need to report immediately to physician

Teach parents about proper diet

Indicators for discharge
Adaptation to health status

Afebrile

Absence of any signs of intestinal obstruction

Tolerating diet

Wound healing

Normal bowel functioning

Examples of community resources

Referral usually not indicated

Health

Pain absent

Afebrile

Tolerating diet

Wound healing

Absence of any signs of intestinal obstruction

Stools formed and brown in color

Activity

Alert and active

Knowledge

Parents understand that intussusception can reoccur and recognize symptoms to immediately report to medical personnel

Parents understand and can implement proper diet

Parents understand and can implement wound care

COMPLICATIONS

Abdominal distention
Bowel necrosis
Dehydration

Hemorrhage
Intestinal obstruction
Perforation
Peritonitis
Pneumonia
Shock
Strangulation with gangrene
Wound infection

Ischemic chest pain (Code: 783.7)

CONCURRENT CRITERIA
Identification of patient's physical and psychosocial needs and/or concerns

Relief from frequent recurrent pain

Fear of coronary care unit environment, increased dependency, change in lifestyle, pain, and/or threat of death

Explanation of nature of condition, cause, management, prognosis, and involvement in care

Understanding of diagnosis and of coronary care unit

Recommended nursing action consistent with diagnosis
Nursing services

Monitor heart rate and rhythm with electrocardiogram (especially during pain—monitor immediately) record within 10 minutes

Give medication as required, if chest pain occurs

Maintain physical and emotional rest

Develop an open relationship for expression of verbal and nonverbal communications

Health education

Prepare patient for transfer from coronary care unit (progress for patient)

Explain function and anatomy of heart and relationship to patient's condition

Teach risk factors

Reinforce explanation of physician's diagnosis, in simple terms, to patient and family

Indicators for discharge
Adaptation to health status

Pain with activity controlled

Understanding of activity, diet, drugs, and risk factors verbalized

Understanding of diagnosis verbalized

Heart rate within normal range and rhythm

Participation in antismoking program, if indicated

Examples of community resources

Pain clinic (if available)
American Heart Association
Visiting Nurse Association or public health nurse

RETROSPECTIVE CRITERIA
Health

Diet tolerated
Chest pain controlled
Heart rate within normal range
Body weight approaching ideal weight

Activity

Ambulatory without increase in chest pain
Self-care

Knowledge

Patient and/or significant other verbalizes understanding of diagnosis, risk factors, diet, drugs, and follow-up care

COMPLICATIONS

Hyperlipidemia
Myocardial infarction
Pulmonary embolism

Jaundice and/or biliary atresia, obstructive, in children (Code: 576)

CONCURRENT REVIEW CRITERIA
Identification of patient's physical and psychosocial needs and/or concerns

Relief of obstruction, pain, nausea and vomiting, diarrhea, itching, and bile in stools and/or urine

Promotion of intake to ensure output of 1,000 ml each day

Maintenance of skin integrity

Adaptation to hospitalization, including emotional support, play therapy, and diversional activities

Education of parents regarding nature of disorder, treatment, and home care

Recommended nursing action consistent with diagnosis
Nursing services

Check patency of nasogastric tube every 2 hours; irrigate if necessary

Monitor intravenous fluids to ensure output of 800 to 1,000 ml every 24 hours

Observe and record condition of incision every 4 to 8 hours

Check stools for character and color; test for bile and check urine for color every 4 to 8 hours

Reposition patient frequently and provide nasopharygeal suctioning, when needed, to avoid pulmonary infection

Apply lotion to child's skin, cover child's hands with mittens; keep child's nails trimmed, since itching may be intense

Monitor vital signs every 1 to 4 hours

Preoperatively, give injections of vitamin K to prevent excessive bleeding

Provide extra comfort measures, if infant is very uncomfortable

Health education

Educate parents regarding child's need for conscientious skin care

Educate parents, preoperatively, regarding surgical procedure

Educate parents regarding home care

Indicators for discharge
Adaptation to health status

Afebrile

Vital signs stable

Wound healing

Food and fluids tolerated

Education regarding home care completed

Normal activity for age and developmental level resumed

Examples of community resources

Referral usually not indicated

RETROSPECTIVE REVIEW CRITERIA
Health

Afebrile

Vital signs stable

Food and fluids tolerated

Wound healing

Stools and urine free of bile

Complications not evident

Activity

Alert, no limitation in movement, resuming normal activity for age

Knowledge

Parents understand and can implement postoperative and discharge care

COMPLICATIONS

Ascites

Esophageal varices

Hemorrhage

Intestinal obstruction

Pancreatitis

Pulmonary infection

Wound infection

Leukemia (Codes: 204, 204.1, 205, 205.1, 206, 206.1)

CONCURRENT CRITERIA
Identification of patient's physical and psychosocial needs and/or concerns

Expression of feelings regarding treatment, prognosis, and indications of presence or absence of specific discomforts and/or pain

Relief from unusual bleeding and/or infections, including presence of petechiae on body, weakness, lassitude, fever, abdominal discomfort, anemia, retinal hemorrhages, and sternal tenderness

Adaptation to changes in body image, such as weight loss, or loss of hair

Continuing emotional support to patient and family because of prognosis, length of illness, and painful procedures

Protection from infections

Recommended nursing action consistent with diagnosis
Nursing services

Observe entire body for petechiae and lesions every 24 hours; *do not give intramuscular injections*

Observe for active bleeding from any body orifice; if any, alert physician immediately

Locate specific areas of pain; control pain

Observe vital signs for elevated temperature every 4 hours

Provide emotional support

Health education

Explain rationale for protecting from injuries and infection

Teach patient to check own body for petechiae or signs of infections

Teach patient/family about the nature of the disease, signs of complications about which to notify physician, and the necessity of periodic observation and lifelong treatment

Explain treatments, medications, and available community resources

Indicators for discharge
Adaptation to health status

Inpatient treatment goals of hospitalization reached

Patient/family knowledgeable about disease, signs of complications, and specific treatment goals

Plans completed for appropriate care and follow-up after discharge

Patient/family adjusted to patient's changes in body image and limited strength for activities

Patient/family understands antineoplastic chemotherapy program administered during hospitalization; knows continuing program regimen

Examples of community resources

Visiting Nurse Association or Public health nurse

American Cancer Society

RETROSPECTIVE CRITERIA
Health

Afebrile
Pain controlled
Complications not evident
No infections
No open skin lesions or signs of hemorrhage
Stable blood counts
Mentally adjusted to need for lifelong treatment and to change in body image

Activity

Ambulation and activities to self-tolerance, with avoidance of fatigue

Knowledge

Patient/family understand diagnosis, medications, plan of care, signs of complications, and resources available

Patient/family understand involvement in treatment plan

Patient/family understand necessity of periodic observation and lifelong treatment

COMPLICATIONS

"Basic crisis"

Bone marrow suppression

Brain hemorrhage

Chemotherapy complications

Chemotherapy transfusions

Gastrointestinal hemorrhage

Gout or uric acid nephropathy

Irradiation therapy complications

Irreversible thrombocytopenia

Overwhelming infection

Pressure on brain stem

Leukemia, acute, in children (Codes: 204, 204.1, 205, 205.1, 206, 206.1)

CONCURRENT CRITERIA
Identification of patient's physical and psychosocial needs and/or concerns

Protection from exposure to infection

Provision of emotional support for parents/child, with understanding of nature of disease, treatment, cost, prognosis, and necessity of follow-up care

Observation and reporting of side effects from chemotherapeutic drugs

Alleviation of pain and discomfort, weakness, malaise, anorexia, petechiae, lymph node swelling, splenomegaly, leukocytosis, and anemia

Adjustment to changes in body image, hospitalization, and decrease in physical activities

Recommended nursing action consistent with diagnosis
Nursing services

Maintain isolation principles; use careful handwashing technique; prevent exposure of child to persons with infections

Provide emotional support to parents/child

Observe, record, and report side effects from chemotherapeutic drugs

Administer sedation as ordered, with gentle handling of child

Protect child from falls; pad side rails, if necessary; use pressure dressings on bone marrow biopsy, injection sites, and venipuncture sites

Health education

Teach name, dosage, purpose, frequency, side effects, and reportable observations of all medications and or chemotherapy

Teach side effects of chemotherapeutic drugs

Instruct on importance of keeping child away from persons with infections

Instruct parents to protect child against injury

Instruct parents to provide as normal an environment as possible for child

Indicators for discharge
Adaptation to health status

Induction of remission or improved control of symptoms

Freedom from infection

Afebrile

Stable condition

Examples of community resources

Visiting Nurse Association or public health nurse

School nurse

American Cancer Society

RETROSPECTIVE CRITERIA
Health

Afebrile

Absence of infection and subcutaneous bleeding

Tolerating chemotherapy

Mentally adjusting to need for lifelong treatment plan and to change in body image

Activity

Ambulatory and active to individual tolerance level, with avoidance of fatigue

Knowledge

Parents know name, dosage, and time schedule for medications and understand side effects

Parents realize necessity of keeping child away from persons with infections and exposure to injurious situations

Parents recognize signs and symptoms of an exacerbation and need for early reporting to medical personnel and can implement treatment plan

Parents understand need for as normal activities as possible appropriate for age, with imposition of limitations to promote normal growth and development

COMPLICATIONS

Adverse reaction to chemotherapy

Bacterial infection

Brain hemorrhage

Disseminated cytomegalic disease

Fungal infection

Gastrointestinal tract hemorrhage

Hyperuricemia

Massive lymph node enlargement interfering with respiration

Overwhelming infection

Septicemia

Severe bone pain

Lymphoma, malignant (Code: 202.2)

CONCURRENT REVIEW CRITERIA
Identification of patient's physical and psychosocial needs and/or concerns

Expression of feelings about treatment and prognosis

Improvement or maintenance of body functions

Concern over and acceptance of changes in body image

Awareness and provision of comfort needs

Relief of symptoms, including pain, malaise, fever, weight loss, and/or sweating

Recommended nursing action consistent with diagnosis
Nursing services

Assess and control pain

Meet nutritional needs

Assist with emotional and spiritual needs, including referring to other hospital resources

Provide safe environment; prevent infections

Provide emotional support for treatment, including palliative irradiation, corticosteroids, or chemotherapy

Health education

Teach prevention of infection

Teach nutrition

Supply information regarding available community resources

Explain continued medical and/or nursing care and complications from chemotherapy

Explain activity limits and goals

Indicators for discharge
Adaptation to health status

Patient/family understands disease, treatment, and signs and symptoms to report to physician

Home care after discharge arranged; resources available

Physical status stable

Examples of community resources

Visiting Nurse Association or public health nurse

American Cancer Society

RETROSPECTIVE REVIEW CRITERIA
Health

Pain controlled

Diet tolerated

Weight gained

Mentally adjusting to change in body image

Activity

Maximum level of mobility reached

Knowledge

Patient/family understands appropriate follow-up care and resources

Patient/family understands disease prognosis, medications, nutrition, and treatment plan

COMPLICATIONS

Absence of medically suitable discharge environment

Complications from chemotherapy
  Alopecia
  Bone marrow depression
  Gastrointestinal disturbances
    Constipation
    Diarrhea
    Mucositis
    Nausea and vomiting
  Tissue breakdown
  Toxicity beyond therapeutic limits

Progressive deterioration with metastasis

Pulmonary embolism

Septicemia

Manic depressive illness and/or mania (Codes: 296.1, 296.33)

CONCURRENT REVIEW CRITERIA
Identification of patient's physical and psychosocial needs and/or concerns

Fears related to social stigma of mental illness

Concern regarding hospitalization, including fear of treatment and of length of stay

Concern for significant others, for loss of time from employment, and over change of role

Restrictions on physical activity

Recommended nursing action consistent with diagnosis
Nursing services

Involve nursing staff in development of treatment plan

Closely observe patient for signs of danger to self, others, or property

Closely observe patient for memory loss or confusion resulting from electroconvulsive therapy

Restrict stimuli affecting patient

Monitor blood pressure every 4 hours

Health education

Explain name, dosage, frequency, side effects, and observations to report of each discharge medication

Inform patient and signficant other of treatment plan and realistic expectations of treatment

Assist patient and significant other in developing healthy and helpful interaction with each other

Indicators for discharge
Adaptation to health status

Free of symptoms and/or problems that necessitated admission

Understanding of illness, indicated treatment and specific treatment, and specific treatment goals

Completion of plan for discharge care

Progressing toward specific treatment goals

Examples of community resources

Outpatient psychiatric nurse

RETROSPECTIVE REVIEW CRITERIA
Health

Absence of psychotic symptomatology

Absence of mania

Regular sleep pattern

Activity

Independent in activities of daily living

Ambulatory

Patient sets goals and makes plans for achieving them

Patient interacts in one-to-one and group relationships

Relationship and communication with significant others reestablished

Knowledge

Patient understands illness and treatment goals

Patient and/or significant other verbalizes understanding of the signs and symptoms of remission and the need to report them to the physician

Patient verbalizes understanding of instructions for taking medications, of signs and symptoms of untoward reactions, and of the need to report these to the physician

COMPLICATIONS

Complications of electroconvulsive therapy

Drug reaction

Psychotic behavior

Mass, breast, with mastectomy (Codes: 174, 198.3, 217, 233)

CONCURRENT CRITERIA
Identification of patient's physical and psychosocial needs and/or concerns

Alleviation of symptoms

Fear of death, loss of femininity, and surgical mutilation

Understanding of surgical procedure and expected pre- and postoperative courses

Adjustment of diagnosis of cancer

Adaptation to altered body image, maintenance of self-esteem, and reestablishment of relationship with males

Recommended nursing action consistent with diagnosis
Nursing services

Provide pre- and postoperative information and emotional support; allow and encourage discussion of impending surgery

Relieve pain through medication, positioning, and other measures

Inspect wound for signs of complications; change dressing as needed to promote wound healing; elevate arm on affected side on 2 to 3 pillows; assist with turning, coughing, and deep breathing every 2 to 4 hours for 48 hours and as needed

Assess and report deviations from normal physiological response parameters to physician; initiate treatment

Provide temporary prosthesis for patient

Health education

Instruct patient in techniques and importance of coughing and deep breathing; reinforce postoperatively

Instruct patient in need for early self-care and ambulation

Discuss and teach patient about adjustment and expected reaction to loss and change in body image

Provide information about and discuss the use of a prosthesis

Provide information about and discuss arm care and exercises

Indicators for discharge
Adaptation to health status

Independent in activities of daily living

Normal physiological responses reestablished

Wound healing

Reach to Recovery volunteer visited

Ability to cope with and acceptance of mastectomy evident

Uses temporary prothesis; knows when and where to obtain permanent prosthesis

Examples of community resources

Reach to Recovery

RETROSPECTIVE CRITERIA
Health

Raises arm above head on affected side

Mentally adjusted to diagnosis, change in body image, and feelings about relationships with males

Wound healing

Mass surgically removed

Pain controlled

Complications not evident

Activity

Ambulatory

Independent in activities of daily living

Implements arm exercises and applies breast prosthesis

Knowledge

Understands wound and arm care, arm exercises, and limited activity level

Has understanding of the surgery performed, prognosis, plan for follow-up care, medications, and ways to explain procedure to family

Knows when and where to obtain permanent prosthesis

COMPLICATIONS

Anxiety and/or depression

Edema of the arm on the affected side

Hemorrhage

Infection of hand and arm

Pneumonia

Swelling of hand and arm

Tissue necrosis

Wound infection

Meniere's syndrome (Code: 385)

CONCURRENT REVIEW CRITERIA
Identification of patient's physical and psychosocial needs and/or concerns

Relief of symptoms, including dizziness, tinnitus, headache, nausea, vomiting, decreased hearing, or uncoordination

Anxiety over loss of hearing, lack of balance, and change in body image

Protection from body injury during an attack

Understanding of diagnostic or therapeutic medical management, including the purpose, preparation, outcome, and specific aftercare

Understanding of surgical management (ultrasonic surgery or cryosurgery), including the purpose, procedure, pre- and postoperative care, special care units, and possible outcomes, including loss of hearing and destruction of labyrinth

Recommended nursing action consistent with diagnosis
Nursing services

Observe for desired effects of each medication, such as diuretics (chlorothiazide), vasodilators (nicotinic acid), and antiemetics (dimenhydrinate)

Maintain adequate hydration, nutrition, and elimination

Provide for safety

Minimize effects of decreased hearing on communication

Postoperatively, maintain vital body functions

Health education

Explain pathology, course, prognosis, and surgical treatment, if appropriate, of disorder

Explain medications, including each drug name, dosage, frequency, desired and side-effects, and precautions

Teach methods to reduce severity of symptoms, including moving slowly, changing position slowly, arranging people and articles so head movement is reduced, darkening room, not reading or watching television

Instruct on low salt diet

Teach safety measures for during an attack and restrictions, such as not driving

Indicators for discharge
Adaptation to health status

Nausea, vomiting, and dehydration absent

Vertigo episodes decreased in severity and frequency

Coordination improved

Examples of community resources

Social services

Visiting Nurse Association or public health nurse

Speech and hearing rehabilitation center

RETROSPECTIVE REVIEW CRITERIA
Health

Symptoms of nausea and vomiting absent

Vertigo decreased in severity and frequency

Coordination improved

Activity

Able to carry out activities of daily living without difficulty

Ambulatory

Adapts communication to minimize effects of decreased hearing

Knowledge

Understands ramifications and possible outcomes of disorder

Understands specifics of medications, such as the name, dosage, frequency, desired and side effects, and restrictions (such as not driving)

Understands and can implement safety measures should an attack occur

Understands and can implement diet

COMPLICATIONS

Deafness

Permanent facial paralysis

Vertigo

Meningitis, bacterial (Code: 320.8)

CONCURRENT REVIEW CRITERIA
Identification of patient's physical and psychosocial needs and/or concerns

Relief of symptoms, including violent headaches, painful and stiff neck, high temperature, nausea, vomiting, photophobia, convulsions, diplopia, tinnitus, positive Kernig's and Brudzinski's signs, clouding sensorium, and stupor

Fear of death, increased dependency, and change in body image

Concern about possible contagion to others

Understanding by family/patient of medical and nursing management, including antibiotic therapy; isolation; the purpose, preparation, and after-care of diagnostic and therapeutic medical procedures; frequent vital sign and neurological checks, fluid therapy, and fever sponges and "packs"

Maintenance of vital body functions and

prevention of deterioration in condition, by providing adequate hydration, nutrition, elimination, ventilation, cardiovascular functioning, and observation for signs of increased intracranial pressure, with nursing intervention if necessary

Protection from injury and complications, through seizure precautions and care, skin care, and measures to prevent pneumonia and urinary tract infections

Recommended nursing action consistent with diagnosis
Nursing services

Implement safety measures during restlessness, seizures, or coma

Maintain vital body functions, including adequate hydration, nutrition, ventilation, elimination, and cardiovascular functions

Closely observe for desired effects and side effects of medications (sulfa drugs, penicillin, methicillin sodium, chloramphenicol, or tetracycline) and therapeutic procedures (lumbar puncture), with prompt nursing intervention should untoward reactions occur

Prevent deterioration of condition and complications caused by immobility, such as circulatory stasis and pneumonia; observe for increased intracranial pressure

Reduce anxiety about disease and concern about possible contagion to others

Health education

Explain purpose, duration, and the method for maintaining initial isolation

Explain means of preventing contagion to others, if source is identifiable

Explain medical and nursing management, including the purpose, preparation, and outcome of the medical regime, special care units (such as isolation wards), medications, intravenous nasogastric tubes, lumbar punctures,

suctioning, positioning, artificial airways, ventilatory devices, and seizure care

Acquaint patient with appropriate community agencies that may be of assistance after discharge

Indicators for discharge
Adaptation to health status

Antibiotic therapy completed

Afebrile

Maximum improvement of neurological deficits after therapy

Family/patient understanding of care necessary for home care during convalescing period

Contact with referral agencies for follow-up care

Examples of community resources

Visiting Nurse Association or public health nurse

Social services

Physical and speech rehabilitation centers

School nurse

RETROSPECTIVE REVIEW CRITERIA
Health

Full range of motion of neck without pain

Headaches absent

Infection alleviated

Afebrile

Maximum improvement achieved for neurological deficits

Complications not evident

Activity

Able to carry out activities of daily living consistent with neurological deficit

Knowledge

Family/patient understands importance of prompt medical attention to bacterial infections

Family/patient understands and can implement rehabilitative care necessary for home management of patient with residual neurological deficits

Family/patient understands care as related to epileptic attacks, including medications, safety precautions, measures for decreasing occurrences, and legal precautions

Family/patient understands the importance of follow-up medical surveillance

Family/patient understands the functions of appropriate community agencies that may be of assistance after discharge

COMPLICATIONS

Adverse drug reaction
Arthritis

Circulatory stasis
Contractures
Cranial nerve damage
Decubitus ulcers
Increased intracranial pressure
Internal hydrocephalus
Myocarditis
Nephritis
Persistent fever
Pneumonia
Septic shock
Urinary tract infection

Meningitis in children (Codes: 027, 036, 045, 046, 320, 323)

CONCURRENT REVIEW CRITERIA
Identification of patient's physical and psychosocial needs and/or concerns

Understanding by family/patient of medical and nursing management, isolation, contagion to others, and discharge care

Relief of symptoms, including irritability with or without nuchal rigidity, anorexia, vomiting, lethargy, increased intracranial pressure, and stiff and painful neck

Reassurance about hospitalization and provision of diversionary activites

Emotional support to patient and family

Fear of invasion of body with needles and other diagnostic equipment

Recommended nursing action consistent with diagnosis
Nursing services

Check vital signs and level of consciousness frequently

Maintain prescribed rate of flow for intravenous fluids; administer intravenous medications as ordered

Restrain patient in a functional position to safeguard intravenous equipment and to prevent aspiration if vomiting occurs

Observe for any seizure activity or signs of increased intracranial pressure

Measure head circumference daily

Health education

Explain to parents the importance of intravenous therapy and how to help maintain it

Explain to parents that irritability is part of illness and usually goes away as child improves

Explain predisposing factors and the importance of reporting symptomatology and of providing early medical care

Teach parents the name, dosage, frequency, side effects, and observations to report of each discharge medication

Indicators for discharge
Adaptation to health status

Afebrile at least 24 hours prior to discharge (100° F or lower)

Appetite returned

Antibiotic therapy completed

Laboratory tests (lumbar puncture and nose and throat cultures) negative

Examples of community resources

Visiting Nurse Association or public health nurse

RETROSPECTIVE REVIEW CRITERIA
Health

Afebrile 24 hours prior to discharge (100° F or lower)
Diet tolerated
Laboratory tests (lumbar puncture and nose and throat cultures) negative
Irritability decreased

Activity

Ambulation appropriate for age and stage of development

Knowledge

Parents understand the name, dosage, frequency, side effects, and observations to report of each discharge medication
Parents know to call physician if child should run any fever before office appointment
Parents understand predisposing factors, such as ear and sinus infections, importance of avoiding colds and crowded places, and importance of early medical care and reporting of symptomatology

COMPLICATIONS

Adrenal hemorrhage
Adverse drug reaction
Brain abscess
Convulsions
Cranial nerve damage
Increased intracranial pressure
Internal hydrocephalus
Myocarditis
Nephritis
Septic shock

Meningitis, fungal (Code: 320.8)

CONCURRENT REVIEW CRITERIA
Identification of patient's physical and psychosocial needs and/or concerns

Relief of symptoms, including listlessness, irritability, anorexia, mild fever, headaches, vomiting, extraocular palsies, convulsions, stiff and painful neck, paralysis, and coma
Understanding by family of cause, prognosis, course of disease, and requirement that all family members and close contacts be screened for infection, such as coccidioidomycosis, histoplasmosis, mucormycosis, blastomycosis, or cryptococcosis, as appropriate for identified organism and coexisiting tuberculosis
Understanding by family/patient of medical and nursing management for long-term care, including drug of choice, rest, high-protein diet, and long-term restricted activity
Protection from deterioration, injury, and complications, such as thrombophlebitis from drug therapy or other adverse drug reactions, pneumonia, decubitus ulcers, or contractures
Explanation of community resources available to assist with care of patient during long-term illness

Recommended nursing action consistent with diagnosis
Nursing services

Maintain patient's safety during restlessness, seizures, coma, or paralysis
Maintain adequate hydration, nutrition, ventilation, elimination, and cardiovascular functions
Prevent problems from immobility, such as circulatory stasis, pneumonia, and increased intracranial pressure
Closely observe for desired and side effects of medication and for untoward reactions from diagnostic and therapeutic procedures
Immediately refer patient to appropriate agencies if signs of residual neurological deficits, such as deafness, blind-

ness, paralysis, hemiplegia, mental retardation, or epilepsy, should occur; implement measures that begin rehabilitation as related to paralysis, hemiplegia, and epilepsy, including range-of-motion exercises, transfer techniques, activities of daily living program, and bowel and bladder control programs

Health education

Teach patient/family cause, course, prognosis, mode of transmission, and importance of being screened for fungal infection

Educate patient/family about appropriate rehabilitation measures that may include positioning and range-of-motion exercises for paralysis or hemiplegia, skin care, transfer techniques, bowel and bladder control program, assistance for activities of daily living, precautions and care for postmeningitis seizures and medication

Instruct patient/family about activity restrictions, diet, and frequency of follow-up medical visits

Explain to patient/family about community agencies available to assist with discharge care

Indicators for discharge
Adaptation to health status

Afebrile
Symptoms relieved
Complications not evident
Health teaching completed
Referral agencies contacted

Examples of community resources

Visiting Nurse Association or public health nurse

Physical, audio, and visual rehabilitation centers

Mental health centers in the event of mental retardation, if in a child

Public school for guidance in learning and for tutoring, if in a child

RETROSPECTIVE CRITERIA
Health

Causative organism identified and controlled
Afebrile
Symptoms diminished or absent
Complications not evident

Activity

Able to carry out activities of daily living consistent with presence of neurological deficits
Ambulatory

Knowledge

Understands cause, course, prognosis, mode of transmission, and importance of all contacts being screened for fungal infection and tuberculosis; has made some plans to implement screening

Understands and can implement at home rehabilitative measures required by neurological deficits

Understands and can implement safety measures, as related to seizures, paralysis, and impaired mental judgment

Understands and knows the name, purpose, dosage, frequency, side effects, and precautions for each discharge medication; understands need for regular medical checkups

Understands community agencies that can assist after discharge

COMPLICATIONS

Abnormal behavior
Adverse drug reaction
Blindness
Circulatory stasis
Convulsions
Deafness
Decubitus ulcers
Hyponatremia
Increased intracranial pressure
Joint contractures
Mental impairment
Persistent fever
Pneumonia
Residual brain damage with paralysis
Thrombophlebitis

Meningitis, syphilitic, acute (Code: 320.8)

Identification of patient's physical and psychosocial needs and/or concerns

Relief of symptoms, including headaches, nausea, vomiting, convulsions, palsies, fever, stiff and painful neck, and possibly stupor

Fear of rejection, contagion, increased dependency, and loss of time from work and school

Explanation that disorder is infectious (early secondary phase) and all contacts must be identified for treatment

Emotional support and assistance to patient/family in dealing with feelings of guilt, shame, embarrassment, and social alienation, as related to venereal disease

Understanding of medical and nursing management, as related to severity of disease, including medications; bed rest; intravenous therapy; nasogastric feedings, if in stupor; possible seizure care; frequent observation and neurological checks for signs of increased intracranial pressure; precautions or initial isolation; purpose, preparation, and outcome of medical procedures, such as lumbar puncture; duration of absence from school or work; restrictions, if any; and measures taken to prevent complications of immobility, especially in case of stupor

Identification of community agencies that must be contacted, as required by law, and those available for assistance with discharge care

Recommended nursing action consistent with diagnosis
Nursing services

Assist patient/family in dealing with feelings

Ensure adequate hydration, nutrition, elimination, ventilation, and cardiovascular functions

Provide relief from or minimize severity of symptoms, by giving fever sponges and ice packs and forcing fluids for temperature elevation; rest, analgesics, control of noxious stimuli, positioning, and comfort measures for pain; and liquids that are easily digested and tolerated for nausea and vomiting

Prevent injury during restlessness, convulsions, or stupor; if in a stupor, implement measures to prevent problems caused by immobility, such as frequent turning, skin care, suctioning, range-of-motion exercises, proper positioning, alignment, and use of supportive devices

Complete health teaching and initiate referrals to community agencies

Health education

Explain ramifications of disease, including the cause, course, and prognosis (usually no residual neurological deficits if treatment is prompt and adequate)

Teach medical management, including the name, dosage, frequency, duration of treatment, side effects, and precautions of each medication and the importance of regular medical follow-up with laboratory studies to determine effectiveness of medications

Provide sex education, including methods of contracting the disease, signs and symptoms of syphilis, and methods of preventing it; explain the necessity of treatment for all persons having had intimate relations with the patient, the necessity of avoiding sexual relations with anyone until the patient is considered to be noninfectious by the physician, and the necessity of avoiding sexual relations with any former sexual partners who remain untreated

If neurological deficits do occur, teach family appropriate care and management of patient, as related to severity of deficits

Indicators for discharge
Adaptation to health status

Report to Department of Public Health completed
Asymptomatic
Complications not evident
Maximum neurological improvement
Appropriate referrals made
Health teaching completed

Examples of community resources

Department of Public Health
Visiting Nurse Association or public health nurse
School health department
Social services

RETROSPECTIVE REVIEW CRITERIA
Health

Asymptomatic
Complications not evident
Maximum neurological improvement
Mentally adjusted to diagnosis and social ramifications of disease

Activity

Able to carry out activities of daily living with little or no assistance
Ambulatory

Knowledge

Understands cause, course, prognosis, transmission, and methods of prevention of disease
Understands the name, dosage, frequency, duration of therapy, side effects, and precautions of each medication and the importance of regular medical follow-up with laboratory studies to determine effectiveness of medications
Understands restrictions on sexual activity until patient is fully recovered and is considered to be noninfectious
Knows importance of keeping appointments for necessary treatment; knows purpose of community agencies contacted for assistance after discharge
Family understands care and management of patient when neurological deficits, such as palsy, epilepsy, paralysis, or mental retardation, remain

COMPLICATIONS

Adverse drug reaction
Convulsions
Cranial nerve damage
Decubitus ulcers
Increased intracranial pressure
Internal hydrocephalus
Joint contractures
Mental impairment
Persistent fever
Residual brain damage with motor paralysis

Meningitis, syphilitic, chronic (Code: 320.8)

CONCURRENT REVIEW CRITERIA
Identification of patient's physical and psychosocial needs and/or concerns

Immediate interruption of disease process to reduce residual neurological damage, including memory changes, deterioration in judgment, personality changes, tremors of the lips, tongue, fingers, and hands, convulsions, and psychosis

Understanding of disease ramifications, including pathology, course, prognosis, and treatment; realization that this stage is not infectious and that mental changes may not be reversible, depending on the progress of the disease and the response to treatment, since organisms at this stage frequently are drug resistant

Explanation of medical and nursing management and availability of community resources

Protection from physical injury, as related to motor deficits and convulsions and from social and economic loss, as related to impaired judgment and deterioration of mental status

Adjustment of family to problems related to altered state of patient, including a lowered mental and emotional level, working at an emotionally and physically nontaxing job, or to the need for custodial care

Recommended nursing action consistent with diagnosis
Nursing services

Closely observe for desired effects and side effects of medication, with prompt intervention should side effects occur

Protect patient from physical injury from convulsions, or impaired motor function and from social and economic injury from impaired judgment and deterioration of mental status

Ensure adequate hydration, nutrition, and elimination

Prevent complications resulting from immobility, including contractures, urinary infections, pneumonia, decubitus ulcers, and pulmonary embolism

Implement measures to reduce severity of headaches; provide rest, and maintain orientation

Health education

Instruct on the name, dosage, frequency, side effects, desired effects, and duration of therapy of each discharge medication, if applicable

Explain to family disease and possible residual deficits requiring decisions for posthospital care

Teach family methods for implementing home care for convulsions, immobility, or mental disability

Inform family/patient about community agencies available to assist with home care

Indicators for discharge
Adaptation to health status

Mental status and neurological signs improved

Discharge environment suitable and realistic for patient's needs

Referrals completed

Health teaching completed

Examples of community resources

Visiting Nurse Association or public health nurse

Mental health clinic

Social worker

RETROSPECTIVE REVIEW CRITERIA
Health

Headaches controlled

Mental status and neurological signs improved

Complications not evident

Activity

Ambulatory

Completes activities of daily living with minimal assistance or supervision

Knowledge

Family/patient understands and knows the name, dosage, frequency, desired effects, side effects, duration of therapy, and precautions, if any, of each discharge medication, if applicable

Family understands disease and ramifications and has made appropriate decisions related to care of patient after discharge

Family understands and can implement appropriate home care for convulsions and impairments related to immobility and provides adequate supervision when mental deficits occur

Family understands community services available for assistance after discharge

COMPLICATIONS

Adverse drug reaction

Charcot's joints

Convulsions

Decubitus ulcers

Deterioration of judgment
Distended bladder
Drug resistent organism
Hypotonia of lower extremities
Impaired motor functions
Joint contractures
Memory or personality changes

Optic atrophy
Pneumonia
Psychosis
Pulmonary embolism
Tremors of lips, tongue, or fingers
Trophic ulcers
Urinary infection

Meningitis, tuberculous (Code: 320.8)

CONCURRENT REVIEW CRITERIA
Identification of patient's physical and psychosocial needs and/or concerns

Relief of symptoms, including listlessness, irritability, anorexia, mild fever, headaches, vomiting, extraocuar palsies, night cries, convulsions, stiff, painful neck, paralysis, positive Kernig's and Brudzinski's signs, and coma

Family understanding of cause, prognosis (usually affects children more often than adults), course, and need to have all family members and close contacts screened for tuberculosis

Understanding of medical and nursing management for long-term care

Protection from deterioration, injury, and complications

Community resources supporting family in care of patient during long-term illness

Fear of body invasion by needles; fear of hospitalization and separation from family

Recommended nursing action consistent with diagnosis
Nursing services

Implement measures to maintain safety during restlessness, seizures, or coma

Implement measures to maintain adequate hydration, nutrition, ventilation, elmination, and cardiovascular functions

Closely observe for desired effects and side effects of medications, such as streptomycin, isoniazid, and paramino-

salicylic acid, and for untoward reactions from diagnostic and therapeutic procedures, such as lumbar puncture

Implement measures to prevent deterioration of condition and complications from immobility, such as circulatory stasis and pneumonia; observe for increased intracranial pressure

Refer immediately to appropriate agencies if signs of residual neurological deficits, such as deafness, blindness, paralysis, hemiplegia, mental retardation, or epilepsy, should occur; implement measures, such as range-of-motion exercises, transfer techniques, activites of daily living, and bowel and bladder control program, to begin rehabilitation with regard to paralysis, hemiplegia, and epilepsy

Health education

Educate family on pathology, course, treatment, mode of transmission, and importance of being screened for tuberculosis

Educate family on rehabilitation measures should patient be bedridden at home after acute phase with residual neurological deficits such as paralysis or hemiplegia requiring range-of-motion exercises, frequent turning, skin care, transfer techniques, bowel and bladder control programs, and methods by which to assist the patient in learning to carry out activites of daily living; teach how to deal with the patient during and after an epileptic seizure; the name, dosage, frequency, side effects, desired effects, and precautions of each discharge medication; methods for reducing the occurrence of seizures; and the legal ramifications

Teach tuberculosis medications, including the name, dosage, frequency, duration of period to be taken, desired effects, side effects, and precautions of each; explain diet, activity restrictions, and need for rest

Explain the importance of regular medical supervision and checkups

Educate family regarding appropriate community agencies for assistance

Indicators for discharge
Adaptation to health status

Afebrile
Symptoms relieved
Complications not evident
Referral agencies contacted
Health teaching completed

Examples of community resources

Visiting Nurse Association or public health nurse

Physical, audio, and visual rehabilitation centers

Mental health centers for mental retardation

Public school for guidance in learning and tutoring

RETROSPECTIVE REVIEW CRITERIA
Health

Afebrile
Asymptomatic
Complications not evident

Activity

Performs activities appropriate for age

Knowledge

Family/patient understands pathology, course, prognosis, and need for close contacts to be screened for tuberculosis

Family/patient understands care for neurological deficits, such as hemiplegia, paralysis, and epilepsy

Family/patient understands convalescent care of a tuberculous patient, including rest, activity restrictions, allowances, and diet

Family/patient understands community agencies that have been contacted to assist them and have appointments when appropriate

COMPLICATIONS

Abnormal behavior
Adverse drug reaction
Circulatory stasis
Contractures
Convulsions
Deafness
Decubitus ulcers
Hyponatremia
Increased intracranial pressure
Mental impairment
Persistent fever
Pneumonia
Residual brain damage resulting in motor paralysis

Meningitis, viral (Code: 045)

CONCURRENT REVIEW CRITERIA

Identification of patient's physical and psychosocial needs and/or concerns

Relief of symptoms, including headaches, painful neck, high temperature, nausea, and vomiting

Concern about possible contagion to others

Family/patient understanding of cause, prognosis, and outcome (including that viral meningitis generally is more benign than other types, with residual effects being rare and that the patient seldom becomes camatose or has decreased levels of consciousness)

Family/patient understanding of medical and nursing management, including antibiotics; the purpose, preparation, and outcome of diagnostic and therapeutic procedures, such as lumbar puncture and subdural taps (if in a child); frequent monitoring of vital signs, and frequent neurological checks, fluid therapy, and close observation for more serious symptoms, such as convulsions, decreased levels of consciousness, diplopia, or positive Brudzinski's and Kernig's signs, that may indicate another form of meningitis

Recommended nursing action consistent with diagnosis
Nursing services

Implement measures to maintain adequate hydration, nutrition, and elimination

Closely observe for desired effects and side effects of medications (primarily penicillin, sulfa drugs, and chloramphenicol)

Implement measures to reduce fever, provide comfort, and reduce pain

Reduce anxiety over nature of disease itself and concern about contagion to others

Health education

Explain type of meningitis, course, and prognosis; if initial observatory isolation required, explain purpose and duration

Teach measures to provide care for person with childhood disease or viral infections in order to prevent complication of viral meningitis; avoid persons with viral infections

Teach the name, dosage, frequency, desired effects, side effects, how long to be taken after discharge (until bottle is empty) and precautions for each discharge medication

Explain need for follow-up visit

Explain duration of absence from school or work, activity restrictions, if any, and diet

Indicators for discharge
Adaptation to health status

Afebrile
Complications not evident
Health teaching completed
Referrals completed

Examples of community resources

Visiting Nurse Association or public health nurse
School nurse

RETROSPECTIVE REVIEW CRITERIA
Health

Headaches controlled
Pain absent
Afebrile
Complications not evident

Activity

Ambulatory
Able to perform activities of daily living

Knowledge*

Knows duration of absence from school or work and activity restrictions, if any, while convalescing

Knows the name, dosage, frequency, desired and side effects, precautions, and how long to be taken for each discharge medication

Understands measures for preventing viral infections, such as proper immunization, diet, general health princi-

---

*In all cases where there is a learning disability and no family, the responsible party assuming health care supervision must be knowledgeable about after-care, and this must be documented on the nurse's notes.

ples, and avoidance of persons who are infected

Knows importance of continued medical surveillance

COMPLICATIONS

Adverse drug reactions
Convulsions
Decubitus ulcers
Increased intracranial pressure
Mental impairment
Persistent fever
Residual brain damage resulting in motor paralysis

Meningocele, myelomeningocele, spina bifida (Codes: 741.9, 756.2)

CONCURRENT CRITERIA
Identification of patient's physical and psychosocial needs and/or concerns

Correction of defect and control of symptoms, including spina bifida without meningeal or spinal cord involvement, requiring no treatment; motor-sensory impairment of the extremities; cyanosis and ulceration of the skin; bowel and bladder disturbances, with symptoms related to severity of meningocele and myelomeningocele; surgery for meningocele and myelomeningocele done within 24 hours of birth up to 2 years

Protection from trauma and infection by proper positioning to prevent irritation, contamination, or rupture of sac; by positioning to prevent wristdrop and footdrop, skin care to prevent skin breakdown; bladder Credé to prevent urinary retention and infection from stasis

Assistance for parents in coping with having a deformed child and with long-term management of associated problems

Understanding by parents of purpose, preparation, and expected and possible

outcomes of diagnostic and therapeutic medical and surgical procedures as well as special after-care and nursing management, so that realistic plans for care can be made

Understanding by parents of community agencies available for assistance in care of child after discharge

Recommended nursing action consistent with diagnosis
Nursing services

Provide supportive and preoperative nursing care, including frequent assessment of condition for irritation, abrasion, rupture, leakage of cerebrospinal fluid, and infection of sac; for motor and sensory functions; for urinary and bowel retention; for hydrocephalus by daily measurement of heal circumference, since hydrocephalus is frequently a secondary complication; for signs and symptoms of meningitis, such as hyperirritability, increased sensitivity to noise and light; for nuchal rigidity and vomiting; implement proper positioning to prevent damage to sac, infection, footdrop, and wristdrop, provide skin

care; ensure adequate elimination by
Credé, suppositories, and diet

Physically prepare child for surgery

Prepare parents for child's surgery with
explanation of surgery, possible residual deficits, special care units, and
nursing care

Postoperatively, provide nursing care,
including close observation for elevated temperature, bladder and bowel
dysfunctions, and other complications;
position with head lower than spine to
maintain pressure of cerebrospinal
fluid within the brain (contraindicated
when child is hydrocephalic); frequently change position to prevent decubitus
ulcers or hypostatic pneumonia; properly align to prevent footdrop, wristdrop, and muscle stretching; provide
adequate hydration and nutrition; observe dressing for leakage or purulent
drainage

Explain to parents community agencies
available for assistance after discharge

Provide health teaching; initiate discharge planning and referrals

Health education

Teach parents about medications, including the name, dosage, frequency, side
effects, action to take should side
effects occur, and precautions for each

Teach parents method and importance of
good skin care

Instruct parents as related to activities,
positioning, and turning

Instruct parents as to bowel and bladder
training program with Crede, adequate
fluids, insertion of suppository, diet
schedule, and methods of controlling
seepage

Instruct parents on application and use of
braces and other adaptive devices

Instruct and guide parents as related to
providing ego-supportive measures to
child, imposing limitations, implementing measures to promote maximum muscle functions within restriction of neurological deficit

Stress importance of frequent, regular

medical, dental, and psychological
checkups, with proper immunizations
to avoid infections and proper surveillance of bladder and bowel functioning

Indicators for discharge
Adaptation to health status

Condition stable
Muscle functions stable or improved
Complications not evident
Health teaching completed
Referrals made

Examples of community resources

Visiting Nurse Association or public
health nurse
Social services
Spina Bifida Association of America
Surgical clinic
Medical clinic

RETROSPECTIVE CRITERIA*
Health

Defect corrected
Wound healing
Symptoms controlled
Muscle functions stable or improved
Complications not evident

Activity

Able to perform activities appropriate for
age and maximum for disability

Knowledge

Parents understand and know the name,
dosage, frequency, side effects, actions
to take should side effects occur, and
precautions for each discharge medication

Parents understand and can implement
care to maintain skin integrity, provide
bowel and bladder training, and promote maximum muscle functions

*Criteria are for newborns up to 2 years. Criteria
must be modified or adapted for patients who are
older or suffering from problems that require additional surgery or that are related to the initial condition.

231

Parents can apply and implement use of braces and other adaptive devices

COMPLICATIONS

Decubitus ulcers
Dehydration
Footdrop or wristdrop
Hydrocephalus
Intestinal obstruction due to severe constipation

Meningitis
Pneumonia or respiratory distress
Shock
Urinary tract infection
Wound infection
Wound rupture with cerebrospinal fluid leakage

Mental retardation of childhood or adolescence
(Codes: DMS II 310-315)

CONCURRENT CRITERIA
Identification of patient's physical and psychosocial needs and/or concerns

Identification of reason for admission, which should be for testing and teaching activities of daily living; otherwise, should seek more definitive treatment of psychiatric symptoms
Assessment of the state of child's/adolescent's physical health
Patient's beliefs, attitudes, fears, and expectations of own behavior and hospitalization
Adaptive measures and methods by which maximum potential can be reached
Emotional support to parents/patient

Recommended nursing action consistent with diagnosis
Nursing services

Explore patient/family's beliefs, attitudes, and expectations of patient and treatment facility
Observe and assess ongoing behavior of patient within 8 hours of admission, every 8 hours for 1 week, then during facility-defined periods; document any changes
Implement behavior-specific interventions, such as life-space interview, seclusion, suicide precaution, or behavior modification
Assist in developing and implementing

an after-care program and family-specific interventions
Implement and assess physical therapies and therapeutic program, including medications, dosages, and procedures

Health education

Explain ward procedures and milieu to patient/family
Discuss treatment goals, therapeutic modalities, and adaptive methods by which maximum potential can be reached with patient/family
Teach family to make use of specific therapeutic modalities, such as behavior modification, principles of psychodynamics, communication theories, and attitude therapy
Discuss, demonstrate, and explain use of any medication
Teach family about mental retardation; demonstrate realistic goal-setting

Indicators for discharge
Adaptation to health status

Evidence of family's knowledge of patient's ability limitations from mental retardation and about setting realistic goals for patient's daily routine at home and school
Evidence of patient beginning reintegration into family, community, and school
Patient/family demonstration of self-care

capability in areas of medicine administration, recognition of feelings, limit-setting, and help-seeking

Completion by treatment facility and family of contact and planning for after-care, with special attention to special education

Examples of community resources

Outpatient psychiatric nurse

Visiting Nurse Association or public health nurse

School nurse

School for special education classes

RETROSPECTIVE CRITERIA
Health

Development and teaching levels determined

No physical illness or complications evident

Activity

Able to perform activities of daily living appropriate for developmental level

Knowledge

Family knows treatment goals, administration of discharge medication, recognition of feelings, limit-setting, and help-seeking

Family knows what after-care plans have been made, understands plans, and how to implement them

COMPLICATIONS

Drug reaction

Neurotic, sociopathic, or psychotic reactions

Multiple sclerosis (Code: 340)

CONCURRENT REVIEW CRITERIA
Identification of patient's physical and psychosocial needs and/or concerns

Control of symptoms, including slurred speech, blurred vision, intention tremor, nystagmus, retrobulbar neuritis, incontinence, spastic paralysis, increased tendon reflexes, bilateral extensor-plantar responses, and changes in mental state

Feelings of anxiety over deterioration; feelings of hopelessness; concern over changes in family role and body image

Patient/family understanding of course, prognosis, and medical management of disease, that is, that the disease process is characterized by periods of exacerbations and remissions with progressive deterioration but that progress of disease can be delayed considerably by proper management

Patient/family understanding of nursing management to maintain independent

activities of daily living for a longer period and to delay the rapidity of deterioration

Protection from injury and complications as related to impairment and residual defects following exacerbation periods, including safety care during seizures, and safeguards against falling, which may be associated with hemiplegia, ataxia, or visual disturbances; against burns, as related to poor judgment; and against social and economic injury, as related to poor judgment

Recommended nursing action consistent with diagnosis
Nursing services

Implement measures to protect against injury, including use of a tongue blade, siderails, supportive measures during a seizure, and canes, while ambulatory, and eyepatches or frosted lenses, to improve vision

Implement measures, by which activities

of daily living can be maintained independently by patient for a longer period of time, by assistive and self-help devices, such as using a raised toilet seat or bedside commode, learning to shower by sitting on a stool or to take a bath by using handrails and a stool in the tub, and using button hooks, modified clothing, and elongated handles on eating utensils

Implement measures to prevent or reduce muscle spasticity by daily stretching exercises to the following muscles: hamstrings, gastrocnemius, hip adductors, biceps, wrist and finger flexor muscles; by passive and range-of-motion exercises; and by sleeping in a prone position; assist with ambulation, when necessary

Implement measures to prevent decubitus ulcers, skin tears, and contractures by assisting patient in frequent turning, maintaining good skin care, using protective devices, such as sheepskin, donuts, and lotions; and providing proper alignment and use of supportive devices

Implement measures to promote or improve bowel and bladder control, improve speech, and overcome incoordination

Health education

Teach family/patient methods of doing active, passive, range-of-motion, and stretching exercises to avoid muscle fatigue and to encourage walking exercises

Teach family/patient to avoid excessive heat or cold to skin when there is impairment of sensation, to inspect pressure areas daily for redness or skin breakdown, to change position frequently, to maintain skin in a clean, dry condition, and to use protective devices, such as sheepskin, lotions, and donuts

Teach patient to use canes or walker, to walk with feet wider apart than usual to provide a broad base of support to counter walking incoordination, and to use plate guards and weighted eating utensils to overcome incoordination of upper extremities

Teach patient/family elements of bowel and bladder programs and have them implement them in the hospital under supervision

Teach the patient transfer techniques; teach the family methods of dealing with the emotional, social, and mental problems created by the disease

Indicators for discharge
Adaptation to health status

Symptoms more manageable
Complications not evident
Patient/family understand disease process and nursing measures to cope with ramifications of it
Health teaching completed
Referrals made

Examples of community resources

Visiting Nurse Association or public health nurse
Multiple Sclerosis Society
Speech and physiotherapy clinics or centers
Mental health clinics
Social services

RETROSPECTIVE REVIEW CRITERIA
Health

Symptoms more manageable
Mentally accepting condition, change of role, and modification of life-style

Activity

Ambulates with feet forming a wider base and with cane or walker
Able to perform activities of daily living with aid of adaptive devices
Performs range-of-motion and stretching exercises without fatigue

Knowledge

Patient/family understands and knows the name of each discharge medication, including the dosage, frequency, desired effect, side effects, and precautions for each

Patient/family understands methods to protect patient from injury, that is, epileptic care; avoidance of extreme temperatures, if limbs have sensory loss, and use of frosted lenses to improve vision

Patient/family understands and can implement methods to prevent muscle spasticity, including massage, daily stretching and range-of-motion exercises, walking, and proper sleeping position

Patient/family understands and can implement measures to prevent decubitus ulcers, skin breakdown, and contractures

Patient/family understands and can implement measures to promote bowel and bladder control, improve speech and vision

Patient/family understands and can implement use of adaptive equipment

COMPLICATIONS

Bowel and bladder incontinence
Convulsions
Decubitus ulcers
Inanition
Incoordination
Joint contractures
Kidney infection
Muscle weakness and spasticity
Slurred speech
Urinary incontinence
Urinary infections
Urinary retention
Visual disturbances

Multiple sclerosis, coordination disturbances (Codes: 77.4, 340)

CONCURRENT REVIEW CRITERIA
Identification of patient's physical and psychosocial needs and/or concerns

Adaptation to progressive sensory-motor loss to paralysis
Relief of incoordination, ataxia, and/or intention tremor
Prevention of bowel and bladder dysfunction
Emotional changes and reactions
Understanding of exacerbations and/or remissions
Maintenance of skin integrity

Recommended nursing action consistent with diagnosis
Nursing services

Help design an activity program not to fatigue patient but to maintain self-care, mobility, and exercise program
Establish bladder and bowel programs
Promote skin care
Give emotional support to decrease depression or personality alterations

Implement social, vocational, and/or recreational counseling
Assess ability for self-care and discharge planning for home care

Health education

Teach family/patient the importance of patient avoiding fatigue but of not being too dependent or inactive
Teach family/patient the disease process, course, prognosis, and medical and nursing management
Teach family/patient care regime and activity program, including use of assistive devices, for patient
Teach family/patient bowel and bladder programs for patient

Indicators for discharge
Adaptation to health status

Potentially long remission
Attainment of patient's goals in self-care
Family/patient understanding of disease process, course, and prognosis

Plans for vocational, social, and/or recreational activities

Family/patient can implement or provide for care at home

Examples of community resources

Visiting Nurse Association or public health nurse

Multiple Sclerosis Society

RETROSPECTIVE REVIEW CRITERIA
Health

Sensory-motor symptoms have improved or have not increased for 1 month

Bowel and bladder function regulated

Mentally accepting emotional changes, reactions, and condition

Minimal amount of fatigue

Activity

Mobility program instigated

Bowel and bladder programs in progress

Self-care program initiated

Home-care program implemented

Uses assistive devices

Knowledge

Patients/family states disease process, course, prognosis, medical and nursing management, and medications

Knows importance of rest and activity within limitations

Knows importance of social and recreational activities

COMPLICATIONS

Convulsions

Decubitus ulcers

Inanition

Joint contractures

Kidney infection

Muscle weakness and spasticity

Paralysis

Pulmonary embolism

Thrombophlebitis

Urinary tract infection

Visual disturbances

Muscular dystrophy (Code: 330.3)

CONCURRENT REVIEW CRITERIA
Identification of patient's physical and psychosocial needs and/or concerns

Management of symptoms, including weakness of proximal musculature of extremities, waddling gait and "climbing up" on body to attain upright position, diminished deep tendon reflexes, joint contractures, scoliosis, lordosis, muscle hypertrophy or atrophy, muscular fibrillation, and hypertrophic polyneuritis

Fear of confinement to chair or bed, change in body image, modification of life expectations or roles, and increased dependency

Emotional support to patient/family to assist in coping with condition and lifelong treatment plan

Maintenance of activity critical to prevent permanent loss of muscle function

earlier than progressive stage of disease demands and to prevent joint contractures; avoidance of infection; maintenance of self-sufficiency within limits of disability

Patient/family understanding of nature of disease; prognosis; medical and nursing management, including supportive measures, physical therapy and orthopedic devices, nutrition and hydration; medications, hereditary considerations, and community agencies for assistance after discharge.

Recommended nursing action consistent with diagnosis
Nursing services

Implement measures to improve or maintain nutrition (but to avoid overweight) and hydration, to reinforce physical therapy activities and to provide supportive measures

Implement measures to maintain activity and muscle functions within the restrictions of the stage of the disease process

Implement measures to assist patient in carrying out activities of daily living; promote a degree of independence consistent with stage of disease process and utilization of orthopedic devices

Implement measures to prevent secondary infections, contractures, and increasing dependency

Provide family counseling regarding emotional and intellectual needs of the patient for normal development and mental health, through setting limitations, avoiding overprotection, forming realistic goals, providing schooling or vocational guidance, and encouraging patient to be as self-sufficient as possible

Health education

Explain ramifications of disease, type of dystrophy, course, and prognosis

Provide genetic counseling

Instruct about diet and avoiding overweight, which strains already weakened muscles

Explain importance and method of stretching and resistive exercises, activities, and use of adaptive and supportive equipment like braces to maintain existing muscle functions as long as possible

Explain role and function of community agencies available for aid

Teach to avoid infections and traumas that might cause patient to be placed on bedrest even for short periods of time, through proper vaccinations and immunizations, avoidance of persons with infections, regular medical checkups, regular dental care, avoidance of excessive fatigue, avoidance of unrealistic goals for the patient

Teach patient self-care methods within limits of disability

Indicators for discharge
Adaptation to health status

Complications not evident
Referrals made
Family/patient teaching adequate for health maintenance outside the hospital

Examples of community resources

Muscular dystrophy association
Visiting Nurse Association or public health nurse
School nurse
Vocational rehabilitation center
Social services

RETROSPECTIVE REVIEW CRITERIA
Health

Symptoms more manageable
Mentally adjusting to condition and change in life-style
Weight approaching ideal weight
Fears relieved or controlled
Complications not evident

Activity

Activity is the same as on admission with use of adaptive or prosthetic equipment
Able to walk with adaptive or prosthetic devices and perform activities of daily living
Performs exercise daily

Knowledge

Family/patient understands ramifications of disease process, as to type, course, prognosis, and medication and have made realistic plans for care after discharge

Family/patient understands genetic basis of disease and realizes chances of other offspring also having the disease

Family/patient understands basic principles of good nutrition and methods of limiting caloric intake in order not to complicate state with overweight

Family/patient understands importance of activities related to preventing more rapid loss of muscle functions and have made a plan for daily stretching and resistive exercises as well as for routinely maintaining other activities

Family/patient understands importance of seeking medical attention to even minor illnesses because of the problem of these minor illnesses decreasing activity, which might in turn hasten muscle function loss

Family/patient understands and can implement use of adaptative and prosthetic equipment

Family/patient understands function of community agencies contacted for aid after discharge

COMPLICATIONS

Atelectasis
Cardiac disease
Decubitus ulcers
Inanition
Infections
Joint contractures
Obesity
Persistent fever
Pes equinus
Pneumonia
Pulmonary embolism
Rapid muscle function loss
Respiratory obstruction

Myasthenia gravis (Code: 733)

CONCURRENT REVIEW CRITERIA
Identification of patient's physical and psychosocial needs and/or concerns

Control of symptoms, including development of fatigue and weakness of muscles, diplopia, ptosis of lids, oculomotor muscle paresis and strabismus, "myasthenic smile," facial musculature devoid of wrinkles, difficulty in use and moving of tongue, high-pitched nasal voice, and difficulty in swallowing, chewing, or speaking

Adjustment to changes in body image and life-style and lifelong treatment plan

Protection from trauma, maintenance of vital body functions during crisis, and prevention of respiratory distress or failure, aspiration, dehydration, malnutrition, and problems from immobility and drug toxicity

Explanation of disorder, including cause, chronicity, course, prognosis, and restrictions

Understanding of purpose, preparation, and outcome of diagnostic and therapeutic medical or surgical procedures and of nursing management for self-care at home

Recommended nursing action consistent with diagnosis
Nursing services

Implement and evaluate plan for maintaining adequate ventilation during crisis or post surgery

Implement and evaluate plans for maintaining adequate hydration and nutrition during crisis, postsurgery, or concurrent with radiation therapy

Implement and evaluate plans for protecting patient from trauma, aspiration, problems resulting from drug toxicity and immobility, injury as related to diplopia, and infection

Implement and evaluate plan for aiding patient in adjusting to changes in body image and life-style

Contact health care agencies involved in providing equipment or assistance necessary for home care

Health education

Explain ramifications of disease process as to type, course, prognosis, safety factors, medication, and realistic plans for care after discharge

Teach patient/family about diagnostic

and therapeutic procedures and medical and surgical management, including medications; diet; activity restrictions; special care unit following thymectomy, including the purpose and considerations related to outcome and restrictions of surgery; and measures to alleviate side effects of radiation therapy or drug toxicity

Teach patient/family about nursing management; tracheal care; tracheal suction (if appropriate); methods of diet modification; activities of daily living as related to changing muscle strength; methods of achieving activities within limits of fatigue and rest periods; crisis management, including use of ventilators, suctioning devices, recognition of signs and symptoms of complications; and avoiding sedatives and respiratory depressing analgesics

Explain nursing management for prevention of problems from immobility such as decubitus ulcers, peneumonia, infections, and sensorium disturbances

Teach patient the importance of avoiding upper respiratory infections because of coughing deficiency of myasthenia gravis and deterred immunological response associated with thymectomy or radiation therapy and of receiving adequate early treatment

Indicators for discharge
Adaptation to health status

Neurological weakness decreased
Complications not evident
Necessary knowledge and equipment to manage home care obtained
Appropriate community agencies contacted for follow-up care

Examples of community resources

Visiting Nurse Association or public health nurse
Hospital equipment agencies
Social services
Vocational rehabilitation center

RETROSPECTIVE REVIEW CRITERIA
Health

Symptoms more manageable
Wound healing, if surgery performed
Mentally adjusting to diagnosis, change in life-style and body image, and prolonged treatment
Complications not evident

Activity

Ambulatory
Able to perform activities of daily living with minimal fatigue

Knowledge

Patient/family knows and understands ramifications of disease process, prognosis, and medical and nursing management, methods to prevent complications, safety factors, and discharge treatment plan

Patient/family understands the importance of administering prescribed medication according to prescribed interval on a fixed regular schedule; understands dosage, desired and side effects, precautions and observations to report to physician

Patient/family understands necessity of avoiding infections and of receiving prompt treatment for upper respiratory infections, if they occur

COMPLICATIONS

Aspiration
Decubitus ulcers
Dehydration
Inanition
Malnutrition
Persistent fever
Pneumonia
Pulmonary embolism
Respiratory failure
Respiratory infection
Sensorium disturbances
Side effects of radiation therapy
Toxic drug reaction
Wound infection

Myeloma, multiple (Code: 203)

CONCURRENT CRITERIA
Identification of patient's physical and psychosocial needs and/or concerns

Management of symptoms including control of pain, reduction of tumor mass, maintenance of good urine output to prevent protein participation, ambulation to combat negative calcium balance, avoidance of exposure to trauma for prevention of fractures, relief from anemia and weight loss

Fear of death, uncontrollable pain, pathological fractures, change in life-style and roles, increased dependency, change in body image, and feelings of hopelessness

Explanation of condition including cause, course, prognosis, restrictions, complications, medical and nursing treatment plans, and community agencies available to assist after discharge.

Emotional support to patient/family to assist in coping with condition and progressiveness of disease to death usually within 1½ to 2 years, treatment plan to control pain, and spouse's need for increased independence in family related matters

Maintenance or improvement of nutrition, hydration, elimination, body's physiological responses and mental health

Recommended nursing action consistent with diagnosis
Nursing services

Monitor pain status related to movement that might indicate pathological fracture; implement pain control measures

Implement nursing measures to improve nutrition, hydration, elimination, physiological body responses, mental health, and prevention of complications

Provide emotional support for patient and family, allowing for verbalization of feelings

Assess mobility and/or need for supportive equipment, such as braces or trapeze

Constantly be aware of malignancy level and signs of increasing malignancy

Health education

Teach importance of adequate nutrition, hydration, elimination, pain control measures, prevention of infection, and discharge treatment plan

Explain indicators for consulting physician after discharge

Explain ramifications of disease, cause, course, progressiveness, prognosis, restrictions, complications, medical and nursing management, medication, and community agencies for care after discharge

Indicators for discharge
Adaptation to health status

Treatment goals of inpatient hospitalization reached

Pain controlled

Independent in activities of daily living or has available assistance from family or other agency

Patient/family knowledge of disease, medication regime, and specific treatment goals adequate for home care after discharge

Referrals made

Examples of community resources

Visiting Nurse Association or public health nurse

Social services

American Cancer Society

RETROSPECTIVE CRITERIA
Health

Weight approaching ideal weight

Urine output at least 2,400 ml per day

Mentally coping with condition

Pain under control or minimized

Admission symptoms resolved or under treatment

Activity

Independent in activities of daily living or has available assistance

Knowledge

Patient/family understands medication regime and importance of adequate nutrition and prevention of infection and trauma

Patient/family understands diagnosis, treatment goals, indicators for consulting physician, and application of supportive equipment

Patient/family aware of community agencies available for aid after discharge

COMPLICATIONS

Bone involvement

Bone marrow suppression

Decubitus ulcers

Hematuria from renal tubule casts

Hemorrhage

Hypercalcemia

Infection

Irradiation therapy complications

Nausea and vomiting

Paraplegia from cord tumor

Pathological fracture and pain

Thrombocytopenia

Urinary tract infection

Vertebral fracture

Myocardial infarction, acute (Code: 410.9)

CONCURRENT CRITERIA
Identification of patient's physical and psychosocial needs and/or concerns

Relief of chest pain, weakness, diaphoresis, nausea, fever, hypotension, shock, leukocytosis, and abnormal cardiac rhythm

Adaptation to reduced toleration for physical activity and changed or altered life-style

Fear of sudden death and rejection of diagnosis

Alleviation of apprehension and anxiety to promote physical and mental rest and to help adjust to special care unit

Explanation of condition, cause, course, prognosis, medical and nursing management, activity restrictions, and discharge care

Recommended nursing action consistent with diagnosis
Nursing services

Begin electrocardiographic monitoring within 5 minutes of admission to coronary care unit

Initiate immediate physical assessment with implementation of nursing actions

Initiate medical protocol

Record and document electrocardiogram rhythm strips

Provide psychological support for patient during adaptation to illness

Provide emotional support and adjustment to coronary care unit

Health education

Explain disease process, including problem, signs, and symptoms

Encourage cooperation with plan of care contributing to recovery

Explain restrictions on physical and sexual activities

Teach diet, medications, medical follow-up, and contributory risk factors

Indicators for discharge
Adaptation to health status

Health education completed

Chest pain and syncope absent

Activity tolerated without signs and symptoms of cardiac stress

Acceptance of diagnosis verbalized

Heart rate controlled within normal range

Examples of community resources

Visiting Nurse Association or public health nurse

Cardiac rehabilitation clinic

American Heart Association

RETROSPECTIVE CRITERIA
Health

Mentally adjusted to condition

Weight approaching ideal weight

Chest pain absent

Heart rate within normal range

Activity

Gradual resumption of activities with no signs of cardiac stress or fatigue

Antismoking program, if indicated

Knowledge

Patient and/or significant other verbalizes understanding of disease process, activity restrictions, diet, medications, and need for medical follow-up

COMPLICATIONS

Adams-Stokes disease

Arrhythmia

Cardiac arrest

Congestive heart failure

Fever

Oliguria, anuria, or acute tubular necrosis

Pericarditis

Premature ventricular contractions

Rupture-perforation of interventricular septum

Shoulder-hand syndrome

Thromboembolism

Nausea and vomiting (Code: 781.2)

CONCURRENT CRITERIA
Identification of patient's physical and psychosocial needs and/or concerns

Relief of nausea and/or vomiting

Identification of underlying cause, such as irritation, inflammation, or mechanical disturbance at any level of the gastrointestinal tract; irritating impulses arising in any diseased viscera, as in cholecystitis; disturbances of semicircular canals, as in seasickness; or toxic action of cardiac drugs such as digitalis

Avoidance of unpleasant psychic stimuli, such as strange odors, foul-smelling or foul-tasting medication, emesis basins, or other unattractive objects

Feelings of hopelessness and apprehension

Understanding of disease process, course, duration, medical and nursing management, and prognosis

Recommended nursing action consistent with diagnosis
Nursing services

Position patient to prevent aspiration of emesis

Maintain "low key" environment through unhurried activities, calmness, and explanation of management of symptoms; encourage patient participation in care

Maintain nutrition and fluid balance

Observe and record nature of onset of vomiting, such as circumstances surrounding the episode and other significant information to aid identification of cause of nausea and vomiting

Give emotional support to patient in coping with disease process

Health education

Teach specific cause of nausea and vomiting; however, if specific reason unidentified, teach means of inhibiting reflex, deep breathing, and life-style for maximum relaxation

Explain symptoms, course of disease, treatment, and what to report to physician

Instruct about diet

Provide medication instruction, including the name, purpose, duration, frequency, side effects, and what to report to physician of each

Indicators for discharge
Adaptation to health status

Nausea and vomiting controlled

Diet and fluids tolerated

Cause and prevention of condition understood

Medication understood, including name, frequency, dosage, side effects, and observations to report to physician

Examples of community resources

Referral usually not indicated

Cessation of nausea and/or vomiting

Toleration of food and fluids

Activity

Ambulatory

Independent in activities of daily living

Knowledge

Patient/family member can verbalize cause, medical regime, and discharge treatment plan

COMPLICATIONS

Acidosis

Alkalosis

Congestive heart failure

Dehydration

Neoplasm, malignant, of colon and rectum, with surgical intervention
(Codes: 154, 154.1, 153-153.9)

CONCURRENT REVIEW CRITERIA
Identification of patient's physical and psychosocial needs and/or concerns

Relief of symptoms, including altered bowel function (constipation or diarrhea), blood in the feces, unexplained anemia, weight loss, and mass in colon or rectum.

Fear of death, surgical invasion of body, change in body image, loss of time from work or school, and diagnosis of cancer

Understanding of the diagnosis, prognosis, surgical procedures, expected pre- and postoperative course, nursing management, community agencies available to assist with discharge treatment plan

Adjustment to bowel elimination through colostomy and care of colostomy

Recommended nursing action consistent with diagnosis
Nursing services

Provide pre- and postoperative information and reassurance; allow and encourage verbalization of fears, feelings, and concerns

Relieve pain through medication, positioning, and other measures

Postoperatively reestablish normal physiological response parameters; provide good nutrition, hydration, and elimination; observe for functioning of colostomy and for signs of complications

Implement self-care activities; encourage skin care and assist with exercises to extremities

Initiate health education, discharge planning and referrals

Health education

Preoperatively, instruct about and explain reason for technique of coughing and deep breathing; reinforce postoperatively

Instruct patient in the need for early self-care, ambulation, and regaining of independence

Teach patient to care for colostomy, including care of stoma and skin, use of colostomy bag, techniques of irrigation, if appropriate, routine time for bowel evacuation, complete emptying after irrigation, regulation of diet to avoid diarrhea, places to purchase equipment, and that most patients with colostomies can live normal lives

Explain condition, cause, course, prognosis, medical and nursing management, and plan for home care

Advise about community agencies available to assist with discharge care

Indicators for discharge
Adaptation to health status

Independent in activities of daily living

Able to perform own colostomy care with minimal assistance or supervision

Beginning to accept surgery and colostomy, if present

Normal physiological responses reestablished, including bowel function

Wound healing

Examples of community resources

Visiting Nurse Association or public health nurse

Ostomy club

American Cancer Society

RETROSPECTIVE REVIEW CRITERIA
Health

Wound healing

Pain controlled

Bowel function established via colostomy

Weight increasing

Mentally accepting change in body image and condition

Tolerating diet without altered bowel function

Activity

Independent in ambulation, activities of daily living, and colostomy care

Knowledge

Understands wound care, activity level permissible, discharge diet, and colostomy care

Understanding of surgery performed and prognosis, course, treatment plan, and observations to report to physician

COMPLICATIONS

Anxiety and/or depression
Bowel obstruction
Constipation or diarrhea
Dehiscence
Hemorrhage
Pneumonia
Pulmonary embolism
Sepsis
Skin irritation around stoma area
Stoma prolapse
Stoma stricture
Urinary obstruction and/or infection
Wound infection

Nephrosis in children (Codes: 250.6, 403, 582, 585.2, 590.2, 753.1)

CONCURRENT CRITERIA
Identification of patient's physical and psychosocial needs and/or concerns

Relief of symptoms, including massive edema, proteinuria, hypoalbuminemia, hyperlipidemia, anorexia, shortness of breath, or hypertension

Fear of death, increased dependency, change in body image, loss of time from school or activities, and change in dietary habits

Prevention of infection

Therapy to induce diuresis, to produce protein-free urine, to elevate the serum albumin to normal levels, and to reduce lipidemia

Understanding of patient/family about condition, cause, course, prognosis, medical and nursing management, community agencies for home care, and restrictions

Adjustment to hospitalization with appropriate diversionary activities

Recommended nursing action consistent with diagnosis
Nursing services

Adhere to careful hand-washing technique; prevent exposure of child to persons with known infections

Observe and record distribution of edema; weigh patient daily; record intake and output; evaluate blood pressure

Provide attractive, appealing diet with limitation of salt, catering to child's likes

Provide meticulous skin care with attention to pressure areas

Initiate health teaching and discharge planning

Health education

Instruct parents on importance of reporting recurrent infections to physician

Instruct parents on necessity of weighing child daily at home and reporting weight gain to physician

Instruct child/parents on allowed and restricted activities

Instruct parents on name, dosage, time schedule, and side effects of medications and on observations to report to physician

Instruct child/parents on diet restrictions

Discuss with parents the child's possible feelings about distorted body image

Indicators for discharge
Adaptation to health status

Clearing of edema and beginning of diuresis

Disappearing of hypertension

Lessening of proteinuria and absence of hematuria

Examples of community resources

Visiting Nurse Association or public health nurse

RETROSPECTIVE CRITERIA
Health

Absence of proteinuria
Mentally accepting fears
Afebrile
Control of edema and beginning of diuresis
Decreasing of hypertension
Complications not evident

Activity

Ambulatory

Knowledge

Parents know name, dosage, time schedule, side effects of medications, and observations to report to physician

Child/parents understand permitted activity level

Child/parents understand and can implement diet restrictions

Parents know importance of weighing

child daily and reporting increase to physician

Parents know importance of reporting recurrent infections to physcian

COMPLICATIONS

Ascites
Hypertension
Infections
Renal failure
Respiratory distress

Nerve injuries, peripheral (Codes: 959.2, E988)

CONCURRENT REVIEW CRITERIA
Identification of patient's physical and psychosocial needs and/or concerns

Relief from motor or sensory impairment or pain

Understanding of medical and surgical treatment as well as nursing management necessary for realistic health maintenance after discharge

Concern over loss of independence, impaired independence, or loss of time from school or work

Rehabilitative measures to regain full functioning ability

Preventive measures concerning problems caused by immobility

Recommended nursing action consistent with diagnosis
Nursing services

Provide preoperative nursing care, including pain control, rest, nutrition, hydration, and elimination; explain surgical procedures, expected outcome, recovery room, estimated period of hospitalization, progressive ambulation, chest physiology exercises, possibility of plaster casts, splints, or braces, and use of crutches

Physically prepare patient for surgery

Implement postoperative nursing care, including pain control, rest, nutrition, hydration, elimination, supervision of prescribed exercises, prevention of immobility problems, wound care, and cast care if indicated

Observe for signs of physical deterioration, such as shock, excessive bleeding, respiratory difficulty, changes in mental status, changes in motor or sensory functions; provide prompt nursing intervention should any signs occur

Assist in use of crutches, braces, or walker

Aid in discharge planning

Health education

Explain measures to reduce pain and promote rest

Instruct about therapeutic and restricted activities

Instruct about cast or wound care, including signs and symptoms of circulatory impairment or wound infection and appropriate action to initiate

Instruct about application of splints, braces, or compression dressings

Instruct about the name, purpose, dosage, frequency, side effects, action to take if side effects occur, and precautions as related to each discharge medication

Advise when to return to physician's office or clinic for follow-up medical care

Teach safety measures

Indicators for discharge
Adaptation to health status

Condition stable
Complications not evident
Health teaching completed
Referrals made

Examples of community resources

Visiting Nurse Association or public health nurse

Orthopedic clinic
Social services
Physiotherapy clinic

RETROSPECTIVE REVIEW CRITERIA
Health

Motor or sensory impairment relieved
Wound healing
Pain controlled
Complications not evident

Activity

Able to ambulate using crutches, canes, or
  braces correctly and safely
Able to apply braces, splints, and
  compression dressings correctly
Implements cast or wound care

Knowledge*

Understands and can implement pain-
  reducing and rehabilitative measures
Understands therapeutic and restricted
  activities and can implement therapeutic ones

---

*If the patient is unteachable and there is no family,
the responsible party assuming health care must
understand after-care, and this must be documented
on nurse's notes.

Understands and can implement cast or
  wound care
Understands the name, purpose, dosage,
  frequency, side effects, action to take if
  side effects occur, and precautions of
  each discharge medication
Understands and can implement safety
  measures
Knows when to return to physician's
  office or clinic for follow-up medical
  care

COMPLICATIONS

Arrhythmias
Atelectasis
Circulatory impairment
Drug reaction
Hemorrhage
Pneumonia
Pulmonary embolism
Respiratory difficulty
Shock
Thrombophlebitis
Urinary incontinence
Urinary infections
Urinary retention
Wound infection

Neurofibroma or neuroma of unspecified site (Code: 225.9)

CONCURRENT CRITERIA
Identification of patient's physical and psychosocial needs and/or concerns

Relief from presenting symptoms
Understanding of extent of involvement,
  prognosis, treatment, and that tumors
  of intraspinal or intracranial segments
  can be fatal
Assistance in coping with disfigurement
  associated with cutaneous manifestations of plexiform neuroma, if present
Genetic counseling
Understanding of community agencies
  available for assistance when necessary

Recommended nursing action consistent with diagnosis
Nursing services

Implement comfort measures
Ensure adequate hydration, nutrition,
  and elimination
Implement safety measures against injuries associated with cranial or spinal
  nerve deficits or with impairment of
  mental process associated with intracranial lesions
Assist patient in adjusting to disfigurement or decreased independence associated with intraspinal or intracranial
  motor and/or sensory deficits

Instigate rehabilitative measures for neurological deficits

Health education

Explain medications, including the name, purpose, dosage, frequency, side effects, action to take should side effects occur, and precautions for each

Teach rehabilitative measures, such as bowel and bladder control programs, use of prosthetic and adaptive devices, measures to reduce or prevent problems from immobility, and measures to improve motor functions as related to spinal and cranial deficits

Teach measures to reduce discomforts, as related to pressure of neuroma, inadequate blood supply, and sensory disturbances

Explain therapeutic and restricted activities

Instruct about safety measures, as related to motor and sensory disturbances of the spinal and intracranial lesions

Indicators for discharge
Adaptation to health status

Condition stable
Neurological deficits stable, controlled, or improved
Complications not evident
Health teaching completed
Referrals made

Examples of community resources

Visiting Nurse Association or public health nurse
Social services
American Cancer Society
Pain clinic
Physical and vocational rehabilitation centers

RETROSPECTIVE CRITERIA
Health

Presenting symptoms relieved
Mentally coping with body disfigurement and condition
Complications not evident

Activity

Able to carry out activities of daily living with or without adaptive or prosthetic devices
Ambulatory

Knowledge

Knows and understands the name, dosage, frequency, side effects, purpose of drug, action to take should side effects occur, and precautions of each discharge medication

Understands safety measures, as related to motor and sensory disturbances

Understands and can implement use of adaptive and prosthetic devices, rehabilitative measures, comfort measures, and measures to maintain adequate hydration, nutrition, and elimination

Understands and can implement measures to prevent problems resulting from immobility

COMPLICATIONS

Drug reaction
Motor or sensory disturbances
Persistent fever
Pneumonia
Spinal cord compression
Thromboembolism
Wound infection

Neurosis, anxiety (Code: DSM II 300.3)

CONCURRENT REVIEW CRITERIA
Identification of patient's physical and psychosocial needs and/or concerns

Expression of concern regarding physical health

Expression of concern regarding impaired social, familial, or occupational functioning

Identification of specific symptoms of anxiety, patients beliefs, attitudes, fears, expectations of own behavior and hospitalization

Recommended nursing action consistent with diagnosis
Nursing services

Observe for symptoms of anxiety and pattern of attacks

Provide medication, when required, for treatment of symptoms

Encourage patient to verbalize feelings

Encourage patient to interact with other patients, family, and/or friends

Make recommendations for treatment plan

Health education

Teach patient and significant other about disease process and body's physiological response to anxiety

Teach methods for dealing with symptoms, such as breathing into a paper bag when hyperventilation occurs

Involve patient and significant other in developing treatment plan and/in having realistic expectations of the plan

Indicators for discharge
Adaptation to health status

Achievement of inpatient treatment goals

Control of admitting symptoms

Establishment of follow-up treatment plan

Examples of community resources

Outpatient psychiatric nurse

RETROSPECTIVE REVIEW CRITERIA
Health

Decrease in verbalization of somatic complaints

Regular sleep pattern

Activity

Able to perform activities of daily living

Sets goals and makes plans for achieving them

Interacts in one-to-one group relationships

Knowledge

Patient verbalizes understanding that nonverbal behavior should confirm verbal expression of feelings

Patient verbalizes understanding of the signs and symptoms of remission and the need to report these to the physician

Patient verbalizes understanding of instructions for taking medications, signs and symptoms of untoward reactions, and the need to report these signs to the physician

COMPLICATIONS

Development of psychotic symptomatology

Drug reaction

Neurosis of childhood or adolescence (Code: DSM II 300)

CONCURRENT CRITERIA
Identification of patient's physical and psychosocial needs and/or concerns

Identification of neurotic problem that precipitated admission, such as attempted suicide, overwhelming anxiety, or school or other phobia

Evaluation of the state of child's/adolescent's (patient's) physical health

Exploration of patient's beliefs, attitudes, and expectations of own behavior and hospitalization

Exploration of family's beliefs, attitudes, and expectations of patient and treatment facility

Evaluation of chronology of patient's/family's development and coping

Recommended nursing action consistent with diagnosis
Nursing services

Provide nursing assessment of patient family and community within 7 days of admission

Instigate ongoing behavioral observation and assessment of patient within 8 hours of admission

Implement behavior-specific interventions such as life-space interview seclusion, suicide precautions , and/or behavior modification

Assist in development and implementation of after-care of patient and family-specific interventions

Implement and assess physical therapies, such as medications, and diagnostic procedures

Health education

Explain to patient/family about ward procedures and milieu

Discuss with patient/family about treatment goals and therapeutic modalities

Teach family to make use of specific therapeutic modalities, such as behavior modification, principles of psycho-dynamics, communication skills, and attitude therapy

Discuss, explain, and teach about any medication, including action, use, dosage, and side effects

Indicators for discharge
Adaptation to health status

Decrease in neurotic symptoms or process that led to hospitalization, including decreased aggressive behavior, expressive anxiety, or phobic responses

Completion of planned medical and/or other evaluation; completion of after-care plan

Evidence of reintegration into family, community, and school

Patient/family demonstration of self-care capability in areas of medication administration, limit-setting, recognition of feelings, and help seeking

Examples of community resources

Outpatient psychiatric nurse
School nurse
Public health nurse

RETROSPECTIVE CRITERIA
Health

Regular sleep patterns
Presenting symptoms controlled
No physical illness or problems

Activity

Self-care
Parents implement limit-setting
Reintegrated into family unit

Knowledge

Patient/family knows what treatment goals were accomplished

Patient/family knows what after-care plans have been made; all understand plans and their parts in them

COMPLICATIONS

Adverse reactions to treatment modalities, such as procedures, drugs, or psychological or social therapies

Suicide

Exacerbation of clinical signs and/or symptoms

Failure of family and/or support system

Neurosis, depressive (Code: DSM II 300.14)

CONCURRENT REVIEW CRITERIA
Identification of patient's physical and psychosocial needs and/or concerns

Protection from harm to self or others

Understanding by patient/family of illness, course, cause, prognosis, and medical and nursing management

Expression of fears related to social stigma of emotional illness

Expression of concerns regarding hospitalization, including fear of treatment, length of stay, and increased dependency

Expression of concern for significant others and loss of time from employment or school

Recommended nursing action consistent with diagnosis
Nursing services

Involve nursing staff in development of treatment plan

Closely observe patient for signs of danger to self, others, or property

Interact with patient to encourage recognition and verbalization of feelings

Health education

Inform patient and significant others of treatment plan and realistic expectations of the plan

Assist patient and significant others in developing healthy and helpful interactions with each other

Indicators for discharge
Adaptation to health status

Free of symptoms and/or problems that necessitated admission

Understanding of own illness, indicated treatment, and treatment goals

Progress toward reaching specific treatment goals

Examples of community resources

Outpatient psychiatric nurse

RETROSPECTIVE REVIEW CRITERIA
Health

Decrease in verbalization of somatic complaints

Free of symptoms and/or problems that necessitated hospitalization

Regular sleep pattern

Activity

Able to perform activities of daily living

Ambulatory

Sets goals; makes plans for achieving them

Interacts in one-to-one and group relationships

Knowledge

Understands own illness, indicated treatment, and treatment goals

Verbalizes understanding that nonverbal behavior should confirm verbal expression of feelings

Verbalizes understanding of the signs and symptoms of remission and when to report to physician

Verbalizes understanding of instructions for taking medications, signs and symptoms of untoward reactions, and what to report to physician

COMPLICATIONS

Attempted suicide

Development of psychotic symptomatology

Drug reaction

Newborn, normal (Code: 650)

CONCURRENT REVIEW CRITERIA
Identification of patient's physical and psychosocial needs and/or concerns

Development of bonding to parents

General observation and assessment of neurological control to determine normality, through Apgar score, quality of cry, muscle tone, reflexes, and feeding and sucking pattern

Assessment and maintenance of basic vital signs, including respiratory function; heart rate, rhythm, murmurs, and volume; temperature; retractions; nasal flaring; grunting, and apical heart rate

Immediate protection from trauma of birth in a warm, infection-free, safe environment

Recommended nursing action consistent with diagnosis
Nursing services

Administer feedings of sterile water every 4 to 6 hours, later glucose, then formula or breast feedings

Keep temperature normal; dry immediately after birth; place in incubator, Isolette, or radiant warmer and adjust temperature to maintain normal body temperature

Suction oropharynx and nasopharynx immediately at birth, as needed, with bulb syringe; suction trachea and stomach with tracheal catheter attached with mucous trap, as necessary

Take Apgar score at 1 and 5 minutes after delivery

Apply cord clamp under hemostat and care for cord by keeping it dry

Auscultate heart rate hourly after delivery, then 4 to 8 hours, and respiratory rate every 30 minutes, then 4 to 8 hours

Encourage parental roles

Health education

Involve parents immediately after delivery; wrap infant; let parents hold; let mother put to breast, if she desires

Demonstrate and have parents return demonstration for the following: bathing, feeding, diaper changing, cord care, circumcision care, and taking rectal temperature

Write instructions, demonstrate, and have parents return demonstration for formula preparation and sterilization; if breast feeding, instruct accordingly

Instruct in dressing infant for warmth; instruct about temperature of home

Instruct in safety of home, such as about diaper pins, other children playing with infant, preventing exposure to infections, keeping bed railing elevated

Discuss paternal roles with parents; identify feelings, such as conflicts, love, or indifference

Indicators for discharge
Adaptation to health status

Care of newborn, such as formula, bath, cord care, and circumcision care understood by parents

Home environment ready for infant—sanitary (to best of knowledge)

Severe contagious infections in home environment or any contagious infection in mother not evident

Follow-up appointments with pediatrician established

Infant taking formula and gaining weight

Examples of community resources

Visiting Nurse Association or public health nurse

Well baby clinic

Health

Temperature normal
Vital signs stable
Fluid intake tolerated
Elimination of urine and stool established
Weight increasing
Umbilical stump dry; clamp removed
Jaundice at acceptable level for age—absent at 24 hours, absent or mild at 48 hours, absent or mild to moderate at 72 hours
Circumcision clean and dry
Phenylketonuria (PKU) test completed or arrangement for test made

Activity

Alert
Responsive

Knowledge

Parents understand infant care and time of follow-up medical visits

COMPLICATIONS

Congenital anomalies
Cyanosis
Fever
Hyperbilirubinemia
Infection
Intolerance of feedings
Physiological depression
Respiratory distress

Omphalocele or gastroschisis in children (Codes: 551.2, 756.8)

CONCURRENT CRITERIA
Identification of patient's physical and psychosocial needs and/or concerns

Prevention of infection of exposed intestinal contents
Prevention of tension on abdominal area
Provision of emotional support for child/family
Maintenance of adequate nutrition
Teaching family about care of incision

Recommended nursing action consistent with diagnosis
Nursing services

Use sterile technique in working with omphalocele or incision
Turn child every 2 hours; position so as not to cause tension on omphalocele or incision and to increase pulmonary ventilation
Aspirate nasogastric or gastrostomy tube every 2 to 4 hours or use continuous suction; record drainage
Assist family in expressing feelings about prolonged hospitalization of child; develop trusting relationship with child
Observe for nausea and vomiting or decreased appetite

Health education

Discuss medical and surgical treatments with family
Teach family about adequate nutrition consistent with diet ordered by physician
Explain positioning of child so as not to cause pressure on abdomen

Indicators for discharge
Adaptation to health status

Defect in abdominal wall or skin closed and healing
Fluids being tolerated
Weight gain beginning
Vital signs stable and afebrile for 24 hours prior to discharge
Normal activities being resumed

Examples of community resources

Referral usually not indicated

RETROSPECTIVE CRITERIA
Health

Vital signs stable and afebrile for 24 hours prior to discharge
Infection or discharge in abdominal area not evident

Abdominal wound healed
Bowel functioning
Formula being tolerated well

Activity

Activities appropriate for age

Knowledge

Family understands and can implement
diet and care of infant

COMPLICATIONS

Dehiscense
Hematoma
Intestinal obstruction
Nausea and vomiting
Pneumonia
Sepsis
Ventilatory insufficiency
Wound infection

Otitis media, acute, in children (Codes: 381, 381.1, 381.9)

CONCURRENT CRITERIA
**Identification of patient's physical and
psychosocial needs and/or concerns**

Relief of symptoms, including ear pain, a
sensation of fullness in ear, hearing
loss, or fever and chills
Adjustment to hospitalization and fears
Drainage and cleaning of the ear canal
Prevention of spread of infection
Teaching about care of ear
Control of pain

**Recommended nursing action consistent
with diagnosis**
Nursing services

Use thorough hand-washing before and
after caring for ear
Observe and record amount and color of
drainage from ear
Use cotton pledgets soaked in saline or
hydrogen peroxide to clean ear canal
If drainage from ear is profuse, cover skin
around ear with zinc oxide, petrolatum,
or cold cream
Observe and report any allergic reactions
to antibiotics

Health education

Explain to child/parents techniques of
medication administration and treatments
Instruct child not to touch drainage from
ear
Teach child/family how to cleanse ears
properly

Instruct parents on signs of ear infections
manifested by child, such as complaints of popping noises or tugs at ears
and need to report them immediately to
medical personnel
Discuss the purpose of a myringotomy
and home care

Indicators for discharge
Adaptation to health status

Vital signs stable and afebrile for 24
hours prior to discharge
Drainage and pain in ear not evident
Family teaching about medications, treat-
ments, and ear care completed
Normal activities being resumed
Food and fluids being tolerated well

Examples of community resources

Referral usually not indicated

RETROSPECTIVE CRITERIA
Health

Vital signs stable and afebrile 24 hours
prior to discharge
Drainage and pain in ear not evident
Food and fluids being tolerated

Activity

Activities appropriate for age

Knowledge

Family understands and can administer
medications or treatments

Child/family know about and can implement care of ear

Family can recognize signs of ear infection, such as child complaining of popping noises or tugging at ear; know importance of prompt reporting of these signs to medical personnel

COMPLICATIONS

Brain abscess	Mastoiditis
Conductive hearing loss	Meningitis
Facial nerve paralysis	Septicemia
Labyrinthitis	

Otitis media, chronic, in children (Codes: 381.3-381.6)

CONCURRENT CRITERIA
Identification of patient's physical and psychosocial needs and/or concerns

Adjustment to hospitalization and fears
Draining and cleaning of ear canal
Prevention of spread of infection
Teaching about medications and treatments
Support for child/family, if surgery is required
Teaching about care of ear

Recommended nursing action consistent with diagnosis
Nursing services

Use thorough hand-washing technique before and after caring for ear
Observe and record amount and color of drainage from ear
Use cotton pledgets soaked in saline or hydrogen peroxide to clean ear canal
If drainage from the ear is profuse, cover skin around ear with zinc oxide, petrolatum, or cold cream
Observe for and report any allergic reactions to antibiotics

Health education

Explain techniques of medication administration and treatment
Instruct child not to touch drainage from ear
Explain to child/family about surgical procedures to be undertaken
Teach child/family how to cleanse ears properly

Indicators for discharge
Adaptation to health status

Vital signs stable and afebrile for 24 hours prior to discharge
Discharge and pain in ear not evident
Teaching of family about medications, treatment, and ear care completed
Normal activity being resumed
Food and fluids being tolerated well

Examples of community resources

Referral usually not indicated

RETROSPECTIVE CRITERIA
Health

Vital signs stable and afebrile for 24 hours prior to discharge
Food and fluids being tolerated

Activity

Activities appropriate for age

Knowledge

Family understands about medications and treatments
Child/family know about and can implement care of ear
Family can implement home postoperative care

COMPLICATIONS

Brain abscess	Meningitis
Facial nerve paralysis	Septicemia
Hearing loss	Sigmoid sinus
Mastoiditis	

Pacemaker, permanent implant (Code: 30.4)

CONCURRENT CRITERIA
Identification of patient's physical and psychosocial needs and/or concerns

Explanation of potential complications, including severe bradycardia, dyspnea, syncope, Adams-Stokes disease, and chest pain

Fear of death, incapacitation, or failure of artificial pacemaker

Adaptation of life-style to activity limitation of pacemaker

Emotional support for understanding disease course, prognosis, operative procedure, and pre- and postoperative courses

Recommended nursing action consistent with diagnosis
Nursing services

Recognize failure of pacemaker to perform properly, by such symptoms as bradycardia, fatigue, hiccups, faintness, pain, decreased blood pressure, decreased urinary output, or electrocardiogram pattern changes

Keep patient at bedrest and limited arm activity for 72 hours postinsertion

Institute rigid skin care to incision site

Obtain order for range-of-motion exercises to affected arm and shoulder on third day

Increase activity as directed by physician

Health education

Explain activity, including importance of consistent limb exercise, sexual activity, as tolerated, avoidance of traveling for 3 months, and vocational adaptation

Teach self-monitoring of pulse daily

Explain recharging battery (if rechargeable battery inserted)

Teach family/patient about care and maintenance of pacemaker and about signs and symptoms of malfunction

Stress importance of medical follow-up and use of medical alert information tag

Indicators for discharge
Adaptation to health status

Pacemaker functioning properly

Understanding of activity restrictions, care of pacemaker, pulse counting, and signs and symptoms of diminishing battery life verbalized

Acceptance of disease and need for pacemaker verbalized

Understanding of electrical safety (that is, avoidance of microwave ovens) verbalized

Examples of community resources

Visiting Nurse Association or public health nurse

Pacemaker clinic

Vocational rehabilitation center

American Heart Association

RETROSPECTIVE CRITERIA
Health

Functioning artificial pacemaker

Clean, healing wound

Complications not evident

Activity

Ambulatory

Self-completion of activities of daily living

Performs exercises

Monitors pulse daily

Knowledge

Patient/family verbalizes understanding of disease process, pacemaker function and maintenance, activity limitations, procedures for taking pulse daily and for determining if pacemaker is functioning appropriately; knows when battery replacement is required; knows name, side effects, dosage, frequency, and desirable actions of medication; and understands when to notify physician of potential difficulty

COMPLICATIONS
Adams-Stokes disease
Bradycardia

Chest pain
Dyspnea
Infection
Pacemaker malfunction
Premature ventricular contractions
Syncope

Pain, joint, and swelling (Codes: 274, 713, 714.1, 788.3, 788.4)

CONCURRENT REVIEW CRITERIA
Identification of patient's physical and psychosocial needs and/or concerns

Relief of severe, persistent pain

Fear of decreased mobility or joint function, loss of time from normal activities, change in role, and increased dependency

Psychological support to ensure emotional rest; intermittent systemic rest periods; articular rest, using support or splints; physical therapy even in presence of pain

Recommended nursing action consistent with diagnosis
Nursing services

Observe and assess joint mobility and function twice daily

Control pain

Organize nursing care to include supervised rest periods, preservation of joint function, prevention of deformity, and administration of medications, especially salicylates

Provide extensive psychological support; encourage emotional rest and expression of feelings

Maintain heat applications through packs or warm tub baths to promote muscle relaxation and pain control, especially prior to exercising

Provide health teaching

Health education

Teach rehabilitation measures of heat application, range-of-motion exercises, prevention of deformities, increasing joint function

Instruct on medication, including the name, dosage, frequency, duration, and side effects to report to physician

Suggest measures to reduce tension, provide emotional rest, and adjust lifestyle to include rest periods

Indicators for discharge
Adaptation to health status

Absence or reduction of joint pain and swelling

Ambulatory

Completion of health teaching

Examples of community resources

Physical rehabilitation center

Visiting Nurse Association or public health nurse

RETROSPECTIVE REVIEW CRITERIA
Health

Absence or control of joint pain

Absence or reduction of joint swelling

Complications not evident

Activity

Ambulatory

Minimal assistance with activities of daily living

Range-of-motion exercises to all joints

Knowledge

Understands importance of and can perform range-of-motion exercises

Understands medication instructions, disease process, symptoms to report to physician, measures to ensure emotional rest, and methods of moist heat applications

COMPLICATIONS

Drug reaction
Joint deformity
Loss of joint function
Septic joint from infection

Pain, low back (Code: 789.1)

CONCURRENT REVIEW CRITERIA
Identification of patient's physical and psychosocial needs and/or concerns

Relief from pain, muscle spasms, and impairment of activity

Concern over loss of time from work or school

Understanding of condition (postural strain or spondylolisthesis) and medical or surgical and nursing management in order to make realistic plans for health maintenance after discharge

Prevention of problems related to immobility

Rehabilitation to regain normal function

Recommended nursing action consistent with diagnosis
Nursing services
For conservative management of low back pain

Implement pain-reducing measures, including bedboards, support under lumbar spine and knees, moist heat to back, avoidance of massage during acute stage (to prevent muscle spasms), analgesics, and rest

Maintain traction (Buck's extension or back strapping with adhesive tape) and positioning for comfort

Ensure adequate hydration, nutrition, and elimination

Prevent complications resulting from inactivity through turning, use of protective devices and gentle massage of bony prominences, improving chest physiology, hydration, and active and passive exercises of extremities

Following acute phase, strengthen back muscles with exercises of diaphragmatic breathing and active contraction of abdominal and gluteal muscles and apply back brace or corset

For surgical management of low back pain

Provide preoperative nursing care for spinal fusion, including pain control; adequate hydration, nutrition, and elimination; and teaching about surgical procedure of hemilaminectomy or of spinal fusion, recovery room, pain control, log-roll turning, breathing and coughing exercises, and estimated period of hospitalization

Physically prepare patient for surgery

Implement postoperative nursing care, including observation for signs of shock, infection, neurological deficits, and physiological responses

Maintain skin integrity and prevent complications from circulatory stasis by frequent log-roll turning, active and passive exercises of extremities, avoiding extreme flexion of knees during early postoperative period, gently massaging bony prominences, and using protective devices

Control pain

Maintain adequate hydration, elimination, and nutrition

Health education
For conservative therapy

Instruct on relation of muscle spasms to position and on methods to reduce pain

Instruct on therapeutic and restricted activities to avoid back strain, spasms, and/or pain

Instruct on and encourage the use of a bedboard at home

Explain the name, dosage, frequency, side effects, action to take if side effects occur, and precautions of each medication

Advise patient when and why it is necessary to return to clinic or physician's office for follow-up visit

For surgical treatment

Advise patient that activities should increase gradually, according to tolerance, after surgery

Instruct on type and duration of therapeutic and restricted activities to avoid flexion strain to the spine, including stair climbing and automobile riding

Teach measures to reduce discomfort

Advise patient when and why it is necessary to return to clinic or physician's office for follow-up visit

Instruct on body mechanics

Explain the name, dosage, frequency, purpose, side effects, action to take if side effects occur, and precautions of each discharge medication

Indicators for discharge
Adaptation to health status

Condition stable
Complications not evident
Ambulatory
Health teaching completed
Referrals made

Examples of community resources

Visiting Nurse Association or public health nurse
Social services
Orthopedic clinic or physical rehabilitation center

RETROSPECTIVE REVIEW CRITERIA
Health

Pain reduced
Muscle spasms absent
Strength of back muscles increased
Wound healing, if surgically treated
Complications not evident

Activity

Ambulatory with proper body mechanics
If brace or corset is prescribed, able to apply

Knowledge

Understands purpose of discharge medications and knows the dosage, frequency, name, side effects, action to take if side effects occur, and precautions of each

Understands and can implement pain-reducing measures

Understands therapeutic and restricted activities and can implement proper body mechanics

Understands when and why it is necessary to return to physician's office or clinic for follow-up visit

COMPLICATIONS

Circulatory stasis
Decubitus ulcers
Infection
Loss of bowel or bladder function
Persistent, severe pain and evidence of persistent nerve root irritation
Pneumonia
Progression of neurological deficits while at bedrest
Recurrent episodes of incapacitating back pain or sciatica
Shock

Pain, low back (including arthritis and disc pathology)
(Codes: 353, 724, 725.1, 726, 728.8, 728.9, 756.1, 788.1, 789.6, 805.4, 805.5, 805.9, 808.9, 846, 847.2, 847.3)

CONCURRENT REVIEW CRITERIA
Identification of patient's physical and psychosocial needs and/or concerns

Relief of severe, persistent pain that may radiate to lower extremities

Fear of sensory-motor dysfunction; decreased flexion or extension of spine

Anxiety and/or depression about condition, dependency, loss of time from normal activities, and change in sexual role

Understanding of disease process, medical and nursing management, duration of hospitalization, and expected outcome of treatment

Recommended nursing action consistent with diagnosis
Nursing services

Provide daily neurological assessment

Assess pain and/or spasms and implement measures to relieve or control

Implement counseling session for sexual counseling as well as for relieving depression and/or anxiety

Review physical and emotional status every 3 days

Monitor traction and/or application of back brace or corset

Maintain patient's knees in flexed position; administer medications; apply heat; avoid fatigue; increase activity as tolerated

Health education

Implement exercise program, including pelvic tilt and quadricep setting

Teach body mechanics, including avoidance of bending or lifting from the waist, and avoidance of activities placing strain on back

Teach body alignment and moving in bed and in chairs

Teach necessary adaptation for activities of daily living

Explain application of back brace or corset

Indicators for discharge
Adaptation to health status

Pain absent or decreased to tolerable level

Neurological involvement not increased

Anxiety or depression absent or controlled

Health teaching completed

Sexual problems resolving

Examples of community resources

Physical rehabilitation center or orthopedic clinic

Social services

Visiting Nurse Association or public health nurse

RETROSPECTIVE REVIEW CRITERIA
Health

Anxiety controlled

Complications not evident

Body in correct alignment

Pain absent or at tolerable level

Neurological involvement not increased

Activity

Able to perform activities of daily living

Applies proper body mechanics when bending or lifting from waist

Implements exercise program

Knowledge

Understands and can perform proper body mechanics, exercise program, and proper body alignment

Understands and can verbalize possible solutions to sexual problems, disease process, and symptoms to report to physician

COMPLICATIONS

Lower extremity nerve root compromise
Neurogenic bladder
Paraparesis
Pulmonary embolism
Sensory-motor dysfunction
Thrombophlebitis

Parkinson's disease (paralysis agitans) (Code: 342)

CONCURRENT CRITERIA
Identification of patient's physical and psychosocial needs and/or concerns

Relief of symptoms, including loss of functional adaptive capabilities, such as walking, feeding, self-care, and dressing; tremors; drooling; speech impairment; or pain in extremities

Expression of feelings of hopelessness and social isolation

Understanding of ramifications of disease, including slow progression, mental ability not being affected, medications to provide relief of symptoms, and medical and nursing management

Understanding of preparation, purpose, and expected outcome of surgery, if thalamotomy is done, including preoperative and postoperative teaching

Family understanding of measures to maintain patient's independence as long as possible

Recommended nursing action consistent with diagnosis
Nursing services

Observe for desired effects and side effects of medication and for drug toxicity, with appropriate nursing intervention, if necessary

Promote adequate activity to prevent immobility through active and passive, stretching, walking, and postural exercises

Provide relief from pain, through massage, warm wet compresses to joints, and warm tub baths, and relief from insomnia

Assist patient in remaining independent through use of adaptive devices

Emphasize positive aspects of illness; assist in dealing with feelings of hopelessness and social isolation

Health education

Explain medications, including the name, desired effects, side effects, signs of drug toxicity, dosage, frequency, precautions, and measures to minimize side effects of each

Provide diet instructions, including elimination of vitamin B_6 from diet when L-dopa is drug of choice for treatment

Teach measures by which patient can avoid fatigue and emotional distress, since these factors increase tremors

Teach exercise regime; emphasize that activity reduces immobility and delays onset of more rapid deterioration of condition

Teach patient/family to implement measures to reduce pain and relieve insomnia of patient

Indicators for discharge
Adaptation to health status

Motor functions improved
Mental status improved
Complications not evident
Referrals made

Examples of community resources

Visiting Nurse Association or public health nurse
Medical clinic
Social services

RETROSPECTIVE CRITERIA
Health

Mentally adjusting to ramifications of condition

Nonintentional tremors decreased or controlled

Motor functions improved

Mental status improved

Complications not evident

Activity

Ambulatory with avoidance of fatigue

Able to carry out activities of daily living with little or no assistance from others

Implements exercise program

Knowledge

Patient/family knows the name, dosage, frequency, desired effects, side effects, and precautions of each discharge medication

Patient/family understands diet restrictions and can list food to be avoided if L-dopa is drug of choice

Patient/family understands measures by which fatigue and emotional distress can be avoided

Patient/family can demonstrate exercises to be done daily by patient and can state how many times a day they are to be done

Patient/family understands and can implement measures to reduce pain and relieve insomnia of patient

COMPLICATIONS

Atelectasis

Contractures

Decubitus ulcers

Pneumonia

Pulmonary embolism

Urinary incontinence

Urinary infection

Urinary retention

Parkinson's disease (rehabilitation) (Code: 342)

CONCURRENT CRITERIA
Identification of patient's physical and psychosocial needs and/or concerns

Relief of symptoms, including dysarthria, aphonia, dysphagia, emotional disturbances, or fatigue

Assessment of amount and degree of rigidity and nonintentional tremors

Adaptation to loss of functional abilities including feeding, self-care, or dressing

Establishment of medication regime

Emotional reaction to disease and to life changes

Recommended nursing action consistent with diagnosis
Nursing services

Assess self-care ability, establish an activities of daily living program with assistive devices

Assess ambulation; establish an ambulation program

Assess speech; establish communication program

Provide emotional support and counseling

Reevaluate every 3 weeks

Monitor medication response and side effects

Health education

Instruct about method, action, and side effects of medications

Teach self-care program and use of any assistive devices

Explain nutritional and fluid needs

Implement speech program, teaching slow rate of speech and taking a deep breath before speaking

Teach disease process, expectations, treatment, and symptoms to report to physician

Indicators for discharge
Adaptation to health status

Meeting activities of daily living goals

Satisfactorily following medication regime

Negotiating ambulation program

Coping with disease process

Comprehending and implementing health teaching

Examples of community resources

Visiting Nurse Association or public health nurse

Parkinson's Disease Association

RETROSPECTIVE CRITERIA
Health

Mentally accepting disease and change in life-style

Decrease in rigidity and nonintentional tremors

Control of presenting symptoms

Adequate hydration

Activity

Mobility with or without assistive devices

Activities of daily living program with minimal assistance

Implements speech program

Knowledge

Knows medication regime and side effects, disease process, and symptoms to report to physician

COMPLICATIONS

Atelectasis

Decubitus ulcers

Depression

Emotional disturbance

Pneumonia

Pulmonary embolism

Urinary incontinence

Urinary infection

Urinary retention

Peptic ulcer, nonsurgical (duodenal or gastric) (Code: 533)

CONCURRENT CRITERIA
Identification of patient's physical and psychosocial needs and/or concerns

Relief of symptoms, including hemorrhage, perforation, obstruction, vomiting coffee ground emesis, nausea, pain that may be relieved by food, heartburn, dehydration, gastric distention, weakness, bloody stools, irritability, pallor, chills, and fever

Understanding of medical and nursing treatment as well as nursing management necessary for realistic planning for health maintenance after discharge

Fear of cancer, loss of time from work or school, or changes in body image, resulting from inability to function at normal capacity

Maintenance of vital body functions, depending on severity of symptoms

Understanding of community agencies available to assist during convalescence

Recommended nursing action consistent with diagnosis
Nursing services

Implement measures designed to interrupt life-threatening processes, including controlling bleeding, replacing fluids to maintain cardiovascular function, conserving body heat, positioning in low or semi-Fowler's position; ensuring ventilation, and promoting rest

Observe for signs of physical deterioration, by frequent monitoring of vital signs, including rectal temperature every 2 hours: apical and radial pulses, respiration, and blood pressure every 15 minutes; bowel sounds; color of emesis; intake and output hourly;

hemoglobin, hemocyte, and electrolyte reports; and changes in mental status

Promote adequate hydration, nutrition, and elimination

Provide emotional support to patient/family with reduction of stressful situations

Health education

Instruct patient on foods included in diet and those to be avoided, acceptable cooking methods; and need for slowly eating small, frequent meals

Instruct patient on the name, purpose, dosage, frequency, side effects, action to take if side effects occur, and precautions of each discharge medication

Instruct concerning therapeutic and restricted activities

Instruct concerning avoidance of alcohol and tobacco

Indicators for discharge
Adaptation to health status

Condition stable
Complications not evident
Health teaching completed
Referrals made

Examples of community resources

Visiting Nurse Association or public health nurse
Surgical clinic

RETROSPECTIVE CRITERIA
Health

Presenting symptoms relieved or controlled

Hydrated
Tolerating diet
Complications not evident

Activity

Able to reduce stressful situations
Ambulatory
Able to carry out activities of daily living
Avoids alcohol and tobacco

Knowledge

Knows the name of each discharge medication; understands the purpose, dosage, frequency, side effects, action to take if side effects occur, and precautions of each

Understands and can carry out diet restrictions and allowances

Understands therapeutic and restricted activities and can implement therapeutic ones

Understands importance of and can implement plan for avoiding tobacco and alcohol

COMPLICATIONS

Drug reaction
Hemorrhage from peptic ulcer
Infections
Intractability to treatment
Perforation
Pneumonia
Pulmonary embolism
Pyloric obstruction
Thrombophlebitis
Wound infection

Periarthritis of major joint (Code: 729.3)

CONCURRENT CRITERIA
Identification of patient's physical and psychosocial needs and/or concerns

Relief of severe, persistent pain; depression; and fatigue

Fear of loss of mobility or muscle weakness

Nutrition to maintain or obtain desired weight

Recommended nursing action consistent with diagnosis
Nursing services

Initiate activities of daily living program to include self-care (dressing and hygiene) and avoidance of fatigue

Implement rehabilitation measures, including muscle-strengthening and range-of-motion exercises and an ambulation program

Instigate counseling sessions to explore anxiety and/or depression

Assess neurological state, mobility, joint functioning, and symptoms of complications

Provide nutrition to maintain or obtain desired weight

Health education

Teach rehabilitation measures to increase mobility, muscle strength, progressive ambulation, and activities of daily living

Instruct about diet to maintain proper nutrition and desired weight

Explain condition, course, prognosis, medical and nursing treatment plans, medications, and symptoms to report to physician

Teach measures to reduce pain and avoid fatigue

Indicators for discharge
Adaptation to health status

Symptoms alleviated

Activities of daily living and ambulation goals achieved

Depression absent or resolved

Pain absent or at tolerable level

Health and rehabilitation teaching completed

Examples of community resources

Visiting Nurse Association or public health nurse

RETROSPECTIVE CRITERIA
Health

Weight approaching ideal weight

Pain absent or at tolerable level

Symptoms alleviated

Depression absent or resolved

Activity

Ambulation with or without assistive devices and avoiding fatigue

Activities of daily living with minimal assistance

Performs exercise program

Knowledge

Knows food selection and meal planning necessary for adequate nutrition and weight

Knows and performs muscle-strengthening and range-of-motion exercises without fatigue

Understands and can verbalize medication instructions, disease process, and symptoms to report to physician

COMPLICATIONS

Fracture of related bony structure

Joint contractures

Reflex sympathetic dystrophy (causalgia)

Thrombophlebitis

Personality disorders and certain other nonpsychotic mental disorders of childhood or adolescence (Codes: DSM 301-304)

CONCURRENT CRITERIA

Identification of patient's physical and psychosocial needs and/or concerns

Identification of maladaptive patterns of behavior, usually behavior dangerous to self, others, or property

State of child's/adolescent's (patient's) physical health

Exploration of patient's beliefs, attitudes, and expectations of own behavior and of hospitalization

Exploration of family's beliefs, attitudes, and expectations of patient and of treatment facility

Determination of chronology of patient's/family's development and coping

Recommended nursing action consistent with diagnosis
Nursing services

Provide nursing assessment (of patient, family, and community) within 7 days of admission

Maintain ongoing behavioral observation and assessment of patient within 8 hours of admission, every 8 hours for 1 week, then during facility-defined periods (document changes)

Implement behavior-specific interventions, such as life-space interview, seclusion, suicide precautions, or behavior modification

Assist in developing and implementing after-care program and family-specific interventions

Implement and assess physical therapies, such as medications or diagnostic procedures

Health education

Explain ward procedures and milieu to patient/family

Discuss treatment goals and therapeutic modalities with patient/family

Teach family to make use of specific therapeutic modalities, such as behavior modification, principles of psychodynamics, communication theories, and attitude prescription

Discuss, demonstrate, and explain about any medication

Indicators for discharge
Adaptation to health status

Decreased incidence of maladaptive behavior (partially decreased assualtive or suicidal [self-destructive] behavior)

Evidence of beginning reintegration into family, community, and school

Patient/family demonstration of self-care capability in areas of medication administration, recognition of feelings, limit-setting, and help-seeking

Examples of community resources

Outpatient psychiatric nurse
School nurse

RETROSPECTIVE CRITERIA
Health

Maladaptive patterns of behavior alleviated
Regular sleep pattern
No physical illness or problems

Activity

Can set limits
Self-care
Family implementation of therapeutic modalities
Reintegration into family unit

Knowledge

Patient/family knows what treatment goals were accomplished

Patient/family knows what after-care plans have been made; understands plans and each family member's part in them

COMPLICATIONS

Adverse reactions to diagnostic or therapeutic modalities (procedures, drugs, or psychological or social therapies)

Exacerbation of clinical signs and/or symptoms

Failure of family and/or social support system

Pneumonia (Codes: 480-486)

CONCURRENT REVIEW CRITERIA
Identification of patient's physical and psychosocial needs and/or concerns

Relief of respiratory distress, including dyspnea, tachypnea, bradypnea, hypoxia, and fatigue

Relief of hyperthermia with associated metabolic problems, tachycardia, and fluid deficit

Identification of behavioral changes, such as apprehension, stupor, delirium, or sympathetic nervous system response (for example, gastrointestinal anorexia)

Relief from coughing, including nonproductive and productive rales and bronchial

Prevention of infections, such as lung abscess, systemic infection, or pleural effusion

Control of pain

Recommended nursing action consistent with diagnosis
Nursing services

Maintain patent airway by checking respiratory rate and rhythm; hyperflexing jaw and elevating head of bed; checking lung sounds; initiating turning, coughing, and deep breathing; reporting pure carbon dioxide greater than 50 mm Hg and pure oxygen less than 60 mm Hg; and administering oxygen as ordered

Evaluate fluid status, by checking temperature for baselines and chilling episodes, recording intake and output, checking cardiac rate and rhythm, and checking hypertension; replace fluids and nutrients consistent with bodily needs and depletions; check weight

Evaluate and secure sensorium status, by maintaining quiet environment, maintaining planned rest periods, explaining therapies, giving antipyretics as needed and ordered, and encouraging patient to verbalize fears and concerns

Assist during spontaneous and induced coughing episodes; provide selected respiratory therapies, such as humidification, oxygen, vaporization, suctioning, positioning, or postural drainage

Obtain blood and sputum cultures; administer antimicrobials as ordered

Administer analgesics as ordered after offering emotional support, encouraging utilization of coping mechanisms, and splinting chest with pillows and positioning

Health education

Teach identification of symptoms, such as respiratory distress, hyperthermia, behavioral changes, cough, infection, and pain

Teach means by which to avoid overexertion, such as rest periods and identification of circadian rhythm

Defer complex teaching during acute phase, remaining open to questions from patient

Teach adequate hydration and nutrition

Teach avoidance of recurrence of disease by avoiding chills, drafts, and communicable diseases

Teach normal technique of ventilation

267

Indicators for discharge
Adaptation to health status

Afebrile below 100° F, orally
Absence of rales
Nonproductive cough
Normal vital signs
Patient understanding of home treatment
Positive plans for discharge

Examples of community resources

Visiting Nurse Association or public health nurse
American Respiratory Association (patient services booklets)

RETROSPECTIVE REVIEW CRITERIA
Health

Afebrile below 100° F, orally for 24 hours prior to discharge
Rales absent
Nonproductive cough
Respiratory distress absent
Pain controlled or absent
Complications not evident

Activity

Ambulatory with prescribed rest periods

Knowledge

Patient/family knowledge of discharge medication, including frequency, dosage, side effects, and observations to report to physician
Patient/family knowledge of droplet infection spread
Patient/family knowledge of importance of reporting signs and symptoms of respiratory infection
Patient/family avoidance of overtiring

COMPLICATIONS

Atelectasis
Drug reaction
Empyema, lung abscess
Septic shock
Suprainfections
Tracheotomy

Pneumonia, bacterial (Codes: 480-486)

CONCURRENT CRITERIA
Identification of patient's physical and psychosocial needs and/or concerns

Relief of symptoms, including sudden onset of shaking chills, fever, stabbing chest pain exaggerated by respiration, cough with rust-colored sputum, tachypnea of 30 to 40 breaths per minute, or herpes simplex lesions
Ventilation and oxygenation of lungs
Increased hydration to help liquefy secretions and maintain output
Fear of not being able to breathe
Control of pain

Recommended nursing action consistent with diagnosis
Nursing services

Monitor respiratory status, breath sounds, and vital signs every 4 hours; admin-

ister oxygen for severe cyanosis or marked dyspnea; supervise inhalation, positive pressure breathing treatments, if ordered, and postural drainage; check sputum characteristics
Observe for signs of complications, with prompt nursing intervention if any occur
Identify and explain condition that predisposed patient to pneumonia, such as viral respiratory diseases, malnutrition, exposure to cold, noxious gasses, alcohol intoxication, depression of cerebral functions by drugs, and cardiac failure
Assist with expectoration of sputum by splinting chest with pillows or having patient sit upright when coughing; turn, cough, deep breathe; and postural drainage

Emotional support and assistance when patient has feeling of not being able to breathe

Health education

Explain disease process, course, treatment, medical and nursing management, prognosis, duration of hospitalization, activity restrictions or gradual convalescence, and symptoms to report to physician

Teach about conditions that predispose to pneumonia and methods to implement to avoid recurrence of disease such as keeping warm, not being chilled, avoiding contact with upper respiratory infections, preventing fatigue, increasing moisture in environment, especially the bedroom

Provide medication instructions including name, dosage, frequency, purpose, and side effects to report to physician

Teach methods to decrease or stop smoking

Indicators of discharge
Adaptation to health status

Afebrile

Symptoms resolved or controlled

Ambulatory without respiratory distress or fatigue

No evidence of complications

Health teaching completed

Examples of community resources

Visiting Nurse Association or public health nurse

RETROSPECTIVE CRITERIA
Health

Afebrile

Absence of pain or difficulty in breathing

Predisposed condition resolved or controlled

Activity

Independent in activities of daily living

Ambulatory, but experiences fatigue

Involved in antismoking program

Knowledge

Understands and can verbalize disease process, conditions that predispose to pneumonia, methods to prevent recurrence, medication instructions, methods to decrease or stop cigarette smoking, techniques of postural drainage, and symptoms to report to physician

COMPLICATIONS

Abdominal distention

Airway obstruction

Atelectasis

Cardiac arrhythmias

Complications of medication (drug fever)

Congestive heart failure

Cyanosis

Dyspnea

Electrolyte imbalance

Empyema

Endocarditis

Fractured ribs

Lung abscess

Malnutrition

Meningitis

Pericarditis

Pleural effusion

Pleuritic pain

Pulmonary edema

Respiratory failure

Shock

Tracheostomy

Urinary retention

Poisoning, lead, in children (Code: 984)

CONCURRENT CRITERIA
Identification of patient's physical and psychosocial needs and/or concerns

Relief of symptoms, including metallic taste in mouth, anorexia, irritability, apathy, abdominal colic, vomiting, diarrhea, constipation, headaches, leg cramps, black stools, oliguria, stupor, convulsions, palsies, coma, or neurological deficit

Assessment of parent/child relationship and quality of home environment to determine possible causes of lead poisoning

Adaptation to hospitalization; alleviation of fear

Referral of diagnosed case to Department of Public Health

Recommended nursing action consistent with diagnosis
Nursing services

Provide gastric lavage, if acute lead poisoning

Observe closely for any changes in neurological status

Obtain careful nursing history, especially in regard to incidence of anorexia, clumsiness, ataxia, vomiting, convulsions, or decreased activity

Assess parent/child relationship to determine "quality of mothering" and/or pica behavior in child

Monitor intake and output to ensure output of 800 to 1,000 ml every 24 hours

Rotate injection sites; massage injection site well after administering medication; observe for signs of drug toxicity

Observe for untoward reactions to medications, such as sense of chest constriction, weakness, fever, hypertension, paresthesia, tachycardia, or respiratory distress

Notify Department of Public Health of diagnosed case

Health education

Educate parents regarding possible causes of lead poisoning, course, prognosis, and medical and nursing management

Explain diagnostic procedures performed, methods of treatment, need for long-term medical follow-up to assess possible residual problems, and seizure care

Indicators for discharge
Adaptation to health status

Afebrile

Stable vital signs

Medically suitable home environment

Completion of parent/child education regarding home care and causes of lead-poisoning

Tolerating food and fluids

Resuming normal activities for age and developmental level

Examples of community resources

Social services

Visiting Nurse Association or public health nurse

Department of Public Health

RETROSPECTIVE CRITERIA
Health

Lead level in blood approaching 60 μg per ml

Afebrile

Free of acute symptoms

Tolerating food and fluids well

Complications not evident

Activity

Resuming normal activities for age and developmental level

Knowledge

Parent/child understanding of home care, medication and causes of lead poisoning

Parent understanding of need for long-term medical and/or public health follow-up to assess possible residual problems

Convulsions
Encephalopathy
Renal failure

Poisoning with narcotics, sedatives, or tranquilizers in children
(Codes: 965, 967, 970.1)

CONCURRENT CRITERIA
Identification of patient's physical and psychosocial needs and/or concerns

Relief of symptoms, including headaches, excitement, nausea, convulsions, depression, pinpoint pupils, slow respiration, apnea, rapid and feeble pulse, shock, coma, or acid-base disturbances
Preservation of an open airway
Stimulation of respiratory ventilation
Maintenance of blood pressure and body temperature
Provision of emotional support for child and family
Understanding about safety in the home environment

Recommended nursing action consistent with diagnosis
Nursing services

Check vital signs and level of consciousness every 30 minutes until alert
Turn and position child on his side with neck hyperextended at least every 2 hours
Stimulate child by talking and by having child deep breathe at least every 10 to 15 minutes
Record intake and output for the first 24 to 48 hours
Use therapeutic communication to relieve anxiety of family and determine the cause and type of poisoning

Health education

Teach family about keeping drugs and other hazardous substances out of the reach of children
Instruct family about what to do in case of another poisoning, such as inform-ing them of emergency phone number and antidote
Discuss procedures being carried out for child with child and parents

Indicators for discharge
Adaptation to health status

Stable vital signs and afebrile for 24 hours prior to discharge
No respiratory difficulty present
Resuming normal activity
Tolerating food and fluids
Completion of family teaching; drugs put out of child's reach

Examples of community resources

Home visit by public health nurse to assess safety hazards
Psychiatric consultation, if poisoning is not accidental
Poison control center

RETROSPECTIVE CRITERIA
Health

Stable vital signs and afebrile for 24 hours prior to discharge
Alert and well oriented
Tolerating food and fluids
Complications not evident

Activity

Resuming normal activity for age

Knowledge

Family understands about and can implement measures to keep medications out of reach of children
Family knows what to do if another poisoning occurs

COMPLICATIONS

Coma
Neurological sequelae

Pneumonia
Renal failure
Shock

Poisoning, unspecified, in children (Codes: 985.9, 989.9, 997.9)

CONCURRENT CRITERIA
Identification of patient's physical and psychosocial needs and/or concerns

Relief of symptoms of poisoning
Maintenance of functioning of vital organs
Supportive care during treatment
Teaching about safety in the home environment
Adjustment to hospitalization

Recommended nursing action consistent with diagnosis
Nursing services

Observe child for signs of shock, convulsions, or metabolic disorders; monitor vital signs and level of consciousness every 30 minutes
Develop a trusting relationship with child and family to provide support, to relieve anxiety, and to determine cause of poisoning
Use simple diversions to keep child resting but as alert as possible
Have equipment readily available in case of respiratory difficulty
Give nothing by mouth unless otherwise ordered by physician

Health education

Explain treatments being undertaken to child and family
Teach family about keeping poisons out of reach of children
Instruct family about what to do in case of another poisoning, including informing them of emergency number of poison control center and of need to bring in any container in which poison was stored

Indicators for discharge
Adaptation to health status

Stable vital signs and level of consciousness for 24 hours prior to discharge
Tolerating food and fluids well
Resuming normal activity for age
Completion of teaching parents about prevention of poisoning and what to do in case of poisoning
Urine output of at least 1,000 ml per day

Examples of community resources

Home visit by public health nurse to assess safety hazards
Psychiatric consultation if poisoning is not accidental
Poison control center

RETROSPECTIVE CRITERIA
Health

Stable vital signs and afebrile for 24 hours prior to discharge
Alert and coherent
Tolerating food and fluids
Urine output at least 1,000 ml per day

Activity

Resuming normal activity for age and developmental level

Knowledge

Family understands about and can implement safety in the environment
Family knows about referral resources
Family knows what to do in case of another poisoning

COMPLICATIONS

Coma
Convulsions

Emotional problems (venting feeling of suicide or demonstrating inappropriate behavior)
Gastrointestinal sequelae
Metabolic disorders

Neurological sequelae
Pneumonitis
Renal failure
Shock

Poisoning, volatile hydrocarbon, in children (Code: 981)

CONCURRENT REVIEW CRITERIA
Identification of patient's physical and psychosocial needs and/or concerns

Restoration and promotion of adequate cardiopulmonary function
Restoration and promotion of normal central nervous system function
Restoration of fluid and electrolyte balance
Adaptation to hospitalization; emotional support to parents
Determination of specific information regarding poison ingested

Recommended nursing action consistent with diagnosis
Nursing services

Determine name and quantity of poison ingested, time elapsed since ingestion, child's weight and age, progression of symptoms, and previous treatment
Monitor vital signs every 15 to 30 minutes; observe for fever, tachycardia, tachypnea, dizziness, confusion, level of consciousness, dyspnea, or diminished breath sounds
Thoroughly wash contaminated skin and hair
Use extreme caution to prevent aspiration, keeping equipment for suctioning and endotracheal intubation available
Provide appropriate play therapy and exploration of treatment to aid patient in adaptation to hospitalization

Health education

Discuss with parents ways to provide a safe environment for child at home but without being overly protective
Encourage consultation with community health resources as needed (that is, in case of permanent injury to child)
Discuss with parents the need for follow-up visits to determine evidence of liver or kidney damage

Indicators for discharge
Adaptation to health status

Asymptomatic
Stable vital signs
Activity appropriate to age and developmental level
Completion of parent education regarding poison prevention and need for follow-up examinations
Completion of referrals to community agencies

Examples of community resources

Visiting Nurse Association or public health nurse
Consultation with community mental health agencies

RETROSPECTIVE REVIEW CRITERIA
Health

Asymptomatic
Stable vital signs
Tolerating food and fluids
Alert and coherent

Activity

Appropriate to age and developmental level

Knowledge

Parents understand poison prevention and need for follow-up examinations
Parents are aware of community agencies available to assist them

COMPLICATIONS

Central nervous system depression
Hypostatic pneumonia
Pneumonitis
Pulmonary edema
Respiration depression
Respiratory obstruction
Shock

Polyarthritis, inflammatory (Codes: 712, 712.1, 712.9, 715, 716.1)

CONCURRENT CRITERIA
Identification of patient's physical and psychosocial needs and/or concerns

Relief of severe persistent pain
Fear of loss of mobility, sensory deficit, change in body image, and loss of time from normal activities
Prevention of muscle weakness; decrease of fatigue
Feeling of depression
Improvement of nutritional status
Vocational and social counseling

Recommended nursing action consistent with diagnosis
Nursing services

Develop activities of daily living program with consideration of pain and fatigue factors
Implement rehabilitation measures, including muscle-strengthening and range-of-motion exercises, an ambulation program, changing position every 2 hours, skin care, and massaging bony prominences
Plan sessions to focus on emotional, vocational, and social needs; refer to community agencies
Reevaluate sensory-motor rehabilitation, weight, and neurological deficits every week
Encourage independence without producing fatigue

Health education

Teach rehabilitation measures of muscle-strengthening and range-of-motion exercises, skin care, an ambulation program, and avoidance of fatigue
Teach disease progress, course, treatment regime, medical and nursing management, and symptoms to report to physician
Explain food selection and meal planning for adequate nutrition and maintaining normal weight
Instruct about the name, dosage, frequency, duration, and side effects to report to physician of each medication

Indicators for discharge
Adaptation to health status

Symptoms alleviated
Activities of daily living and ambulation goals achieved
Pain absent or at tolerable level
Depression absent or resolved
Health teaching completed
Fatigue relieved

Examples of community resources

Visiting Nurse Association or public health nurse
Physical and vocational rehabilitation centers

RETROSPECTIVE CRITERIA
Health

Pain absent or at tolerable level
Joints mobile
Symptoms alleviated
Complications not evident

Activity

Performs activities of daily living
Ambulatory with or without assistive devices
Implements rehabilitative measures

274

Knowledge

Understands and can verbalize disease process, symptoms to report to physician, medication instructions, rehabilitative measures, and nutrition instructions

COMPLICATIONS

Decubitus ulcers
Marked weakness of extremity muscles

Myopathy
Peripheral neuropathy
Quadriparesis
Reduced sensation in hands or feet
Severe back pain
Vertebral compression fracture

Polymyositis (Code: 716.1)

CONCURRENT CRITERIA
Identification of patient's physical and psychosocial needs and/or concerns

Relief of symptoms, including muscle tenderness and discomfort, weakness in arms and legs, oropharyngeal weakness, arthralgia, and possible muscle atrophy

Explanation of the nature of the condition, prognosis, and medial and nursing management

Reassurance that rarely does the disease progress to the point of being permanently bedridden

Reduction of anxiety and fear during diagnostic process as related to possibility of muscular dystrophy

Concern over changes in body image and role and over increased dependence

Awareness of community agencies for assistance with discharge care

Recommended nursing action consistent with diagnosis
Nursing services

Maintain or improve nutrition, hydration, elimination, respiratory function, and muscle functions

Implement safety measures

Assist patient/family in coping with changes in patient's role and body image and with patient's increased dependence

Implement comfort measures, including analgesics, physical comfort measures, relief of waking-imagined analgesia, and techniques of distraction

Observe for undesirable effects of medication, since steroid therapy is primary drug of choice; provide prompt nursing intervention when any occur

Health education

Explain the name, dosage, frequency, and duration of drug therapy, acceptable and expected side effects (such as facial mooning, weight gain, edema, acne, increased frequency of urination, nocturia, insomnia, headaches, and fatigue), and measures to take to reduce these side effects; should weight gain be an extreme problem, reduce calories and contact physician

Stress importance of *not* discontinuing steroid therapy abruptly without physician's knowledge

Instruct about immediate notification of physician if unacceptable side effects occur, including hypertension, thromboembolic complications, arteritis, infection, glaucoma, corneal lesions, musculoskeletal effects, adrenal insufficiency, nausea, vomiting, thirst, abdominal pain, convulsions, or depression

Teach to wear medical alert information stating medication name, dosage, and frequency and physician's name and phone number for use in emergencies

Explain measures to avoid exposure to

infection and/or avoid fractures resulting from increased calcium urinary output and osteoporosis

Instruct about high protein, high carbohydrate diet, including foods high in potassium while on steroids

Teach activity restrictions, avoidance of fatigue, use of pacing techniques, range-of-motion and active and passive exercises, and avoidance of circulatory stasis or decreased muscle function

Indicators for discharge
Adaptation to health status

Muscle function improved
Complications not evident
Health teaching completed
Referrals made

Examples of community resources

Visiting Nurse Association or public health nurse
Social services
Physiotherapy clinic
Medical clinic

RETROSPECTIVE CRITERIA
Health

Change in body image accepted
Special diet tolerated
Muscle function improved
Complications not evident

Activity

Ambulatory
Able to carry out activities of daily living with or without assistance of other people or of prosthetic devices
Wears medical alert tag

Knowledge

Patient/family knows and understands the name, dosage, and frequency of each discharge medication; the duration of drug therapy; the importance of taking medicines continually unless stopped by physician; expected and unacceptable side effects; measures to reduce severity of expected side effects, and precautions

Patient/family understands importance and rationale of avoiding infections and seeking prompt medical treatment for even minor illnesses

Patient/family understands that patient should wear a medical alert tag and knows where to get one

Patient/family understands importance of having a kit with cortisone medication on person at all times in event of accident and precipitated adrenal failure

Patient/family understands and can implement proper diet and understands methods by which food can decrease severity of "acceptable" side effects of steroid therapy

Patient/family understands therapeutic and restricted activities and can implement therapeutic ones

Patient/family understands and can implement adaptive measures when neurological deficits remain; patient can apply prosthetic devices unassisted

Patient/family understands purpose of appropriate community agencies assist in care after discharge

COMPLICATIONS

Adrenal failure
Adverse drug reaction
Arteritis
Atelectasis
Corneal lesions
Convulsions
Depression
Dysphagia
Gastrointestinal ulcers
Glaucoma
Hypertension
Infection
Muscle destruction
Nausea and vomiting
Normocytic anemia
Ocular palsies
Pneumonia
Pulmonary embolism
Thirst
Thromboembolism
Wound infection

Polyneuritis (Code: 354)

CONCURRENT CRITERIA
Identification of patient's physical and psychosocial needs and/or concerns

Relief of symptoms, including numbness, hyperesthesia, pain, decreased perception of heat and/or cold, muscle weakness, or paralysis

Understanding of cause, prognosis, and medical and nursing management of condition

Protection from trauma; prevention of complications, including falls, burns, decubitus ulcers, or joint contractures

Identification of causative toxic agents to avoid, such as alcohol, viruses, or heavy metals

Recommended nursing action consistent with diagnosis
Nursing services

Maintain bed rest during acute phase
Provide adequate diet and hydration
Control pain
Prevent complications and remove from exposure to toxic agents

Health education

Explain diet, medications, and prognosis
Explain relationship of alcohol and heavy metals to condition, if appropriate

Indicators for discharge
Adaptation to health status

Afebrile
Muscle strength improved

Complications not evident
Medications and diet understood
Referrals made

Examples of community resources

Visiting Nurse Association or public health nurse
Alanon, if appropriate
Vocational rehabilitation center

RETROSPECTIVE CRITERIA
Health

Afebrile
Complications not evident
Muscle strength improved

Activity

Able to care for self with minimal assistance

Knowledge

Understands need for adequate diet
Recognizes correlation of alcohol ingestion and condition
Recognizes type of employment as factor for causing condition

COMPLICATIONS

Decubitus ulcers
Joint contractures
Pulmonary embolism
Thrombophlebitis

Pressure sores (decubitus ulcers) (Code: 707)

CONCURRENT CRITERIA
Identification of patient's physical and psychosocial needs and/or concerns

Open wounds healed
Protection from potential or existing infection
Knowledge of skin care and decubitus ulcer formation
Maintenance of nutritional status
Emotional reaction to wound

Recommended nursing action consistent with diagnosis
Nursing services

Remove pressure by use of a water bed or foam mattress, positioning and turning, and/or other special devices
Use sterile technique for decubitus ulcer care
Promote circulation in wound area
Assess wound progress daily
Provide emotional support and counseling

Health education

Teach patient/family about skin care and skin inspection
Teach patient/family decubitus ulcer prevention regime, such as use of assistive devices to alleviate pressure, prevention of trauma, exercise and massage, and turning and positioning
Explain nutritional needs and dietary recommendations

Indicators for discharge
Adaptation to health status

Wound healing
Ability to follow skin care regime, inspect skin, and follow prevention regime demonstrated
Signs of nutritional deficiency not evident

Examples of community resources

Visiting Nurse Association or public health nurse

RETROSPECTIVE CRITERIA
Health

Circulation to affected areas improved
Wound healing
Signs of nutritional deficiency not evident

Activity

Patient/family can give skin inspection
Patient/family understands and can implement positioning and turning

Knowledge

Understands and can implement skin care regime and prevention regime
Understands and can provide nutritional needs

COMPLICATIONS

Dehiscence of wound
Necrosis of skin
Wound infection

Psychophysiological disorders of childhood or adolescence
(Code: DSM II 305)

CONCURRENT CRITERIA
Identification of patient's physical and psychosocial needs and/or concerns

Identification of incapacitating and/or life-threatening psychophysiological disturbance; identification of reasons for psychiatric hospitalization rather than medical/surgical (pediatric) service

Assessment of the state of the child's/adolescent's (patient's) physical health

Exploration of patient's beliefs, attitudes, and expectations of own behavior and of hospitalization

Exploration of family's beliefs, attitudes, and expectations of patient and of treatment facility

Determination of chronology of patient's/family's development and coping

Recommended nursing action consistent with diagnosis
Nursing services

Initiate nursing assessment of patient, family, and community within 7 days of admission

Maintain ongoing behavioral observation and assessment of patient within 8 hours of admission, every 8 hours for a week, then during facility-defined periods (document changes)

Implement behavior-specific interventions, such as life-space interviews, seclusion, suicide precautions, or behavior modification

Assist in developing and implementing an after-care program and family-specific interventions

Implement and assess physical therapies, such as medications or diagnostic procedures

Health education

Explain ward procedures and milieu to patient/family

Discuss treatment goals and therapeutic modalities with patient/family

Teach family to make use of specific therapeutic modalities, such as behavior modification, principles of psychodynamics, communication theories, and attitude prescription

Discuss, demonstrate, and explain about any medication

Indicators for discharge
Adaptation to health status

Decrease in intensity of psychophysiological disturbance

Evidence of reintegration into family, community, and school

Patient/family demonstration of self-care capability in areas of medication administration, recognition of feelings, limit setting, and help seeking

Examples of community resources

Outpatient psychiatric nurse
School nurse

RETROSPECTIVE CRITERIA
Health

Life-threatening psychophysiological disturbance alleviated

No physical illness or problems

Activity

Activity appropriate for age
Able to set limits on behavior
Reintegrated into family unit

Knowledge

Patient/family knows what treatment goals were accomplished

Patient/family knows what after-care plans have been made; understands plans and each family member's part in them

COMPLICATIONS

Adverse reactions to diagnostic or therapeutic modalities (such as procedures, drugs, and psychological or social therapies)

Exacerbation of clinical signs and/or symptoms

Failure of family and/or social support system

Psychosis associated with organic brain syndrome (Codes: 290-294)

CONCURRENT REVIEW CRITERIA
Identification of patient's physical and psychosocial needs and/or concerns

Management of symptoms, including loss of adaptability, coarseness of personality, decrease in mental function, irritability, confusion, stubborness, and depression

Pleasant, friendly surroundings with continued usefulness within limits of ability

Control of agitation; minimization of night confusion; reestablishment of sleep pattern

Understanding by family of condition, cause, course, prognosis, medical and nursing management, and possibility of need for custodial care

Recommended nursing action consistent with diagnosis
Nursing services

Closely observe for change in impairment of orientation, memory, intellectual function, or judgment

Administer prescribed medication to control disordered behavior

Provide a safe physical environment

Frequently provide reality orientation

Make recommendations for the treatment plan

Health education

Inform patient/significant other of treatment plan and realistic expectations of the plan

Help patient/significant other understand the disease process and treatment

Explain measures used to provide safe physical environment after discharge

Teach techniques of reality orientation for postdischarge care

Indicators for discharge
Adaptation to health status

Patient able to sleep at night

Absence of disordered behavior

Absence of further impairment in orientation, memory, intellectual function, and judgment

Patient manageable at a lower level of care

Examples of community resources

Outpatient psychiatric nurse

Visiting Nurse Association or public health nurse

Long-term care facility

RETROSPECTIVE REVIEW CRITERIA
Health

Absence of psychotic symptomatology

Regular sleep pattern

Activity

Performs activities of daily living with minimal assistance

Interacts in one-to-one and group relationships

Knowledge

Patient/significant other verbalizes understanding of the signs and symptoms of remission and the need to report these to the physician

Patient/significant other verbalizes understanding of instructions for taking medications, signs and symptoms of untoward reactions, and the need to report these to the physician

COMPLICATIONS

Drug reaction
Exacerbation of clinical signs and/or symptoms

Psychosis associated with organic brain syndrome of childhood or adolescence (Codes: DSM II 291-294)

CONCURRENT CRITERIA
Identification of patient's physical and psychosocial needs and/or concerns

Understanding of nature of impaired reality testing, inappropriate effect, and/or disordered behavior; also, definition of possible organic basis of syndrome and reversibility

Identification of child's/adolescent's (patient's) physical health

Exploration of patient's beliefs, attitudes, and expectations of own behavior and of hospitalization

Exploration of family's beliefs, attitudes, and expectations of patient and of treatment facility

Determination of chronology of patient's/family's development and coping

Recommended nursing action consistent with diagnosis
Nursing services

Initiate nursing assessment of patient, family, and community within 7 days of admission

Provide ongoing behavioral observation and assessment of patient, within 8 hours of admission, every 8 hours for a week, then during facility-defined periods (document changes)

Implement behavior-specific interventions, such as life-space interview, seclusion, suicide precautions, and behavior modification

Assist in developing and implementing after-care program and family-specific interventions

Implement and assess physical therapies, such as medications or diagnostic procedures

Health education

Explain ward procedures and milieu to patient/family

Discuss treatment goals and therapeutic modalities with patient/family

Teach family to make use of specific therapeutic modalities, including behavior modification, principles of psychodynamics, communication theories, and attitude prescription

Discuss, demonstrate, and explain about any medication

If known, discuss with family the etiology of organic brain syndrome, such as lead poisoning, drug or toxic liquid ingestion, or posttraumatic reaction

Indicators for discharge
Adaptation to health status

Sufficient contact with reality and decreased disordered behavior that patient no longer requires continuous hospitalization or continuous observation

Evidence of reintegration into family, community, and school

Patient/family demonstration of self-care capability in areas of medication administration, recognition of feelings, limit setting, and help seeking

Examples of community resources

Outpatient psychiatric nurse
School nurse
Visiting Nurse Association or public health nurse

Health

Decrease in disordered behavior
In contact with reality
Regular sleep pattern
No physical illness or problems

Activity

Activities appropriate for age
Reintegrated into family unit

Knowledge

Patient/family knows what treatment goals were accomplished

Patient/family knows what after-care plans have been made; understands plans and each family member's part in them

COMPLICATIONS

Adverse reactions to diagnostic or therapeutic modalities (such as procedures, drugs, or psychological or social therapies)
Exacerbation of clinical signs and/or symptoms
Failure of family and/or social support system

Psychosis in children (Code: 295.8)

CONCURRENT CRITERIA
Identification of patient's physical and psychosocial needs and/or concerns

Identification of existence of set of symptoms, including autism, symbiotic psychosis, or existence of other behavior indicating impairment of behavior, though, affect, motility, and relationships to the degree of psychosis
State of child's/adolescent's (patient's) physical health
Exploration of patient's beliefs, attitudes, and expectations of own behavior and of hospitalization
Expression of family's beliefs, attitudes, and expectations of patient and of treatment facility
Determination of chronology of patient's/family's development and coping

Recommended nursing action consistent with diagnosis
Nursing services

Initiate nursing assessment of patient, family, and community within 7 days of admission
Maintain ongoing behavioral observation and assessment of patient within 8 hours of admission, every 8 hours for a week, then during facility-defined periods (document changes)
Implement behavior-specific interventions, such as life-space interview,

seclusion, suicide precautions, and behavior modification
Assist in developing and implementing after-care program and family-specific interventions
Implement and assess physical therapies, such as medications or diagnostic procedures

Health education

Explain ward procedures and milieu to patient/family
Discuss treatment goals and therapeutic modalities with patient/family
Teach family to make use of specific therapeutic modalities, such as behavior modification, principles of psychodynamics, communication theories, or attitude prescription
Discuss, demonstrate, and explain about any medications

Indicators for discharge
Adaptation to health status

Evidence of beginning or sufficient contact with reality that continuous hospitalization is no longer required
Evidence of reintegration into family, community, and school
Patient/family demonstration of self-care capability in areas of medication administration, recognition of feelings, limit setting, and help seeking

Examples of community resources

Outpatient psychiatric nurse
School nurse
Visiting Nurse Association or public health nurse

RETROSPECTIVE CRITERIA
Health

Impaired behavior alleviated
No physical illness or problems
Regular sleep pattern

Activity

Activities appropriate for age
Independent in activities of daily living
Interaction with peers and adults as appropriate for age

Knowledge

Patient/family knows what treatment goals were accomplished
Patient/family knows what after-care plans have been made; understands participation of each family member in plans

COMPLICATIONS

Adverse reactions to diagnostic or therapeutic modalities (such as procedures, drugs, or psychological or social therapies)
Exacerbation of clinical signs and/or symptoms
Failure of family and/or social support system

Psychosis, depressive (Codes: 296.1, 296.2, 296.34)

CONCURRENT REVIEW CRITERIA
Identification of patient's physical and psychosocial needs and/or concerns

Relief of psychosis, loss of confidence and self-esteem, especially after discharge
Readjustment of personal relationships and reestablishment of social and economic aspects of life; clarification of precipitating causes
Measures to strengthen personality
Fears related to social stigma of emotional illness, concern regarding treatment (such as electroconvulsive therapy), or concern for significant others, loss of time from employment or school, and role changes

Recommended nursing action consistent with diagnosis
Nursing services

Closely observe patient's behavior for indications of danger to self, others, or property
Closely observe for tolerance to medication
Closely observe for memory loss and/or confusion resulting from electroconvulsive therapy
Frequently interact with patient to encourage verbal expression of feelings
Recommend treatment plan

Health education

Inform patient and significant others of treatment plan and realistic expectations of the plan
Assist patient and significant others in developing healthy and helpful interactions with each other

Indicators for discharge
Adaptation to health status

Absence of symptoms and/or problems that necessitated admission
Understanding of own illness, indicated treatment, and treatment goals
Completion of plan for posthospital care
Progress toward specific treatment goals

Examples of community resources

Outpatient psychiatric nurse
Visiting Nurse Association or public health nurse

RETROSPECTIVE REVIEW CRITERIA
Health

Personality strengthened

Decrease in verbalization of somatic complaints, such as headaches, nausea, vomiting, or fatigue

Regularity of sleep pattern, with 6 to 8 hours of uninterrupted sleep each night

Activity

Performing activities of daily living

Setting goals and making plans for achieving them

Interacting in one-to-one and group relationships

Improving nutrition, as evidenced by eating and retaining prescribed diet

Knowledge

Patient verbalizes understanding that nonverbal behavior should confirm verbal expressions of feelings

Patient verbalizes understanding of the signs and symptoms of remission and when to report to the physician

Patient verbalizes understanding of instructions for taking medications, signs and symptoms of untoward reactions, and the need to report these to the physician

COMPLICATIONS

Attempted suicide

Complications of electroconvulsive therapy, such as memory loss and/or confusion

Drug reaction

Psychosis, other (acute confusional state of adolescence)
(Code: DSM II 298.2)

CONCURRENT CRITERIA
Identification of patient's physical and psychosocial needs and/or concerns

Identification of confusion of psychotic proportions, such that adolescent (patient) is acute danger to self/others

State of patient's physical health

Exploration of patient's beliefs, attitudes, and expectations of own behavior and of hospitalization

Exploration of family's beliefs, attitudes, and expectations of patient and of treatment facility

Determination of chronology of patient's/family's development and coping

Recommended nursing action consistent with diagnosis
Nursing services

Implement nursing assessment of patient, family, and community within 7 days of admission

Maintain ongoing behavioral observation and assessment of patient within 8 hours of admission, every 8 hours for a week, then during facility-defined periods (with documentation of changes)

Implement behavior-specific interventions, such as life-space interview, seclusion, suicide precaution, and behavior modification

Assist in developing and implementing after-care program and family-specific interventions

Implement and assess physical therapies, such as medications or treatment procedures

Health education

Explain ward procedures and milieu to patient/family

Discuss treatment goals and therapeutic modalities with patient/family

Teach family to make use of specific therapeutic modalities, such as behavior modification, principles of psychodynamics, communication theories, and attitude prescription

Discuss, demonstrate, and explain about
any medication

Indicators for discharge
Adaptation to health status

Sufficient contact with reality that living
with family is possible

Evidence of reintegration into family,
community, and school

Patient/family demonstrates self-care capability in areas of medicine administration, recognition of feelings, limit
setting, and help seeking

Examples of community resources

Outpatient psychiatric nurse
School nurse
Visiting Nurse Association or public
health nurse

RETROSPECTIVE CRITERIA
Health

Psychotic behavior controlled
No physical illness or problems
Regular sleep pattern

Activity

Interaction with peers and adults as
appropriate for age
Activities appropriate for age
Independent in activities of daily living

Knowledge

Patient/family knows what treatment
goals were accomplished
Patient/family knows what after-care
plans have been made; understands
plans and each family member's part in
them

COMPLICATIONS

Adverse reaction to diagnostic or therapeutic modalities (procedures, drugs, or
psychological or social therapies)
Exacerbation of clinical signs and/or
symptoms
Failure of family and/or social support
system

Purpura, thrombocytopenic (Code: 287.1)

CONCURRENT CRITERIA
Identification of patient's physical and psychosocial needs and/or concerns

Relief of symptoms, including petechiae,
epistaxis, bleeding gums, vaginal
bleeding, gastrointestinal bleeding, hematuria, and/or easy bruising
Explanation of disease process, treatment, course, medical and nursing
management, duration of hospitalization, and expected outcome of care
Feeling of hopelessness; fear of change in
life-style and loss of time from normal
activities
Gentle contact in order to prevent
prolonged bleeding, which occurs after
minor traumas

Recommended nursing action consistent with diagnosis
Nursing services

Make systematic observations to assist in
identifying etiology, presence of hemorrhage, and presence of potential
trauma
Give psychological support for expression of feelings of helplessness and for
concern about change in body image
and loss of time from normal activities
Provide bed rest and prevention of
trauma
Implement oral hygiene before and after
meals to decrease incidence of bleeding
gums

Measure intake and output for maintenance of electrolyte balance

Administer steroid therapy; explain possible side effects and the need to avoid suddenly stopping steroids without physician's order

Health education

Instruct about the name, purpose, dosage, frequency, side effects to report to physician, and medical alert information of each medication

Explain disease process, cause, and treatment; medical and nursing management; steroid therapy or splenectomy; and symptoms to report to physician

Stress importance of a safe environment; instruct about measures to avoid trauma, such as not participating in contact sports, not having elective surgery or tooth extractions, not being exposed to potential toxins, and not taking unnecessary medications

Teach patient/family to develop a lifestyle that maximizes safety and permits productivity

Indicators for discharge
Adaptation to health status

Hemorrhage ceased
Cause of bleeding identified
Blood count stable
Mental status improved
Health teaching completed
Environment evaluated for safety

Examples of community resources

Visiting Nurse Association or public health nurse
Vocational rehabilitation center

RETROSPECTIVE CRITERIA
Health

Platelet count rising
Bleeding stopped or controlled
Feelings of hopelessness resolved or improving

Activity

Ambulatory
Performs activities of daily living with minimal assistance

Knowledge

Understands and can verbalize medication instructions, disease process, methods by which to avoid trauma, safety precautions, and observations to report to physician

COMPLICATIONS

Drug reaction
Hemorrhage, such as cerebral, nasal, gastrointestinal, or urinary tract
Paralysis from pressure of hematoma on nerve tissue
Shock
Splenectomy*

---

*If condition surgically treated, criteria set must be modified for splenectomy.

Pyloric stenosis, congenital hypertrophic (Code: 750.1)

CONCURRENT CRITERIA
Identification of patient's physical and psychosocial needs and/or concerns

Relief of condition, vomiting, and malnutrition

Provision of adequate nutritional intake

Reestablishment of fluid and electrolyte balance

Proper positioning to lessen occurrence of vomiting and to prevent aspiration

Understanding by parents of condition, cause, course, prognosis, medical and nursing management, and discharge care

Recommended nursing action consistent with diagnosis
Nursing services

Monitor intravenous fluids given to restore hydration and to correct hypokalemic alkalosis

Observe, record, and report symptoms of dehydration by monitoring skin turgor and urine and stool output

Position infant on right side or abdomen to facilitate emptying of stomach; elevate head after feeding to prevent aspiration of mucus or emesis

Weigh daily to ascertain degree of dehydration and malnutrition

Avoid excessive handling of infant to minimize vomiting

Physically prepare infant for surgery; explain surgery to parents

Health education

Explain feeding schedule and proper feeding technique, such as slow, careful feeding, frequent burping, and proper positioning of infant after feeding; instruct on dietary needs

Explain need to avoid excessive handling, but teach careful handling to meet emotional needs of infant

Explain importance of reporting excessive vomiting to physician

Instruct on home care of incision, if applicable

Psychologically prepare parents for infant's surgery by explaining all procedures and equipment

Indicators for discharge
Adaptation to health status

Tolerating diet for age

Absence of wound complications

Wound healing

Stable weight status

Afebrile

Examples of community resources

Visiting Nurse Association or public health nurse, if additional teaching required

RETROSPECTIVE CRITERIA
Health

Afebrile

Tolerating feedings

Wound healing

Stable weight status

Complications not evident

Activity

Normal infant activity

Knowledge

Parents understand and can implement feeding techniques and dietary needs

Parents can implement home care for incision, if applicable

COMPLICATIONS

Dehydration from malnutrition

Electrolyte imbalance

Hemorrhage

Operative perforation of duodenum

Pneumonia

Wound infection

Radiculopathies and herniated lumbar disc (Code: 725)

CONCURRENT CRITERIA

Identification of patient's physical and psychosocial needs and/or concerns

Relief of symptoms, including intractable pain or paralysis and possibly sensory disturbances, such as tactile or temperature

Understanding of diagnostic and therapeutic medical or surgical procedures, special care units, specific after-care, and purpose and expected outcome of procedures

Concern over absence from work and decreased independence

Understanding of measures to prevent or avoid recurrence of injury

Understanding of community agencies available for assistance during convalescent period

Recommended nursing action consistent with diagnosis

Nursing services

Implement comfort measures, including applying heat to area according to prescribed intervals, positioning as recommended by physician (semi-Fowler's or prone position), changing position from side to side by log-roll technique; using child's or fracture bedpan to decrease discomfort during elimination, avoiding use of trapeze, administering analgesics, providing diversional therapy, and using waking-imagined analgesics; massaging is not generally recommended because of stimulation of muscle spasms

Reduce discouragement and fear of increased dependence or possible future surgery

Prevent footdrop or problems related to immobility, including thrombophlebitis, hypostatic pneumonia, decubitus ulcers, anorexia, urinary infection, and dehydration

Observe for therapeutic and side effects

of medications, with prompt nursing intervention should side effects occur

Apply supportive devices (braces or corsets) for ambulation

Maintain proper traction (such as Buck's extension) by positioning and by assuring that weights hang free

Provide preoperative nursing care, teaching, and psychological and physical preparation of patient undergoing a laminectomy or a spinal fusion

Implement postoperative nursing care, including closely observing for physical deterioration or change in condition by frequently monitoring vital signs and observing dressing or cast for evidence of excessive wound drainage, with prompt nursing intervention should signs of shock or excessive bleeding occur

Implement comfort measures, including proper techniques in turning patient, using sufficient personnel to avoid twisting or piecemeal turning, arching, or sagging of the hips or shoulders; using log-roll technique in turning, providing proper support of legs and back in turning; administering analgesics half an hour prior to turning procedure, if possible; administering muscle relaxants; using diversional techniques for pain relief; and ensuring proper rest periods

Ensure adequate elimination

Assist in rehabilitation, including exercises for maintaining muscle tone in feet, quadriceps setting, flexion and extension of knees, and application of brace for ambulation

Health education

Instruct about the name, dosage, purpose, frequency, side effects, action to take should side effects occur, and precautions of each discharge medication

Explain application of brace

Identify therapeutic and restricted activities

Teach body mechanics to prevent future back injury

Explain community agencies available to assist during convalescent period

Indicators for discharge
Adaptation to health status

Pain controlled
Condition stable
Complications not evident
Referrals completed

Examples of community resources

Social services
Visiting Nurse Association or public health nurse

RETROSPECTIVE CRITERIA
Health

Wound healing
Mentally accepting condition
Symptoms relieved or improved
Complications not evident

Activity

Ambulatory and able to apply prosthetic device (brace or corset) by self correctly

Implements rehabilitative measures, especially use of body mechanics

Knowledge

Understands and knows name of discharge medications, purpose, dosage, frequency, side effects, action to take if side effects occur, and precautions

Understands therapeutic activity and restricted activity

Understands and can carry out proper body mechanics

Understands community agencies available for assistance

COMPLICATIONS

Hemorrhage
Paralysis
Persistent fever
Pulmonary embolism
Shock
Thrombophlebitis
Wound infection

Renal failure in children (Codes: 403, 585, 585.1, 586.2)

CONCURRENT CRITERIA
Identification of patient's physical and psychosocial needs and/or concerns

Relief of symptoms, including sudden onset of oliguria, proteinuria, hematuria, anorexia, nausea, vomiting, lethargy, and/or elevated blood pressure

Play therapy and/or diversional activities to help child adjust to hospitalization

Restricted fluid intake

Provision of aseptic environment or reverse isolation to prevent infections

Emotional support for parents/child with explanation of medical and nursing management

Recommended nursing action consistent with diagnosis
Nursing services

Strictly monitor intake and output

Observe for changes in physiological responses, including blood pressure, hematuria, oliguria, proteinuria, nausea, vomiting, diarrhea, or fluctuations in weight

Provide emotional support to parents/child concerning condition and treatments

Adjust fluid intake to provide only for body's needs during oliguric stage

Promote clean environment and restrict

visits from persons with known infections

Health education

Instruct on diet restrictions of nitrogen, potassium, phosphate, sulfate, and protein

Explain allowed and restricted activities

Instruct on the name, purpose, dosage, frequency, side effects, and action to initiate if side effects occur of each medication

Explain medication methods to evaluate renal function and signs and/or symptoms of decreased renal function

Indicators for discharge
Adaptation to health status

Controlled hypertension

Normal urinary output

Stable condition

Patient coping with changed body image

Acceptance of diet restrictions

Examples of community resources

Visiting Nurse Association or public health nurse

RETROSPECTIVE CRITERIA
Health

Mentally accepting condition and change in body image

Controlled hypertension

Adequate urinary output or maintenance on dialysis

Stable condition

Complications not evident

Activity

Ambulatory

Independent in activities of daily living appropriate for age

Knowledge

Parents/child understands and can implement proper diet

Parents/child knows restricted and allowed activities

Parents know medication schedule

Parents can implement care of shunt, if child is on dialysis

Parents/child aware of possible change in feelings about body image and provision for necessary emotional support

COMPLICATIONS

Anemia

Congestive heart failure

Encephalopathy

Hypertension

Potassium intoxication

Pulmonary edema

Sepsis

Uremia

Water intoxication

Respiratory infections, group, in children

Bronchitis (Codes: 464, 464.1, 489, 590)
Pneumonia (Codes: 480-486)
Upper respiratory infections (Codes: 460, 465)

CONCURRENT CRITERIA
Identification of patient's physical and psychosocial needs and/or concerns

Relief of symptoms, including chills, fever, productive cough, chest pain exaggerated by respiration, tachypnea, and dehydration

Ventilation and oxygenation of lungs

Increased hydration to help liquefy secretions and maintain output

Control of pain

Psychological support for fear of not being able to breathe

Child/parents adjustment to hospitalization and disease process

Recommended nursing action consistent with diagnosis
Nursing services

Monitor respiratory status every 2 hours, vital signs, breath sounds, skin color and turgor, and respiratory difficulty; administer oxygen for severe cyanosis or marked dyspnea; supervise intermittent positive pressure breathing treatment, as ordered, postural drainage, and suction or aspiration of mucus with bulb syringe; evaluate sputum

Force fluids with between meal feedings to 2 liters per day

Administer medication; observe for reactions to antibiotic therapy

Provide psychological support to child/ parents for adjustment to hospital environment; provide diversional activities; aid in planning for postdischarge care

Turn and position child every 2 hours to allow maximum respiratory expansion; gently clean around nostrils to prevent excoriation; use cool liquids, gargle solution, or throat lozenges to relieve throat soreness

Health education

Instruct on the name, dosage, frequency, purpose, duration, and side effects to report to physician of each medication

Explain about disease process, treatment, course, medical and nursing management, and symptoms to report to physician

Explain function and importance of Croupette or vaporizer in providing adequate humidification

Instruct about importance of maintaining good nutritional status as one means of preventing upper respiratory infections

Teach about methods of preventing spread of respiratory diseases, such as covering mouth when coughing, using disposable tissues, disposing of sputum

Explain methods to implement to avoid recurrence of disease, such as keeping warm, not being chilled, avoiding contact with other persons with respiratory diseases, preventing fatigue, and increasing moisture in environment, especially in bedroom

Indicators for discharge
Adaptation to health status

Afebrile

Symptoms resolved or controlled

Ambulatory without respiratory distress or fatigue

Complications not evident

Health teaching completed

Examples of community resources

Visiting Nurse Association or public health nurse

RETROSPECTIVE CRITERIA
Health

Afebrile

Hydrated

Clear, unlabored respiration for 24 hours prior to discharge

Regular sleep pattern

Activity

Minimal assistance with activities of daily living

Planned rest periods to prevent fatigue

Knowledge

Child/parents understand and can verbalize medication instructions, disease process, humidification needs, nutritional instructions, methods to prevent spread of respiratory diseases, means to avoid recurrence, and symptoms to report to physician

COMPLICATIONS

Atelectasis

Dehydration

Drug reaction

Otitis media from upper respiratory infection

Pleural effusion

Pneumonia from upper respiratory infection

Respiratory obstruction

Secondary infection

Septicemia

Rheumatic fever, acute, in children (Codes: 390-392)

CONCURRENT CRITERIA
Identification of patient's physical and psychosocial needs and/or concerns

Relief of symptoms, including carditis, Sydenham's chorea, subcutaneous nodules, erythema marginatum, polyarthritis, fever, malaise, weight loss, anorexia, abdominal pain, recurrent epistaxis, and "growing pains" in joints

Bed rest

Anxiety about restriction of activities; fear of permanent physical impairment; adjustment to change in life-style; fear of death

Understanding of nature of disorder; disease process, course, and prognosis; medical and nursing management; prevention of recurrence

Control of pain

Psychological support for parents/patient

Recommended nursing action consistent with diagnosis
Nursing services

Enforce bed rest during acute phase; provide quiet diversional activities

Monitor physiological responses, including temperature, apical resting pulse, respiratory rate, weight, nutrition, elimination, hydration, presence of infections, skin integrity, oral mucous membranes, joint function and motion, and pain

Maintain proper positioning and body alignment

Provide nursing care without increasing child's fatigue

Provide psychological support to child/parents regarding disease process, restriction of activities, home care, continuation of schoolwork, fears, and/or concerns

Initiate referrals for continuation of care after discharge

Administer medication; observe for effects, both desirable and undesirable, of medication

Health education

Explain disease process, course, prognosis, medical and nursing management, symptoms to report to physician, and necessity of follow-up medical supervision

Instruct on the name, purpose, dosage, frequency, duration, side effects to report to physician of each medication; if steroids ordered, stress importance of not discontinuing suddenly

Instruct in measures to prevent recurrent rheumatic fever by avoiding persons having upper respiratory infections or sore throats; in prophylactic antibiotic therapy, and in the need for prompt therapy within 24 hours of streptococcal infections

Explain activity restrictions; stress importance of planned rest periods, gradual resumption of activities, and avoidance of excessive physical exertion

Teach principles of maintaining good nutrition and providing appetizing meals

Indicators for discharge
Adaptation to health status

Active disease process controlled

Complications not evident

Health teaching completed

Referrals made

Examples of community resources

Teacher for homebound child

Visiting Nurse Association or public health nurse

RETROSPECTIVE CRITERIA
Health

Temperature 98.6° F

Sedimentation rate decreased

Resting pulse rate under 100 beats per minute

Electrocardiogram normal or abnormalities fixated

Nutritional state maintained or improving

Complications not evident

Activity

Maximum assistance with activities of daily living available

Ambulation limited

All activities restricted

Diversional activities to maintain quiet environment; prevent fatigue

Knowledge

Child/parents understand and can verbalize medication instructions, disease process, symptoms to report to physician, prevention of recurrence, nutrition instructions, community agencies available to assist with discharge care, and activity restrictions

COMPLICATIONS

Cardiac arrhythmias
Cardiac invalidism
Congestive heart failure
Myocardial infarction
Pericarditis
Permanent heart valve deformity
Pulmonary embolism
Rheumatic pneumonitis

Schizophrenia (Codes: 295-295.7, 295.9)

CONCURRENT CRITERIA
Identification of patient's physical and psychosocial needs and/or concerns

Relief or control of symptoms, including inappropriate responses in thinking, speech, and behavior; alterations of moods; irrelevant, irrational, or delusional speech; depersonalization; delusions of grandeur or persecution; preoccupation with religion or sex; loss of logical reasoning; and flight of ideas and hallucinations

Need for protective environment

Identification of health status, including personal hygiene and nutrition

Identification of presence or absence of disordered behavior, affect, thought, or perception

Expression of attitude regarding hospitalization

Recommended nursing action consistent with diagnosis
Nursing services

Closely observe patient behavior

Provide for maintenance or improvement of health status

Administer medications to control behavior, when indicated

Perform reality testing

Make recommendations for treatment plan

Health education

Inform patient/significant other of treatment plan and realistic expectations of the plan

Assist significant other in understanding the nature of the illness and its manifestations

Indicators for discharge
Adaptation to health status

Achievement of inpatient treatment goals

Absence of admitting symptoms

Establishment of follow-up treatment plan

Transfer to another institution, such as a state hospital

Examples of community resources

Occupational therapy
Long-term psychiatric facility
Outpatient psychiatric nurse

RETROSPECTIVE CRITERIA
Health

Symptoms controlled
Absence of psychotic symptomatology
Regularity of sleep pattern

Activity

Able to perform activities of daily living
Sets goals and makes plans for achieving them
Interacting in one-to-one and group relationships

Knowledge

Patient verbalizes understanding that nonverbal behavior should confirm verbal expression of feelings

Patient/significant other verbalizes understanding of the signs and symptoms of remission and the need to report these to the physician
Patient verbalizes understanding of instructions for taking medications, signs and symptoms of untoward reactions, and the need to report these to the physician

COMPLICATIONS

Anxiety
Complication of electroconvulsive therapy
Drug reaction

Schizophrenia, adolescent type (Code : DSM II 295.8B)

CONCURRENT CRITERIA
Identification of patient's physical and psychosocial needs and/or concerns

Understanding of nature and extent of psychiatric symptoms
State of adolescent's (patient's) physical health
Exploration of patient's beliefs, attitudes, and expectations of own behavior and of hospitalization
Exploration of family's beliefs, attitudes, and expectations of patient and treatment facility
Determination of chronology of patient's/family's development and coping

Recommended nursing action consistent with diagnosis
Nursing services

Provide nursing assessment of patient, family, and community within 7 days of admission
Maintain ongoing behavioral observation and assessment of patient within 8 hours of admission every 8 hours for a week, then during facility-defined periods (document changes)

Implement behavior-specific interventions, including life-space interview, seclusion, suicide precaution, and behavior modification
Assist in developing and implementing after-care program and family-specific interventions
Implement and assess physical therapies, such as medications or diagnostic procedures

Health education

Explain ward procedures and milieu to patient/family
Discuss treatment goals and therapeutic modalities with patient/family
Teach family to make use of specific therapeutic modalities, including behavior modification, principles of psychodynamics, communication theories, or attitude prescription
Discuss, demonstrate, and explain about any medication

Indicators for discharge
Adaptation to health status

Sufficient contact with reality to function in home with family supervision

Evidence of reintegration into family, community, and school

Patient/family demonstration of self-care capability in areas of medication administration, recognition of feelings, limit setting, and help seeking

Examples of community resources

Outpatient psychiatric nurse
School nurse

RETROSPECTIVE CRITERIA
Health

Symptoms controlled
Logical reasoning and in contact with reality
No physical illness or problems

Activity

Activities appropriate for age
Reintegration into family unit

Knowledge

Patient/family knows what treatment goals were accomplished
Patient/family knows what after-care plans have been made; understands plans and each family member's part in them

COMPLICATIONS

Adverse reactions to diagnostic or therapeutic modalities (procedures, drugs, or psychological or social therapies)
Exacerbation of clinical signs and/or symptoms
Failure of family and/or social support system

Special symptoms of childhood or adolescence (Code: DSM II 306)

CONCURRENT REVIEW CRITERIA
Identification of patient's physical and psychosocial needs and/or concerns

Understanding of exact nature of child's/adolescent's (patient's) behavior (symptom) that necessitated hospitalization (primarily, potential and/or history of destructive behavior to self, others, or property)
Assessment of patient's state of physical health
Determination of patient's beliefs, attitudes, and expectations of own behavior and of hospitalization
Identification of family's attitudes, beliefs, and expectations of patient, treatment facility, and staff
Determination of chronology of patient's/family's development and coping prior to admission

Recommended nursing action consistent with diagnosis
Nursing services

Provide initial nursing assessment of patient, family, and community within 7 days of admission; give special attention to data on special symptoms, for example, speech development if speech disturbance apparent
Maintain ongoing behavioral observation and assessment within 8 hours of admission
Implement behavior-specific interventions, such as suicide precautions with self-destructive behavior or life-space interview with aggressive behavior
Assist in development and implementation of total after-care plans and family-specific interventions
Implement, assist, and evaluate physical therapies, such as drugs or diagnostic procedures

Health education

Explain ward procedures and milieu to patient/family
Discuss treatment goals and therapeutic modalities with patient/family
Teach family to make use of specific therapeutic modalities, such as principles of behavior modification, behavior

dynamics, communication theories, or attitude prescription

Explain and discuss any medication, including its action, usage, dosage, and side effects

Indicators for discharge
Adaptation to health status

Decreased incidence of special symptoms, such as decreased speech, sleep, or eating disturbances and decreased enuresis, encopresis, and cephalalgia

Evidence of reintegration into family, community, and school

Patient/family demonstration of self-care capability in areas of recognition of feelings limit setting, medication administration, and help seeking

Completion of evaluation or treatment plan; completion of outpatient care plan

Examples of community resources

Outpatient psychiatric nurse

School or public health nurse

RETROSPECTIVE CRITERIA
Health

Symptoms decreased
No physical illness or problems
Regular sleep pattern
Complications not evident

Activity

Interacting with adults and peers
Activities appropriate for age
Independent in activities of daily living

Knowledge

Patient/family knows what treatment goals were accomplished

Patient/family knows what after-care plans have been made; understands plans and each family member's role in them

COMPLICATIONS

Adverse reactions to diagnostic or therapeutic modalities (procedures, drugs, or psychological or social therapies)

Exacerbation of clinical signs and/or symptoms

Failure of family and/or social support system

Spinal cord injury or disease, cervical, with quadriplegia
(Codes: 349.4, 806, 806.1, 958, 958.9)

CONCURRENT REVIEW CRITERIA
Identification of patient's physical and psychosocial needs and/or concerns

Adaptation to quadriplegia and activities of daily living

Control of sensory deficits, bladder and bowel dysfunctions, and potential respiratory dysfunction

Adaptation and counseling for social, vocational, recreational, and sexual needs

Emotional support

Maintenance of nutritional needs and skin care; prevention of complications

Relief from pain and spasticity

Recommended nursing action consistent with diagnosis
Nursing services

Change patient's position every 2 hours; force fluids

Instigate passive range-of-motion exercises every 6 hours

Inspect skin and massage bony prominences every 2 hours

Establish bowel program (daily or every 2 to 3 days) and bladder program (every 3 to 4 hours)

Implement activities of daily living program for self-care with or without assistance and/or assistive devices (to include transferring, dressing, hygiene, feeding, and ambulation)

Provide counseling session focusing on sexual, social, vocational, and recreational needs

Identify pattern of pain and/or spasticity; establish protocol for nursing intervention

Monitor breathing patterns at rest and following exercise; utilize optimum ventilatory techniques to assist respiration

Health education

Teach patient activities of daily living program and use of assistive devices

Teach patient necessity and methods of examining skin for decubitus ulcers; teach prevention and treatment of decubitus ulcers

Teach patient food selection and meal planning to maintain adequate nutrition and fluid balance

Teach patient bowel and bladder programs and where to purchase supplies

Teach patient ventilatory techniques to enhance respiration

Indicators for discharge
Adaptation to health status

Patient's self-care goals attained

Social, vocational, and recreational activities planned

Bowel and bladder programs functional

Home care implemented or provided for by patient/family

Physical and emotional conditions stabilized; complications absent or resolved

Examples of community resources

Visiting Nurse Association or public health nurse

Vocational rehabilitation counselor

Physical rehabilitation center

RETROSPECTIVE REVIEW CRITERIA
Health

Physical and emotional condition stabilized; complications absent or resolved

Bowel and bladder programs functional

Activity

Activities of daily living, self-care, and ambulation programs performed with or without assistance and/or assistive devices

Home care program instigated

Knowledge

Understands and can implement skin inspection technique and decubitus ulcer prevention

Understands prevention of urinary or respiratory infections

Knows and can provide adequate types and quantities of food and fluids

COMPLICATIONS

Acute chest pain
Altered sex role
Decubitus ulcers
Fever
Joint contractures
Kidney stones
Osteoporosis and/or fractures
Painful, swollen calf
Pulmonary embolism
Thrombophlebitis
Urinary tract infection

Spinal cord injury or disease, dorsal or lumbar, with paraplegia
(Codes: 806.2-806.5, 958.1, 958.2, 958.9)

CONCURRENT REVIEW CRITERIA
Identification of patient's physical and psychosocial needs and/or concerns

Adaptation to paraplegia and activities of daily living

Control of sensory deficits, and bladder and bowel dysfunctions

Adaptation and counseling for social, vocational, recreational, and sexual needs

Emotional support

Maintenance of nutritional needs and skin care

Mobility

Relief from pain and spasticity

Prevention of medical problems, including urinary tract infections, osteoporosis and/or fractures, spinal shock, or orthostatic hypotension

Recommended nursing action consistent with diagnosis
Nursing services

Change patient's position every 2 hours

Instigate range-of-motion exercises every 6 hours, with passive ones for affected joints and active ones for unaffected joints, and muscle-strengthening exercises every 8 hours

Inspect skin and massage bony prominences every 2 hours

Implement a progressive ambulation program and an activities of daily living program (to include dressing, hygiene, feeding, transferring, and wheelchair use)

Provide counseling sessions focusing on sexual, social, vocational, and recreational needs

Establish bladder program (every 3 to 4 hours during waking hours) and bowel program (daily or every 2 to 3 days)

Identify pattern of pain and/or spasticity; establish protocol for nursing intervention

Health education

Teach patient activities of daily living program and use of assistive devices

Teach patient necessity and methods of examining skin for decubitus ulcers; teach prevention and treatment of decubitus ulcers

Teach patient food selection and meal planning to maintain adequate nutrition and fluid balance

Teach patient bowel and bladder programs and where to purchase supplies

Indicators for discharge
Adaptation to health status

Patient's activities of daily living and ambulation programs attained

Social, vocational, and recreational activities planned

Bowel and bladder programs functional

Home care implemented or provided for by patient/family

Physical and emotional conditions stabilized; complications absent or resolved

Examples of community resources

Vocational rehabilitation counselor

Visiting Nurse Association or public health nurse

Physical rehabilitation center

RETROSPECTIVE REVIEW CRITERIA
Health

Physical and emotional conditions stabilized; complications absent or resolved

Bowel and bladder programs functional

Activity

Activities of daily living, self-care, and ambulation programs performed with or without assistive devices

Knowledge

Knows and can provide adequate types and quantities of food and fluids

Understands and can implement skin inspection technique and decubitus ulcer prevention

Understands self-care program and modified methods of mobility

COMPLICATIONS

Acute chest pain

Altered sex role

Decubitus ulcers

Fever

Joint contractures

Kidney stones

Orthostatic hypotension

Osteoporosis and/or fractures

Painful, swollen calf

Pulmonary embolism

Spinal shock

Thrombophlebitis

Urinary tract infection

Sterilization, female, surgical, for family planning, elective (Code: 13)

CONCURRENT REVIEW CRITERIA
Identification of patient's physical and psychosocial needs and/or concerns

Relief from physical or psychosocial stresses imposed by future pregnancies

Understanding of surgical procedures and implication of same as related to childbearing

Assistance in coping with change in body image

Concern about changes in femininity and sexual image as result of surgery

Preventive measures against problems related to immobility

Recommended nursing action consistent with diagnosis
Nursing services

Provide preoperative care and patient teaching, including explanation of surgical procedure, recovery room, intravenous equipment, dressings, expected duration of hospitalization, deep-breathing and coughing exercises, presence of any discharge, and therapeutic and restricted exercises; validate *informed consent* for operation; physically prepare patient for surgery

Implement postoperative nursing care, including maintaining adequate hydration, nutrition, and elimination; reducing pain; and preventing problems from decreased activity

Provide emotional support measures to aid patient in dealing with change in body image

Health education

Teach the name, dosage, purpose, frequency, side effects, action to take if side effects occur, and precautions of each discharge medication

Instruct patient regarding therapeutic and restricted activities

Instruct patient on proper wound care, if any is necessary

Instruct patient when and why it is necessary to return for medical follow-up care

Indicators for discharge
Adaptation to health status

Condition stable

Wound healing

Complications not evident

Health teaching completed

Referrals made

Examples of community resources

Surgical clinic

Social services

Health

Condition stable
Wound healing
Complications not evident

Activity

Ambulatory
Able to implement proper wound care, if any is necessary

Knowledge

Knows the name, purpose, dosage, frequency, side effects, action to take if side effects occur, and precautions of each discharge medication
Understands and can implement necessary wound care
Understands therapeutic and restricted activities and can implement therapeutic ones
Knows when and why it is necessary to return to the clinic or physician's office for follow-up medical care

COMPLICATIONS

Arrhythmias
Atelectasis
Decubitus ulcers
Drug reaction
Hemorrhage
Pneumonia
Pulmonary embolism
Temperature of 100° F or over
Thrombophlebitis
Urinary incontinence
Urinary retention
Urinary tract infection
Wound infection

Tendon injuries (Codes: 731-731.9)

CONCURRENT CRITERIA
Identification of patient's physical and psychosocial needs and/or concerns

Relief from pain and disability
Understanding of medical and/or surgical treatment and nursing management, so that realistic plans for health maintenance after discharge can be made
Concern over loss of time from work or school and over loss of independence
Rehabilitative measures to regain functioning ability
Preventive measures as related to problems from immobility, depending on area of involvement

Recommended nursing action consistent with diagnosis
Nursing services

Implement nursing measures consistent with medical management, including pain-reducing measures such as elevation of the affected part, application of heat or cold as prescribed, application of elastic bandages or adhesive, and administration of analgesics, sedatives, hypnotics, or tranquilizers and adequate hydration, nutrition, elimination, and rest
Provide preoperative nursing care and teaching, including explaining surgical procedure, recovery room, expected duration of hospitalization, possibility of use of plaster casts or splints, possibility of use of brace; instruct on and demonstrate crutchwalking or use of walker, as may be appropriate, and deep-breathing and coughing exercises; explain postoperative pain-reducing measures that will be used; physically prepare patient for surgery
Implement postoperative nursing care, including wound care and cast care, if cast or splint is used; prevent problems caused by immobility; closely observe for circulatory impairment as related to casts, splints, or compression dressings; provide prompt nursing interven-

tion should circulatory impairment occur

Closely observe for signs of physical deterioration, such as shock, excessive bleeding, respiratory difficulty, or changes in mental status; provide prompt nursing intervention should any complications occur

Implement measures to assist the patient in using crutches, braces, or walker properly and safely

Supervise prescribed exercises as well as exercises of unaffected extremities to maintain strength and function and to prevent problems resulting from immobility

Initiate appropriate referrals

Health education

Instruct on measures to reduce pain and to promote rest

Instruct on safety measures and measures designed to prevent accidents

Teach cast care, if the patient is discharged with a cast, including signs and symptoms of circulatory impairment and appropriate action to take

Instruct on application of braces, Ace bandages, and splints and on use of crutches

Explain the name, dosage, purpose, frequency, side effects, action to take if side effects occur, and precautions concerning each discharge medication

Advise when and why it is necessary to return to physician's office or clinic for follow-up medical care

Instruct on therapeutic and restricted activities

Indicators for discharge
Adaptation to health status

Condition stable
Complications not evident
Health teaching completed
Referrals made

Examples of community resources

Visiting Nurse Association or public health nurse

Physiotherapy clinic or orthopedic clinic
Social services

RETROSPECTIVE CRITERIA
Health

Pain relieved or controlled
Wound healing
Mentally adjusting to change in body image and increased dependency
Complications not evident

Activity

Ambulatory with assistive devices
Able to apply and use braces, compression bandages, splints, crutches, and walker correctly and safely

Knowledge

Knows the name of each discharge medications; understands the purpose, dosage, frequency, side effects, action to take if side effects occur, and precautions of each

Understands therapeutic and restricted activities and can implement therapeutic ones

Understands and can implement pain-reducing measures and measures to promote rest

Understands and can implement cast care

Understands and can implement safety measures

Understands when and why it is necessary to return to physician's office or clinic for follow-up medical care

Understands and can implement any necessary wound care

COMPLICATIONS

Arrhythmias
Atelectasis
Decubitus ulcers
Drug reaction
Hemorrhage
Joint contractures
Pneumonia
Pulmonary embolism
Shock
Temperature of 100° F or over at time of discharge

Thrombophlebitis
Urinary incontinence
Urinary retention
Urinary tract infection
Wound infection

Testicle, undescended, orchiopexy for (Code: 752.1)

CONCURRENT REVIEW CRITERIA
Identification of patient's physical and psychosocial needs and/or concerns

Promotion of adequate urinary output (800 to 1,000 ml per 24 hours)
Promotion of wound healing and care of suture line
Education regarding operative procedure and minor, postoperative limitation in activity
Fear of genital mutilation
Adaptation to hospitalization

Recommended nursing action consistent with diagnosis
Nursing services

Force fluids (or monitor intravenous fluids) to ensure output of 800 to 1,000 ml per 24 hours
Observe and record condition of suture line every 4 to 8 hours: observe for signs of infection
Check tension mechanism (traction suture) to be certain it remains intact (for approximately 7 days postoperatively)
Provide thorough cleansing of genital area after voiding or defecation
Provide appropriate play therapy (such as clay, materials with which to draw, and puppets) to aid patient in expression of mutilation fears as well as to aid in adaptation to hospital environment

Health education

Instruct patient/parents in methods by which to cleanse genital area after elimination
Instruct patient/parents on reasons for traction suture and need for this tension mechanism to remain intact at all times
Instruct parents regarding normalcy of mutilation fears with this type of surgery and with various age groups

Indicators for discharge
Adaptation to health status

Afebrile
Vital signs stable
Wound healing
Patient/parent education regarding postoperative care completed
Food and fluids being tolerated
Normal activities for age and developmental level being resumed

Examples of community resources

Visiting Nurse Association or public health nurse
Psychiatric social worker, if mutilation fears are intense and unresolved

RETROSPECTIVE REVIEW CRITERIA
Health

Mentally accepting surgical invasion of body
Afebrile
Wound healing

Activity

Alert
Movement not limited

Knowledge

Patient/parents understand ways to promote wound healing
Patients/parents understand normalcy of mutilation fears

COMPLICATIONS
Parents' fears regarding possible sterility
of patient
Unresolved fears of mutilation
Wound infection

Thrombophlebitis (Codes: 451, 451.1)

CONCURRENT CRITERIA
Identification of patient's physical and psychosocial needs and/or concerns

Adaptation to immobility
Relief from pain, heaviness of extremities, and edema
Adjustment to alteration in appearance
Fear of embolism formation
Explanation of nature, course, prognosis, and management of condition and involvement in care

Recommended nursing action consistent with diagnosis
Nursing services

Elevate lower extremities
Apply moist heat packs until inflammatory process subsides
Reassure and support patient in adaptation to condition
Observe for any proximal progression of inflammatory process; report immediately if any evident
Maintain constant relationship between time of administration of anticoagulant and time of laboratory tests for coagulation activity
Provide elastic stockings as indicated (for example, while edema is present postoperatively)

Health education

Explain walking as a preferred activity (postoperatively and prophylactically)
Teach avoidance of constricting clothing (such as garters) above the knees
Explain purpose and teach application of elastic stockings
Explain the purpose, dosage, and untoward effects of anticoagulant medication
Explain predisposing factors (such as obesity, prolonged bed rest, or pregnancy)

Indicators for discharge
Adaptation to health status

Patient purposely avoids placing legs in dependent positions for extended periods of time
Patient ambulates without pain in legs
Patient demonstrates knowledge of the purpose, dosage, and untoward effects of anticoagulant medication
Patient/family member demonstrates correct application of elastic stockings

Examples of community resources

Referral usually not indicated

RETROSPECTIVE CRITERIA
Health

Stabilized on anticoagulant medication
No inflammatory process evident

Activity

Ambulatory without pain
Applies elastic stockings

Knowledge

Knows to avoid constrictive clothing
Knows to avoid placing legs in dependent positions
Knows the purpose, dosage, and untoward effects of anticoagulant medication

Understands purpose and can implement application of elastic stockings

COMPLICATIONS

Drug reaction, side effects of anticoagulant medication

Massive lower extremity edema
Pulmonary embolism
Skin necrosis

Thrombosis of abdominal aorta and/or arteries of lower extremities, acute (Code: 444)

CONCURRENT CRITERIA
Identification of patient's physical and psychosocial needs and/or concerns

Relief from pain
Adaptation to sudden change to more dependent status
Fear of loss of limbs or of death
Fear of diagnostic procedures

Recommended nursing action consistent with diagnosis
Nursing services

Check for changes in peripheral pulses and ischemia demarcation line hourly; report within 5 minutes if problem evident
Relieve pain, using narcotics for symptoms and papaverine for arterial spasms
Maintain room temperature at a constant 78° to 80° F
Implement use of foot cradle

Health education

Teach foot care with return demonstration
Explain the purpose of anticoagulation medication
Explain diagnostic and operative procedures, including sensations to be experienced
Discuss potential for mobility, where amputation has occurred
Explain postsympathectomy neuralgia of buttocks and thighs, if applicable

Indicators for discharge
Adaptation to health status

Satisfactory return demonstration of foot care
Demonstration of reliability in self-administration of anticoagulant medication
Image change accepted by patient/family

Examples of community resources

Visiting Nurse Association for adaptation assistance in home

RETROSPECTIVE CRITERIA
Health

Extremity pain absent
Urine output at or above admission levels

Activity

Ambulatory

Knowledge

Patient demonstrates knowledge of foot care; stump care, where applicable; crutchwalking, where applicable; and medication regime and effects

COMPLICATIONS

Changes in vascular bed size
Drug reaction
Gangrene of extremity
Persistent edema

Tonsillectomy and adenoidectomy in children (Codes: 28, 463, 500, 501, 502)

CONCURRENT CRITERIA
Identification of patient's physical and psychosocial needs and/or concerns

Relief of recurrent acute or chronic infections, snoring and mouth breathing, large tonsils, or poor eating habits
Observation and reporting of indications of hemorrhage
Alleviation of operative pain
Provision of emotional support
Adaptation to hospitalization and surgical invasion of body

Recommended nursing action consistent with diagnosis
Nursing services

Provide preoperative nursing, including providing emotional and physical preparation for child, completing preoperative tests, and reporting abnormalities to physician
Implement postoperative nursing to ensure adequate fluid intake; alleviate discomfort or pain with ice collar and/ or pain medication, as ordered by physician; observe for and report signs of hemorrhage
Provide emotional support to child/ parents for adaptation to hospitalization
Implement play therapy and/or diversional activities

Health education

Teach parents signs of hemorrhage and to report these immediately to physician

Instruct on diet and stress importance of adequate fluid intake
Instruct on activity level and need for protection from infection

Indicators for discharge
Adaptation to health status

Able to tolerate oral fluids
Afebrile
Bleeding and severe constant pain in ear absent

Examples of community resources

Referral usually not indicated

RETROSPECTIVE CRITERIA
Health

Afebrile
Pain controlled by oral analgesics
Bleeding absent
Oral fluids being tolerated

Activity

Ambulatory

Knowledge

Parents understand and can implement diet
Parents recognize signs of hemorrhage; know action to take

COMPLICATIONS

Cervical lymph node abscess
Hemorrhage
Peritonsillar abscess
Rheumatic fever, pneumonia, nephritis, or osteomyelitis may follow streptococcal tonsillitis

Toxemia of pregnancy (Code: 637.9)

CONCURRENT CRITERIA
Identification of patient's physical and psychosocial needs and/or concerns

Relief of symptoms, including headache, vertigo, malaise, nervous irritability, visual impairment, epigastric pain, nausea, convulsions, and/or coma; proteinuria; hypertension preceding convulsion and hypotension thereafter; frothing at the mouth; twitching of muscle groups; oliguria or anuria; and papilledema

Fear of loss of fetus or of own life

Quiet, restful environment without stressful situations

Limited fluids

Explanation of condition, reasons for early termination of pregnancy, medical and nursing management, and expected outcomes

Recommended nursing action consistent with diagnosis
Nursing services

Implement absolute bed rest in a single room, with no visitors, not even the husband, and quiet, nonstimulating environment

Observe physiological responses, including blood pressure, respiration, temperature, seizure activity or coma, proteinuria, massive edema, visual disturbances, nausea or vomiting, weight, elimination, hydration, nutrition, fetal heart rate; prevent emotionally stressful situations

Provide psychological support if pregnancy is to be terminated; provide for expression of fear of loss of fetus or of own life

Implement seizure precautions

Provide 1 gm salt, high carbohydrate, moderate protein, low-fat diet; explain rationale of diet to patient

Health education

Explain condition, course, prognosis, reasons for early termination of pregnancy, medical and nursing management, expected outcomes, and posthospitalization symptoms to be reported to physician

Give diet instruction about hospitalization and discharge diets

Teach infant care based on size of infant at birth and condition of infant; if normal infant, instruct about bathing, feeding, clothing, cord care, diapering, normal growth and development, and when to provide medical follow-up

Instruct on the name, purpose, dosage, frequency, duration, and side effects to report to physician of each medication

Indicators for discharge
Adaptation to health status

Pregnancy delivered

Complications not evident

Symptoms of toxemia resolved or controlled

Health teaching completed

Referrals made

Examples of community resources

Visiting Nurse Association or public health nurse

RETROSPECTIVE CRITERIA
Health

Blood pressure within normal range

No protein in urine

Pregnancy delivered

Activity

Independent in activities of daily living

Ambulatory

Able to care for infant

Knowledge

Understands and can verbalize course of condition, diet and medication instructions, infant care, and symptoms to report to physician

COMPLICATIONS

Cesarean section
Coma
Convulsions
Hemorrhage
Infection
Ophthalmic complications
Premature baby
Premature separation of the placenta with hemorrhage
Shock
Transfusion reaction

Tracheal or bronchial foreign body in children (Code: 934)

CONCURRENT CRITERIA
Identification of patient's physical and psychosocial needs and/or concerns

Emotional support for child/family
Maintenance of adequate respiratory ventilation
Promotion of healing of respiratory tract
Provision of instruction about safety in environment

Recommended nursing action consistent with diagnosis
Nursing services

Establish a therapeutic relationship with child/family in which anxiety can be expressed
Monitor child for respiratory difficulty every 15 minutes following removal of obstruction
Monitor oxygen therapy equipment every hour for oxygen concentration, humidification, or malfunctions
Observe for reestablishment of swallowing reflex and, when it is reestablished, force fluids to 2 liters per day
Use simple diversions to help child remain calm and quiet

Health education

Explain to child/family the procedures and equipment being used
Teach family about providing a safe environment in the home by keeping small objects, such as toys with small, movable parts, safety pins, and small candies, out of reach of child

Indicators for discharge
Adaptation to health status

Respiratory distress absent
Afebrile and vital signs stable for 24 hours prior to discharge
Food and fluids being tolerated orally
Normal activities being resumed
Family teaching about a safe environment completed

Examples of community resources

Home visits by public health nurse to assess safety hazards

RETROSPECTIVE CRITERIA
Health

Afebrile and vital signs stable for 24 hours prior to discharge
Respiratory distress absent
Food and fluids being tolerated orally

Activity

Child resuming normal activities for age

Knowledge

Family knows about and can implement a safe environment by keeping small objects, such as toys with small movable parts, safety pins, and small candies, out of child's reach

COMPLICATIONS

Atelectasis
Bronchial obstruction
Lung abscess
Obstructive emphysema
Pulmonary infection

Transient situational disturbances (Code: DSM II 207)

CONCURRENT CRITERIA
Identification of patient's physical and psychosocial needs and/or concerns

Concern regarding social, familial, or occupational functioning

Identification of mental status

Determination of situation precipitating need for hospitalization

Recommended nursing action consistent with diagnosis
Nursing services

Observe patient for symptoms

Maintain frequent interactions with patient, encouraging patient to recognize and verbalize feelings

Encourage socialization by patient

Make recommendations for patient's treatment plan

Health education

Inform patient and significant other of treatment plan and realistic expectations of the plan

Assist patient and significant other in developing healthy and helpful interactions with each other

Indicators for discharge
Adaptation to health status

Inpatient treatment goals achieved

Follow-up treatment plan established and understood by patient and significant other

Symptoms and/or problems that necessitated admission manageable on outpatient basis

Examples of community resources

Outpatient psychiatric nurse

Visiting Nurse Association or public health nurse

RETROSPECTIVE CRITERIA
Health

Symptoms manageable

Sleep pattern regular

Activity

Performs activities of daily living

Sets goals; makes plans for achieving them

Interacts in one-to-one and group relationships

Knowledge

Patient verbalizes understanding that nonverbal behavior should confirm verbal expression of feelings

Patient verbalizes understanding of instructions for taking medications, signs and symptoms of untoward reactions, and the need to report these to the physician

COMPLICATIONS

Attempted suicide

Drug reaction

Transient situational disturbances in children (Codes: DSM II 307-307.2)

CONCURRENT CRITERIA
Identification of patient's physical and psychosocial needs and/or concerns

Identification of child's/adolescent's (patient's) behavior of danger to self and others and source of stress triggering behavior

State of patient's physical health

Exploration of patient's beliefs, attitudes, and expectations of own behavior and of hospitalization

Exploration of family's beliefs, attitudes, and expectations of patient and treatment facility

Determination of chronology of patient's/family's development and coping

Recommended nursing action consistent with diagnosis
Nursing services

Provide nursing assessment of patient, family, and community within 7 days of admission

Provide ongoing behavioral observation and assessment of patient within 8 hours of admission every 8 hours for a week, then during facility-defined periods

Implement behavior-specific interventions, such as life-space interview, seclusion, suicide prevention, and behavior modification

Assist in developing and implementing after-care program and family-specific interventions

Implement and assess physical therapies, such as medications and dosage procedures

Health education

Explain ward procedures and milieu to patient/family

Discuss treatment goals and therapeutic modalities with patient/family

Teach family to make use of specific therapeutic modalities, such as behavior modification, principles of psychodynamics, communication theories, and attitude prescription

Discuss, demonstrate, and explain about any medication

Indicators for discharge
Adaptation to health status

Decreased incidence of nonadaptive behavior; identification of and decrease in some environmental stress

Evidence of reintegration into family, community, and school

Patient/family demonstration of self-care capability in areas of medication administration, recognition of feelings, limit setting, and help seeking

Examples of community resources

Outpatient psychiatric nurse
School nurse
Visiting Nurse Association or public health nurse

RETROSPECTIVE CRITERIA
Health

Nonadaptive behavior controlled
No physical illness or problems
Regular sleep patterns

Activity

No limitations
Performs activities of daily living at age-appropriate level
Interacts with peers and adults on age-appropriate level

Knowledge

Patient/family knows what treatment goals were accomplished
Patient/family knows what after-care plans have been made; understands

plans and each family member's part in them

COMPLICATIONS

Adverse reactions to diagnostic or therapeutic modalities (such as procedures, drugs, or psychological or social therapies)

Exacerbation of clinical signs and/or symptoms

Failure of family and/or social support system

Trigeminal neuralgia and atypical facial pain (Code: 351)

CONCURRENT CRITERIA
Identification of patient's physical and psychosocial needs and/or concerns

Relief from pain

Understanding of medical and nursing management of disease

Understanding of surgical procedure (if treatment of choice) and its purpose, preparation, and after-care, including special units, such as recovery room, and possible outcomes, such as corneal keratitis (inflammation) and partial facial numbness

Improvement of nutritional status

Assistance in dealing with fear related to anticipated attacks

Recommended nursing action consistent with diagnosis
Nursing services

Reduce pain and frequency of attacks by preventing drafts; avoiding approaching bed rapidly or jarring bed; avoiding measures that "trigger" pain, such as shaving or washing affected side of face; offering medium termperature, pureed foods or liquids that can be consumed through a straw; teaching pain-coping measures, such as distraction, behavioral therapy techniques, and waking-imagined analgesia; providing physical comfort measures and analgesics; and avoiding narcotics when phenytoin is given

Improve nutritional state

Improve oral hygiene without triggering attacks

Observe for desired effects and side effects of medications and alcohol injection blocks of the trigeminal nerve

For surgical treatment, implement postoperative nursing care and measures to prevent complications or injury, including closely observing vital signs and signs of change in condition, with necessary nursing intervention; maintaining fluid and electrolyte balance and adequate elimination; relieving pain; providing wound care; preventing hypostatic pneumonia, infection, and problems caused by circulatory stasis; preventing corneal damage; and preventing burns caused by loss of sensation on affected side of face

Health education

Teach pain-reducing methods, including comfort measures and waking-imagined analgesia

Explain the name, purpose, desired and side effects, dosage, frequency, precautions, and actions to take if side effects occur of each medication

Teach methods by which to maintain adequate hydration, nutrition, and oral hygiene without triggering attacks

Provide preoperative and postoperative teaching, including explaining procedure, recovery room, possible outcome of surgery (numbness to eye and possibly to face), intravenous solutions, deep breathing, coughing, frequent turning, early ambulation, postoperative diet (graduated types and steps from liquids to solids), wound care, eye care, and measures to prevent burning face via hot foods and to circumvent initial difficulty in eating caused by loss of sensation on one side of the face

Indicators for discharge
Adaptation to health status

Pain absent or frequency of attacks diminished
Complications not evident
Referrals made
Nutrition improved

Examples of community resources

Pain clinic
Visiting Nurse Association or public health nurse
Surgical clinic

RETROSPECTIVE CRITERIA
Health

Pain absent or frequency of attacks diminished
Nutrition improved
Complications not evident

Activity

Ambulatory
Able to carry out activities of daily living

Knowledge

Understands methods of reducing pain and frequency of attacks should they recur after discharge
Knows the names, action, frequency, dosage, side effects, precautions, and actions to take should side effects occur of each prescribed medication
Understands and can implement measures to maintain hydration and nutrition without triggering attacks
Understands and can implement methods to protect eye from infection or trauma postsurgery
Understands and can implement methods of protecting affected side of face from burns postsurgery

COMPLICATIONS

Adverse drug reaction
Facial paralysis
Paroxysms of pain

Tumors, abdominal, in children (Code: 232.1)

CONCURRENT CRITERIA
Identification of patient's physical and psychosocial needs and/or concerns

Relief of pain, discomfort, and symptoms of acute abdominal distress (nausea, vomiting, distention, or diarrhea)
Maintenance of functions (activity, respiration, digestion, elimination, sleep)
Understanding by family/child of conditions, prognosis, treatment and implications for care
Assistance in adaptation to hospitalization
Fear of mutilation, death, or increased dependency

Recommended nursing action consistent with diagnosis
Nursing services

Provide preoperative assessment of size, position, and resultant symptoms of mass in order to provide proper positioning for body comfort and function
Provide preoperative observation, recording, and prompt remediation of any acute symptoms (nausea, vomiting, pain, diarrhea, or distention) via nursing measures or administration of medication as ordered
Implement preoperative maintenance of adequate nutrition, hydration, and

elimination; provide diet prepared to meet individual preferences; give oral and intravenous fluids

Provide regular monitoring of vital signs—discomfort; intravenous therapy—injection site and rate of flow; quality of respiration, color, body temperature, and activity level; exposure to possible infection; and intake and output

Promptly order preoperative laboratory procedures; administer ordered treatment and medication; surgically prepare abdominal site; instruct patient about postoperative turning and breathing procedures

Provide postoperative maintenance and monitoring of vital signs, hydration, body temperature, incision site and dressing, color, affect, sensory-motor responses, distention, pain, intravenous site and rate, nutrition, and other activities on a progressive basis to encourage independent function and early ambulation

Postoperatively maintain patency of intravenous catheter, nasogastric tube, Foley catheter, and/or any other drainage tubes, irrigating as necessary

Provide postoperative relief of pain and abdominal distress via nursing measures and medication

Postoperatively prevent infection via antibiotics, hygiene, and bed placement

Health education

Explain condition, prognosis, treatment, implications for care, medical and nursing management, and treatment plan for discharge

Teach measures to relieve pain, prevent infections, promote wound healing, and prevent complications

Instruct about dosage, frequency, route, name, side effects, observations to report of discharge medications

Indicators for discharge
Adaptation to health status

Afebrile

Vital signs stable and within normal limits

Wound healing

Foods and fluids being tolerated

Activity normal for age and developmental level being resumed

Home care potential adequate for current health status

Examples of community resourses

Visiting Nurse Association or public health nurse, if parent needs assistance in wound care or emotional support—dependent on patient's activity and prognosis

RETROSPECTIVE CRITERIA
Health

Vital signs stable within normal limits

Wound healed; infection not evident

Pain controlled

Food and fluids tolerated

Elimination normal

Mentally accepting surgical invasion of body

Activity

Resumption of normal activity for age and developmental level

Knowledge

Parental understanding of wound care, activity level permissible, condition, prognosis, treatment plan, medications, and prevention of infections or complications

COMPLICATIONS

Bone marrow depression
Pneumonia
Postoperative intestinal obstruction
Sepsis

Tumors, brain, medically treated (Code: 225)

CONCURRENT CRITERIA
Identification of patient's physical and psychosocial needs and/or concerns

Relief from symptoms, including headaches; vomiting; mental clouding; lethargy; muscle rigidity; decreased coordination; weakness; convulsions; impairment of sphincter control; aberrations in smell, vision, and hearing; memory loss; personality changes; hemiparesis; or aphasia

Anxiety over changes in body image and in role and over possible death

Family/patient understanding of the nature of the disorder, the course of treatment, and prognosis, with realistic planning for discharge care

Understanding of diagnostic and therapeutic management

Awareness of community agencies appropriate for assistance with care after discharge

Recommended nursing action consistent with diagnosis
Nursing services

Observe signs and symptoms of toxicity to chemotherapeutic agents and radiation therapy, with prompt nursing intervention, including temporarily withholding medication until physician is contacted, when severe toxic reactions (such as muscle incoordination, hypertension, peripheral neuritis, drug fever, or paresthesia) are present

Observe tissue irritation, sepsis, or hemorrhage as related to intraarterial perfusion and radiation therapy causing stress ulcers of the stomach, bone marrow depression, thrombocytopenia, and tissue necrosis, with nursing intervention should any of these complications occur

Maintain adequate hydration, nutrition, and electrolyte balance

Implement measures to minimize the discomforts of the less serious side effects of chemotherapeutic agents and radiation therapy, including small, frequent bland feedings when nausea occurs, oral hygiene with soft nonabrasive items, and wigs and scarves when alopecia occurs

Implement measures to protect the patient against infection as related to bone marrow depression and radiation therapy, including implementation and maintenance of isolation when arterial perfusion of chemotherapeutic agents is used

Health education

Explain purpose, procedure, and care of medical, dianostic, and therapeutic procedures, such as home care of intraarterial perfusions; teach name, action, dosage, frequency, and side effects of each discharge medication and frequency of medical and laboratory checkups

Explain importance of prompt medical treatment of all colds or secondary infections and the avoidance of persons with infectious illnesses

Explain methods and importance of maintaining good nutrition and hydration, and the importance of contacting the physician should vomiting occur

Explain measures to reduce pain and manage emotional, behavioral, and role changes

Indicators for discharge
Adaptation to health status

Symptoms relieved or controlled
Complications not evident

Examples of community resources

Visiting Nurse Association or public health nurse

Speech, vision, physical, or vocational rehabilitation centers

Cancer clinic
American Cancer Society

Health

Symptoms relieved or controlled
Anxiety reduced
No evidence of complications

Activity

Ambulatory
Self-completion of activities of daily living

Knowledge

Understands and can implement therapeutic procedure of intraarterial perfusion of chemotherapeutic procedure at home; understands and can implement the care of the injection (or perfusion) site

Understands and knows the name of medications to be discharged with, including dosage, frequency, route, purpose, side effects, precautions, methods of minimizing side effects, and what to do if more serious adverse reactions occur

Understands and can implement care of the skin at the radiation therapy site

Understands the importance of avoiding infection and the need for immediate medical attention should signs and symptoms occur

Understands the importance of and methods used to maintain maintain good nutrition and hydration

Understands the importance of keeping regular appointments with physician for medical surveillance

Understands the importance of self-maintenance of activities of daily living and of ambulation for as long as possible

COMPLICATIONS

Atelectasis
Chemotherapy complications
Decubitus ulcers
Disturbed mental state
Drug reaction
Equilibrium and coordination disturbances
Inanition
Infections
Joint contractures
Persistent fever
Pneumonia
Pulmonary embolism
Seizures
Sensory and motor abnormalities
Speech deficit
Visual alterations

Tumors, brain, with surgical intervention (Code: 225)

CONCURRENT CRITERIA
Identification of patient's physical and psychosocial needs and/or concerns

Relief from symptoms, including headaches, vomiting, mental clouding, lethargy, muscle rigidity, decreased coordination, weakness, convulsions, aberrations in smell, vision, and hearing, memory loss, personality changes, impairment of sphincter control, hemiparesis, or aphasia

Anxiety over change in body image and in role and over possible death

Patient/family understanding of the nature of the disorder, the course of treatment and prognosis, with realistic planning for discharge care

Understanding of diagnostic and therapeutic surgical management

Awareness of community agencies appropriate for assistance with care after discharge

Recommended nursing action consistent with diagnosis
Nursing services

Implement preoperative nursing measures, including supportive measures for neurological deficits; physically prepare patient for surgery; assess baseline, including vital signs; mental status; visual, hearing, and speaking status; bowel and bladder control; gait; focal seizures; and sensory-motor loss in extremities

Implement postoperative nursing care, including comfort measures; maintenance of adequate ventilation, hydration, and elimination; reduction of cerebral edema; and reinforcement of dressing

Observe for change of condition, through frequent neurological assessments for increased intracranial pressure, support measures for seizures, and observations for cerebrospinal fluid leakage, with proper nursing intervention should deterioration occur

Assess for postoperative complications; implement appropriate actions

Implement measures to prevent complications, including aseptic wound care, frequent turning and positioning, prompt physician notification of signs of increased intracranial pressure, hemorrhage, or perforation of gastrointestinal mucosa

Health education

Provide preoperative and postoperative teaching about intravenous administration, equipment, special care units, purpose of and estimated period of time in care units, surgical procedure, prognosis, anticipated outcome as related to neurological residual deficits, procedure of suctioning, and importance of turning, chest physiotherapy, and frequent neurological assessments

Provide family education about rehabilitative measures based on residual neurological deficits, including range-of-motion exercises, transfer techniques, use of adaptive equipment and prosthetic devices, bowel and bladder control programs, speech therapy, visual corrective devices, physical therapy, vocational rehabilitation, and seizure care

Teach family/patient regarding community agencies available to assist with care after discharge

Indicators for discharge
Adaptation to health status

Wound healing
Condition stable
Complications not evident

Examples of community resources

Visiting Nurse Association or public health nurse
Speech, hearing, vision, physical, or vocational rehabilitation centers to meet neurological deficits
American Cancer Society

RETROSPECTIVE CRITERIA
Health

Anxiety under control
Symptoms relieved
Wound healing
No evidence of complications or complications under treatment

Activity

Able to complete activities of daily living with minimal assistance (exception: residual neurological deficits exceed performance of activities of daily living and anticipated improvement does not justify extending stay in acute care setting)

Ambulatory with assistance or prosthetic devices (exception: neurological deficits prevent ambulation and anticipated improvement does not justify extending stay in acute care setting)

Knowledge

Understands and knows the names, dosage, frequency, purpose, side effects, precautions, and action to take should side effects occur of each discharge medication

Understands wound care

Understands care as related to residual neurological deficits, such as for epilepsy—care during and after seizure, measures to reduce frequency of attacks, legal implications, and medications; for muscle weakness—range-of-motion exercises, stretching, and resistive exercises; for paralysis—transfer techniques and use of adaptive equipment; for speech—speech therapy; for visual corrective devices—eye patch or frosted lens; for sphincter problems—bowel and bladder control program; provide skin care

Understands function and role of community agencies available for assistance with care after discharge

COMPLICATIONS

Aneurysm
Arachnoiditis
Atelectasis
Decubitus ulcers
Disturbed mental state
Equilibrium and coordination disturbances
Inanition
Increased intracranial pressure
Intracranial abscess
Joint contractures
Persistent fever
Pneumonia
Pulmonary embolism
Seizures
Sensory and motor abnormalities
Speech deficit
Subdural hematoma
Visual alterations
Wound infection

Tumors of central nervous system (Codes: 192.2, 225, 225.3)

CONCURRENT CRITERIA
Identification of patient's physical and psychosocial needs and/or concerns

Concern about diagnosis, treatment, and prognosis

Assessment of body functions in relation to location of tumor

Concern about limitations, both physical and psychosocial

Indication of presence or absence of increasing intracranial pressure

Recommended nursing action consistent with diagnosis
Nursing services

Monitor neurological signs and symptoms

Monitor pain status

Observe for cerebral spinal fluid leakage from nose or from spinal or cranial wound

Observe for potential complications

Provide emotional support

Health education

Teach prevention of complications

Discuss use of available resources

Explain limits and goals of rehabilitation

Explain rationale to treatments and medications

Teach indicators for consulting patient's physician

Indicators for discharge
Adaptation to health status

Rehabilitation goals achieved

Ability to function at home satisfactory

Plan for appropriate care and follow-up after discharge made

Disease and specific treatment goals understood by patient/family

Examples of community resources

American Cancer Society

Visiting Nurse Association or public health nurse

RETROSPECTIVE CRITERIA
Health

Neurological signs and symptoms stabilized

Activity

Maximum functional level achieved

Knowledge

Patient/family understand appropriate follow-up care and resources

COMPLICATIONS

Aneurysm
Arachnoiditis
Cardiopulmonary problems
Cerebrovascular accident
Decubitus ulcers
Disturbed mental state
Inanition
Intracranial abscess
Subdural hematoma
Wound complications

Tumors of peripheral nervous system (Code: 225.5)

CONCURRENT CRITERIA
Identification of patient's physical and psychosocial needs and/or concerns

Relief of symptoms and explanation that symptoms vary according to area of involvement, such as the eighth cranial nerve for tinnitus, deafness, vertigo, and mild ataxia or uncoordination; the ninth cranial nerve for pain; the tenth cranial nerve for paralysis, hoarseness, dyspnea, dysphagia, and sensory disturbances; the eleventh cranial nerve for inability to move head to unaffected side, drooping shoulder, and spastic muscles; the twelfth cranial nerve for hemiplegia and paralysis of tongue, sensory disturbances (sensory-motor disturbances for all cranial nerves as may be affected); and spinal nerves for sensory-motor disturbances in trunk or extremity area that nerve supplies

Understanding of diagnostic, surgical, and nursing management of disorder so that realistic plans can be made for any care required after discharge

Explanation that lesion is benign, metastatic, or a primary malignancy

Assistance in coping with change in body image, increased dependence, if lesion affects mobility status, or ability to use upper extremities

Fear of death

Maintenance of adequate hydration, nutrition, and elimination

Referral to community agencies for rehabilitation measures and assistance that may be appropriate after discharge, as related to possible residual neurological deficits

Recommended nursing action consistent with diagnosis
Nursing services

Implement safety measures as related to sensory-motor function disturbances and area or organ affected

Maintain adequate hydration, nutrition, elimination, and activity

Maintain communication, as related to a hearing or speaking deficit

Provide preoperative care, including physical preparation of patient, and postoperative nursing measures, including closely observing for signs and symptoms of physical deterioration; minimizing side effects of radiation therapy, if used on malignant lesion; implementing rehabilitation measures, such as muscle-strengthening and range-of-motion exercises, positioning, and application of prosthetic and adaptive devices; and implementing approaches to correct, minimize, or circumvent problems of visual, auditory, and speech disturbances

Prevent problems from immobility, including urinary tract and respiratory infections, pulmonary embolism, constipation, anorexia, contractures, or decubitus ulcers

Health education

Explain the name, dosage, frequency, purpose, side effects, action to take should side effects occur, and precautions of each medication

Instruct about application and use of prosthetic and adaptive devices for activities of daily living

Instruct about therapeutic diet with special feeding or eating techniques and adaptive utensils, therapeutic and restricted activites, and bowel and bladder control programs

Instruct about and explain reasons for measures to prevent problems resulting from immobility, if residual neurological deficits curtail mobility

Explain about community agencies available to assist in care after discharge

Indicators for discharge
Adaptation to health status

Wound healing
Condition stable
Complications not evident
Health teaching completed
Referrals made

Examples of community resources

Visiting Nurse Association or public health nurse
Social services
American Cancer Society
Vocational, speech, and physiotherapy rehabilitation centers

RETROSPECTIVE CRITERIA
Health

Symptoms relieved or controlled
Wound healing

Therapeutic diet tolerated
Complications not evident

Activity

Able to carry out activities of daily living with or without assistance or adaptive or prosthetic devices
Ambulatory

Knowledge

Knows and understands the name, dosage, frequency, side effects, purpose, action to take should side effects occur, and precautions of each discharge medication

Understands and can implement safety measures related to sensory-motor disturbances

Understands use of and is able to apply adaptive and prosthetic devices

Understands and can implement rehabilitative measures

Understands and can implement comfort measures

Understands and can implement measures to maintain adequate hydration, nutrition, and elimination

Understands and can implement measures to prevent problems caused by immobility

COMPLICATIONS

Anorexia
Decubitus ulcers
Joint contractures
Persistent fever
Respiratory infection
Thromboembolism
Urinary tract infection
Wound infection

Tumors of skin or soft tissue with surgical intervention (Code: 92.1)

CONCURRENT CRITERIA
Identification of patient's physical and psychosocial needs and/or concerns

Removal of growth that may be sore or painful from ulceration or rapid growth

Fear of malignancy, recurrence of growth, and surgical procedure

Understanding of condition, course, treatment, and medical and nursing management

Recommended nursing action consistent with diagnosis
Nursing services

Provide preoperative nursing care, including maintaining nutrition, elimination, hydration, and other body functions; explaining surgical procedure, recovery room, and pathological analysis of growth; and giving psychological support

Physically prepare patient for surgery

Implement postoperative nursing care, including monitoring physiological response parameters, controlling pain, turning patient, instigating coughing and deep breathing, inspecting and caring for wound, and giving psychological support concerning outcome of pathological analysis

Health education

Teach measures to decrease exposure of skin to such chronic irritations as the sun, chemicals, or friction

Explain condition, course, treatment, medical and nursing management, and signs and/or symptoms of complications or recurrence to report to physician

Teach the name, dosage, frequency, duration, and side effects to report to physician of each medication

Instruct about wound care, stressing the importance of incision care, if located on face, neck, or visible area of body

Indicators for discharge
Adaptation to health status

Growth surgically removed

Normal physiological responses reestablished

Measures to reduce chronic exposure to skin irritation understood

Examples of community resources

Tumor registry if malignant
American Cancer Society

RETROSPECTIVE CRITERIA
Health

Wound healing
Growth removed
Normal physiological responses reestablished
Mentally coping with fears

Activity

Independent in activities of daily living
Ambulatory

Knowledge

Understands and can implement wound care; understands and can verbalize medication instructions, course of condition, measures by which to prevent chronic exposure to skin irritation, and symptoms to report to physician

COMPLICATIONS

Hemorrhage
Metastasis
Sepsis

Tumors of spinal cord, benign (Code: 225.3)

CONCURRENT REVIEW CRITERIA
Identification of patient's physical and psychosocial needs and/or concerns

Relief of symptoms, including radicular pains and paresthesias, aggrevated by exertion, coughing, and straining; localized muscle weakness or paralysis; muscle atrophy of involved body part; paraplegia; sensory loss; and bowel and bladder sphincter disturbances

Fear and anxiety over change in body image and in role and possible malignancy or cancer

Family/patient understanding of disorder, course, and prognosis, so realistic plans can be made for necessary care after discharge

Understanding of diagnostic and therapeutic surgical management of the tumor

Awareness of community agencies that can assist with care after discharge, if necessary

Recommended nursing action consistent with diagnosis
Nursing services

Provide preoperative nursing measures, such as supportive measures for neurological deficits, and positioning, turning, and maintaining correct alignment to prevent contractures, hypostatic pneumonia, and decubitus ulcers; maintenance of proper hydration, elimination, and nutrition; protection from injury by avoidance of hot water bottles if sensation is lost, side rails if paralysis is present; use of sterile technique during catheterizations; and reduction or relief of pain

Physically prepare patient for surgery and radiation therapy, if used prior to surgery

Reduce discomforts of radiation syndrome, including nausea, skin depigmentation, alopecia, and sore mouth

Establish baseline status by checking vital signs and neurological status by checking gait and motor strength and functions, check skin for edema, decubitus ulcers, rashes, bruises, and dehydration; assess elimination for constipation, diarrhea, retention of urine, and incontinence; observe for muscle spasticity

Implement postoperative nursing care, including comfort measures; ventilation; hydration; nutrition; elimination; and assessment for deterioration or for postoperative complications of shock, respiratory obstruction or distress, infection, and hemorrhage, with appropriate nursing intervention; prevent postoperative complications in convalescent phase, such as wound infection, thrombophlebitis, pulmonary embolism, contractures, urinary tract infection, urinary retention, urinary incontinence, and decubitus ulcers

Implement rehabilitative measures, including transfer techniques, active and passive exercises, and bowel and bladder control programs

Assist patient/family in coping with possible changes in body image and in role

Health education

Explain medications, including the name, dosage, frequency, purpose, side effects, precautions, and measures to minimize or reduce side effects of each discharge medication

Teach wound care

Teach measures to improve or prevent deterioration in muscle functions

Teach safety measures, such as use of canes or walker; if having problems with gait; protection from burns, if experiencing loss of sensation, and use of side rails

Teach prevention of complications during prolonged convalescence, through administration of skin care, extension of activity, avoidance of infectious persons, if on radiation therapy, and maintenance of adequate hydration, nutrition, and elimination

Indicators for discharge
Adaptation to health status

Afebrile
Sensory-motor functions improved
Complications not evident
Referrals made

Examples of community resources

Visiting Nurse Association or public health nurse
Social services
Physical and vocational rehabilitation centers

RETROSPECTIVE REVIEW CRITERIA
Health

Afebrile
Benign tumor removed
Wound healing
Mentally accepting condition
Sensory-motor functions improved
Complications not evident

Activity

Ambulatory unassisted or with prosthetic devices, such as canes, braces, or walker
Able to carry out activities of daily living

Knowledge

Understands and can implement wound care, if necessary
Understands and knows the names, dosage, frequency, purpose, side effects, precautions, and action to take should side effects occur of each discharge medication
Able to implement measures to improve muscle functions or to prevent deterioration
Understands and can implement safety measures
Understands and can implement measures to prevent complications, through administration of skin care and activity prescriptions, avoidance of infections, and maintenance of adequate hydration, nutrition, and elimination

COMPLICATIONS

Atelectasis
Decubitus ulcers
Hemorrhage
Inanition
Joint contractures
Neurological deficit
Paralysis
Persistent fever
Pneumonia
Pulmonary embolism
Respiratory obstruction or distress
Shock
Thrombophlebitis
Urinary incontinence
Urinary retention
Urinary tract infection
Wound infections

Tumors of spinal cord, malignant (Code: 192.2)

CONCURRENT CRITERIA
Identification of patient's physical and psychosocial needs and/or concerns

Relief of symptoms, including radicular pains and paresthesias aggravated by exertion, coughing, or straining; localized muscle weakness or paralysis; muscle atrophy; paraplegia; sensory loss; and bowel and bladder sphinter problems

Fear of malignancy and death

Aid in coping with malignancy and in facing eventual death

Realistic hope for family/patient but also awareness that surgery and radiation therapy are generally considered to be palliative

Understanding of diagnostic and therapeutic surgical management and nursing management designed to promote maximum comfort and functioning ability within limitations of stage of progression of neoplasm

Recommended nursing action consistent with diagnosis
Nursing services

Provide preoperative nursing care, including supportive measures for neurological deficits; positioning, turning, and maintenance of correct alignment to prevent contractures, pneumonia, and decubitus ulcers; maintenance of hydration, elimination, and nutrition; reduction of pain with techniques of distraction, waking-imagined analgesia, physical comfort measures, and analgesics; protection from injuries resulting from sensory loss or muscle weakness; delay of further deterioration or of complications, such as muscle atrophy, urinary tract infection, or thrombophlebitis

Physically prepare patient for surgery and radiation therapy, if used prior to surgery

Reduce discomforts of radiation syndrome, including nausea, skin discoloration, alopecia, or sore mouth

Assess baseline status by checking vital signs, gait, and motor strength and functions; check skin for edema, decubitus ulcers, rashes, bruises, or dehydration; assess elimination for constipation, diarrhea, retention of urine, or incontinence; note type of paralysis as related to muscle flaccidity or spasticity

Prepare patient for radiation therapy (when no surgery is planned); provide care after therapy, including skin care, reduction of nausea, relief of discomforts in mouth, reduction of embarrassment over skin discoloration and alopecia, and protection against infection

Assist patient/family in coping with patient's malignant condition and with facing eventual death

Implement postoperative nursing care, including comfort measures; adequate ventilation, hydration, nutrition, and elimination; assessment for deterioration, with appropriate nursing intervention should shock, respiratory obstruction or distress, infection, hemorrhage, or pulmonary embolism occur

Prevent complications, such as wound infection, thrombophlebitis, contractures, urinary tract infection, urinary retention, urinary incontinence, and decubitus ulcers, during convalescent phase

Encourage independence in activities of daily living, within restrictions of a particular stage of disease, by using transfer techniques, active and passive exercises, and bowel and bladder control measures

Initiate appropriate referrals

Health education

Explain medications, including the name, dosage, frequency, purpose, side effects, measures to minimize or reduce side effects, and precautions of each discharge

Instruct on wound care medication

Teach measures to improve muscle functions and to prevent deterioration; teach safety measures to assist with gait problems and protection from falls and burns

Explain measures to prevent complications from immobility and radiation therapy as disease continues, including administration of skin care, extension of activity, avoidance of infections, and maintenance of adequate hydration, nutrition, and elimination

Advise about community agencies available to assist with discharge care

Indicators for discharge
Adaptation to health status

Afebrile
Sensory-motor functions improved
Complications not evident
Referrals made

Examples of community resources

American Cancer Society
Visiting Nurse Association or public health nurse
Rehabilitation centers
Social services

RETROSPECTIVE CRITERIA
Health

Afebrile
Symptoms relieved or controlled
Malignant tumor surgically removed
Wound healing
Mentally accepting condition
Sensory-motor functions improved
Complications not evident

Activity

Ambulatory
Independent in activities of daily living with or without adaptive devices

Knowledge

Knows and understands the name, purpose, dosage, frequency, side effects, how to reduce side effects, and precautions of each discharge medication

Understands and can implement wound care, if any

Understands and can implement skin care; range-of-motion, flexion and extension, and resistive exercises; transfer techniques; safety measures; and measures to maintain adequate nutrition, hydration, and elimination

Understands and can implement comfort measures to reduce discomforts of radiation syndrome

Understands the functions of appropriate community agencies available for assistance after discharge

COMPLICATIONS

Atelectasis
Complications of radiation therapy
Decubitus ulcers
Edema
Hemorrhage
Inanition
Joint contractures
Metastatic involvement
Muscle atrophy
Paralysis
Persistent fever
Pneumonia
Pulmonary embolism
Radiation therapy complications
Respiratory obstruction or distress
Shock
Thrombophlebitis
Urinary incontinence
Urinary retention
Urinary tract infection
Wound infection

Tumors of sympathetic nervous system (Code: 225.6)

Identification of patient's physical and psychosocial needs and/or concerns

Relief or control of symptoms, including disturbances in cardiac rate, vasomotor impairment, secretion of digestive juices, and disturbances in thycogenolysis and epinephrine secretion, resulting in excessive sweating, no sweating, edema of the skin, trophic ulcers, muscle atrophy from inadequate blood supply, pain, hypotension, hypertension, hypoglycemia, hyperglycemia, anorexia, starvation, nausea, and vomiting

Understanding of pathology as related to cause, prognosis, treatment, and management in order to make realistic plans for care after discharge

Adjustment to changes in body image, life-style, and role and to possibility of death as related to inaccessible malignant tumor

Maintenance or improvement of hydration, nutrition, and elimination

Explanation of community agencies available to assist after discharge and of application of rehabilitative measures

Recommended nursing action consistent with diagnosis
Nursing services

Implement safety measures as related to syncope associated with disturbances in cardiac rate, hypotension, hypoglycemia, or impairment of motor function because of weakness

Maintain adequate hydration, nutrition, and elimination by providing small, frequent feedings of easily digested foods, administering antiemetics, observing for dehydration, frequently offering fluids, accurately measuring intake and output, and implementing bowel and bladder control programs

Provide preoperative nursing care, physically and psychologically, and postoperative nursing care, including closely observing for physical deterioration and implementing measures of rehabilitation for residual neurological deficits, such as poor vasomotor functions, muscle weakness from inadequate blood supply, flushing, and skin being easily traumatized

Initiate referrals

Provide emotional support to patient/family

Health education

Explain medications, including the name, purpose, dosage, frequency, side effects, and action to take should side effects occur of each

Instruct about maintaining adequate hydration and nutrition, including special diets as related to hypo- or hyperglycemia, constipation, and digestive disturbances

Instruct about maintaining or improving muscle functions

Instruct about minimizing effects of vasomotor impairment, including flushing or vasoconstriction and pain from inadequate blood supply and decreased temperatures

Explain surgical procedure and medical and nursing management

Instruct about use of adaptive or prosthetic devices

Indicators for discharge
Adaptation to health status

Control or relief of symptoms
Complications not evident
Condition stable
Referrals made

Examples of community resources

Visiting Nurse Association or public health nurse
Social services

Physical rehabilitation center
American Cancer Society

RETROSPECTIVE REVIEW CRITERIA
Health

Pain controlled
Symptoms relieved or controlled
Wound healing
Muscle functions improved
Complications not evident

Activity

Independent in activities of daily living
with or without adaptive or prosthetic
devices
Ambulatory

Knowledge

Knows and understands the name, dosage, frequency, side effects, purpose,
action to take if side effects occur, and
precautions of each discharge medication
Understands and can implement safety
measures as related to sensory-motor
disturbances

Understands and can apply adaptive or
prosthetic devices
Understands and can implement rehabilitative measures
Understands and can implement comfort
measures
Understands and can implement measures to maintain adequate hydration,
nutrition, and elimination
Understands and can implement measures to prevent problems resulting
from immobility

COMPLICATIONS

Dehydration
Hypoglycemia
Hypotension
Impaired vasomotor function
Neurological deficits
Persistent fever
Pneumonia
Syncope
Thromboembolism
Wound infection

Urinary problems, group, in children
Congenital obstructive uropathy (Codes: 753.2, 753.6)
Urinary tract infection (Codes: 590, 595)
Vesicoureteral reflux/revision (Code: 593.5)

CONCURRENT CRITERIA
Identification of patient's physical and psychosocial needs and/or concerns

Promotion of wound healing and care of
incision
Promotion of intake to ensure output of
1,000 to 1,500 ml per day
Expression of fears of mutilation
Adaptation to hospitalization
Patient/parents education regarding nature of reflux and type of surgical
correction

Recommended nursing action consistent with diagnosis
Nursing services

Check patency of all catheters every 2
hours
Measure and record the amount, color,
and odor of urinary output every 2
hours
Check dressing every 2 hours; change
dressing frequently to keep suture line
dry; observe for signs of infection
Encourage fluid intake of at least 1,000
ml per 24 hours

Provide play therapy to aid patient in expression of mutilation fears and in adaptation to hospital environment (with, for example, clay, drawing materials, and puppets)

Never clamp ureteral catheters

Health education

Patient/parents education regarding need for increased fluid intake

Patient/parents education regarding need to keep suture line dry and signs and symptoms of infection of suture line

Patient/parents education regarding home care and need for medical follow-up

Indicators for discharge
Adaptation to health status

Afebrile

Vital signs stable

Wound healing

Patient/parent education regarding home care and need for medical follow-up completed

Food and fluids being tolerated

Normal activities for age and developmental level resuming

Examples of community resources

Referral usually not indicated

RETROSPECTIVE CRITERIA
Health

Afebrile

Vital signs stable

Wound healing

Food and fluids being tolerated

Activity

Alert

No limitation in activities appropriate for age and developmental level

Knowledge

Patient/parents understand home care and need for medical follow-up

COMPLICATIONS

Adverse reaction to diagnostic or therapeutic agent

Hematoma

Septicemia

Urinary tractinfection

Wound dehiscence

Wound infection

Varicose veins

Simple (Code: 454)

With ulceration (Code: 454.9)

CONCURRENT CRITERIA
Identification of patient's physical and psychosocial needs and/or concerns

Adjustment to alteration in appearance (edema, ulcers, and stasis dermatitis of lower extremities)

Explanation of possibility of compromised venous return

Fear of possible surgery

Prevention of embolism formation

Relief of discomfort, including aching, heaviness, and cramping, of lower extremities

Recommended nursing action consistent with diagnosis
Nursing services

Provide elastic stockings; apply before patient gets out of bed

Encourage walking and lying down as opposed to sitting, standing

Elevate patient's lower extremities when not ambulatory (at least 8 hours per day)

Provide nonconstricting clothing and bandages above knees

Protect edematous extremity from injury

Health education

Demonstrate proper application of elastic stockings

Explain relationship of dependent extremities to compromised venous return

Explain relationship of compromised venous return to development of ulcers, edema, and stasis dermatitis of lower extremities

Explain predisposing factors (such as pregnancy and obesity)

Teach purpose and effects of anticoagulant medication

Indicators for discharge
Adaptation to health status

Demonstration of proper application of elastic stockings

Purposeful elevation of legs when sitting

Demonstration of understanding of avoidance of constricting clothing

Examples of community resources

Visiting Nurse Association or public health nurse

Temporary homemaker service

RETROSPECTIVE CRITERIA
Health

Relief of symptoms

Mentally adjusted to change in body image

Wound healing

Venous return improved

Skin intact

Inflammatory process not evident

Activity

Ambulatory with elastic stockings

Knowledge

Understands and can implement application of elastic stocking

Understands and can implement positioning with legs elevated

Knows purpose and effects of anticoagulant medication

COMPLICATIONS

Edema
Infection
Pulmonary embolism
Skin ulceration
Stasis dermatitis
Venous thrombosis

Vertigo (Code: 780.5)

CONCURRENT REVIEW CRITERIA
Identification of patient's physical and psychosocial needs and/or concerns

Relief of symptoms, including general feelings of insecurity, mental confusion, spinning, light headedness, unsteadiness, and transitory tinnitus, nausea, vomiting, and nystagmus

Understanding of cause, if identifiable, such as infection, lesion of cranial nerves; related to trauma or drugs like tobacco and alcohol, or to a cardiovascular disorder; understanding of course, prognosis, and outcome (neurological deficits)

Protection from bodily injury during an attack

Understanding of diagnostic and therapeutic medical management, including the purpose, preparation, outcome, and specific after-care

Understanding of surgical management, including the procedure (craniotomy or cryosurgery), preoperative and postoperative care, special care units, and possible neurological deficits

Recommended nursing action consistent with diagnosis
Nursing services

Observe for desired and side effects of medication (antiemetics, vasodilators, antibiotics, diuretics, tranquilizers, or vitamins)

Implement measures to provide for safety

Implement measures to maintain adequate hydration and diet

Implement measures to maintain vital bodily functions and to prevent physical deterioration postoperatively, if appropriate

Health education

Explain pathology, course, prognosis, and surgical treatment, if appropriate, to family/patient

Teach the name, dosage, frequency, desired and side effects, and precautions of each medication

Teach safety measures

Explain low-salt diet

Indicators for discharge
Adaptation to health status

Absence of dehydration

Decreased episodes of vertigo

Improvement in coordination

No evidence of complications

Referrals made

Examples of community resources

Visiting Nurse Association or public health nurse

Social services

Vocational rehabilitation center

Physical rehabilitation agency

RETROSPECTIVE REVIEW CRITERIA
Health

Hydrated

Coordination improved

Afebrile

Vertigo decreased in severity and frequency

Activity

Able to perform activities of daily living without help

Ambulatory without impairment of balance

Knowledge

Family/patient understands cause, course, and outcome of disorder

Family/patient understands restrictions about driving while on medication; understands effect of alcohol and tobacco on vertigo

Family/patient understands and knows the name, dosage, frequency, side effects, desired effects, and precautions of each medication

Family/patient understands safety measures should vertigo recur

Family/patient understands diet, if on special diet

COMPLICATIONS

Adverse drug reaction

Dehydration

Persistent fever

SECTION THREE

Complications

Critical nursing management recording and reporting	Health education	Specific instruction for data retrieval
Abscess, anorectal		

Monitor, record, and report temperature elevation every 4 hours
Observe and record redness or edema of rectum
Observe and record rectal dressing for bleeding, drainage, odor, or other problems
	Instruct patient/family about signs and symptoms of infection	Nurse's notes for:
		  Observation for redness or edema of rectum
		  Observation of dressings for presence of blood, drainage, odor, or other problems
		Graphic record for temperature above 101.4° F

Abscess, brain		

Observe, record, and report the presence of any of the following: headache, weakness of arm or leg, depression of vision, focal epileptic seizures, fever and leukocytosis, or change in mental alertness
Support patient during seizures, taking proper safety precautions and actions
Implement measures to reduce fever and force fluids, if not contraindicated
Observe for signs of increased intracranial pressure; report immediately
Implement comfort measures to reduce pain
	Prepare family for possible outcomes
	In the event of postabscess epilepsy, teach patient/family principles of reducing occurrence of seizures by avoiding alcohol, excessive fatigue, and emotional stress; stress the importance of staying on anticonvulsant medication and the name, dosage, frequency, side effects, and precautions of each medication; also teach regarding legal implications
	In the event of residual postabscess hemiparesis, teach family range-of-motion exercises, methods of strengthening quadriceps muscles, methods of assisting patient in carrying out activities of daily living
	In the event of speech deficit, teach family means of improving speech and methods of communication
		Nurse's notes for:
		  Observation of headache, weakness of arm or leg, depression of vision, focal epileptic seizures, fever and leukocytosis, and changes in mental alertness
		  Frequency, characteristics, and precautions of seizures
		  Monitoring of fever and implementation of measures to reduce fever
		  Frequent observation for signs of increased intracranial pressure
		  Notification of physician of any signs of increased intracranial pressure
		  Explanation of comfort measures instituted to reduce pain
		  Preparation of family for possible outcomes
		  Instruction of patient/family about postabscess epilepsy, treatment of postabscess hemiparesis or speech deficit
		Temperature graph for temperature above 101.4° F
		Intake record for forced fluids to help reduce fever
		Medication record for comparison of frequency of analgesic (narcotic) with comfort measures implemented to reduce pain

Continued.

Critical nursing management recording and reporting	Health education	Specific instruction for data retrieval
Abscess, intraperitoneal		
Observe, record, and report the presence of pain, the absence of bowel sounds, and fever	Defer complex teaching during acute phase but respond openly to questions	Nurse's notes for:
		Description of location, duration, intensity, and frequency of pain
Notify physician within 10 minutes of investigation of patient's complaints of pain		Auscultation for bowels sounds with absence of sounds
Implement nothing by mouth order		Notification of physician within 10 minutes of investigation of patient's complaints of pain
Auscultate for bowel sounds every hour		Notation of nothing by mouth order
Provide periods of uninterrupted rest		Deferring of complex teaching during acute phase
		Graphic record for temperature above 101.4° F
Acidosis, diabetic		
Observe, record, and report nausea, vomiting, excessive thirst, "fruity" or acetone breath odor, hyperpnea, fever, increased somnolence, soft eyeballs, warm dry skin, rapid thready pulse, low blood pressure, polyuria, dehydration, distorted vision, mental changes, unconsciousness, or tachycardia	Instruct patient/family on signs and symptoms of diabetic hyperglycemia and appropriate action to take	Nurse's notes for:
		Description of the signs and symptoms of impending diabetic acidosis (nausea, vomiting, excessive thirst, "fruity" breath odor, hyperpnea, fever, increased somnolence, soft eyeballs, warm dry skin, rapid thready pulse, and low blood pressure)
Notify physician of symptoms and/or signs of diabetic acidosis	Reinforce teaching about diet and the importance of adhering to it; have patient plan several different meals to ensure understanding	Notification of physician of impending diabetic acidosis
Monitor and report an elevated blood sugar (above 200 mg per 100 ml of blood), plasma ketone, low carbon dioxide, or marked sugar and acetone in the urine	Reinforce the need to test the urine before each meal; have the patient/family return demonstration	Assessment of precipitating cause of diabetic acidosis (signs of infection, diet abuses, activity level variations, incorrect administration of hypoglycemic agents)
Monitor urine for glucose and acetone before meals and bedtime	Reinforce teaching concerning hypoglycemic agent—particularly dosage and administration; have patient/family demonstrate ability to carry out sterilization and administration techniques correctly	Administration of parenteral fluids according to physician's orders
Assess precipitating cause of diabetic acidosis (for example, infection, diet abuses, activity level variations, and incorrect administration of hypoglycemic agent)	Reinforce teaching concerning relationship of infections and activity level to diabetes control	Instruction of patient/family about diabetes, hyperglycemia, diet adherence, urine testing, hypoglycemic agents, and prevention of infection

Critical nursing management recording and reporting	Health education	Specific instruction for data retrieval
Administer parenteral fluids as ordered (type and amount per 24 hours)		Diabetic flow sheet for urine testing, insulin administration, diet consumption, and activity level
Maintain a record of intake and output every 8 hours		Intake and output record for accurate record every 8 hours
Administer insulin according to established order		Medication record for insulin administration
		Laboratory reports for blood sugar above 200 mg per 100 ml of blood, positive plasma ketones, low carbon dioxide, and marked sugar and acetone in the urine

Airway obstruction in children

Observe, record, and report the presence of cyanosis or dyspnea and a change in respiratory rate and depth	Explain to child/parents treatment being performed and precautions while oxygen is being used	Nurse's notes for: Description of cyanosis, dyspnea, and change in respiratory rate and depth
Position patient on side with neck hyperextended		Positioning on side with neck hyperextended
Notify physician immediately		Notification of physician within 15 minutes
Observe respiratory rate, depth, and difficulty and skin color every 15 minutes until stable, then every 2 hours		Implementation of measures to keep child quiet
Monitor vital signs every 15 minutes until stable		Explanation of procedures to child/parents
Administer oxygen; monitor concentration		Graphic record of vital signs and respiratory rate, depth, and difficulty every 15 minutes until stable, then every 2 hours
Keep child quiet and calm through use of simple diversions		
Keep equipment for respiratory assistance in room		Oxygen record for administration of oxygen and for monitoring of oxygen concentration
Explain treatments to child/parents		

Alkalosis, hypochloremic

Observe, record, and report the presence of dehydration, dry mucous membranes, loss of tissue turgor, and latent or manifest tetany	Instruct patient/family about potential complications of hypochloremic alkalosis and rationale for treatment	Nurse's notes for: Description of mucous membranes, tissue turgor, tetany
		Notification of physician

Continued.

Alkalosis, hypochloremic—cont'd

Notify physician within 1 hour

Monitor vital signs hourly until stable

Measure intake and output hourly until symptoms relieved

Instruction of patient/family about complications and rationale for treatment

Intake and output record for hourly monitoring

Graphic record for hourly monitoring of vital signs

Amputation of lower extremity for diabetes*

Implement measures to assist patient/family in coping with changes in patient's body image

Record and report postoperative observations, including shock, hemorrhage, phantom pain, changes in mental status, joint contractures, motor or sensory impairment, or infection

In the event of shock from hemorrhage, apply a tourniquet and administer parenteral fluids to replace fluid loss, record vital signs every 15 minutes until stable, then hourly for 8 hours, then every 4 hours

Instruct patient/family on reason for amputation; explain surgical procedures; recovery room; intravenous therapy, possible traction or rigid plaster dressing; exercises to strengthen arm muscles, quadriceps, and other muscles in preparation for crutchwalking; deep-breathing exercises; postoperative measures to control discomfort; and frequency of postoperative procedures (such as vital signs)

Nurse's notes for:

Description of measures implemented to assist patient/family with change in patient's body image

Effectiveness of preoperative teaching and care

Postoperative observation for shock (evidenced by decreased or falling blood pressure; vertigo; restlessness; anxiety; tachycardia with weak, thready pulse; shallow respiration; extreme weakness; lethargy; cool, pale, clammy, or cyanotic skin; urinary output below 30 ml per hour; or excessive body fluid loss from wound); hemorrhage; phantom pain; changes in mental status; joint contractures; sensory-motor impairment; and wound infection (evidenced by purulent drainage or odor)

Notification of physician if signs and symptoms of shock are observed

Application of tourniquet and administration of parenteral fluids, if shock is present

---

*This may be necessary because of vascular insufficiency, gangrene, osteomyelitis, or a chronically severe nonhealing skin cancer that resists grafting.

Critical nursing management recording and reporting	Health education	Specific instruction for data retrieval
		Graphic record for recording of vital signs every 15 minutes until stable, if shock is present

Anastomotic leak or stricture of esophagus

Observe, record, and report the presence of midsternal or substernal pain, choking, heartburn, regurgitation without vomiting, dysphagia, or elevation in temperature	Instruct patient/family about importance of bland diet; small, frequent meals, eaten slowly; and use of semi-Fowler's position	Nurse's notes for:
Notify physician of symptoms	Encourage patient to avoid smoking, taking aspirin, bending or stooping, and getting constipated	Observation of choking, pain, vomiting, or dysphagia
Evaluate at meal time for choking, or, if chest tube in place, for feeding draining from chest tube		Notification of physician of symptoms
Serve small, frequent meals, usually bland with low residue		Encouragement to take fluids with meals
Encourage intake of fluids with meals		Instruction about diet and the use of small, frequent meals
Maintain intake and output		Utilization of semi-Fowler's position after meals
Utilize semi-Fowler's position after meals and at bedtime to avoid supine position		Intake/output record for monitoring

Aneurysm, intracranial, or subarachnoid hemorrhage

Observe, record, and report the presence of increased pulse rate that later becomes slow and bounding; widening pulse pressure; irregular respiration; decreased sensorium; pink or red, dry, warm skin; unequal or unreactive pupils; decreasing level of consciousness; increasing loss of motor power; headache on effort; vomiting that may be projectile; bulging fontanelle in infant	Defer teaching during acute phase	Nurse's notes for: Description of pulse rate; widening pulse pressure; irregular respiration; red or pink, dry, warm skin; unequal or unreactive pupils; decreasing level of consciousness; increasing loss of motor power; headache on effort; vomiting that may be projectile
Elevate head of bed 30 degrees, if no skull fracture present		Elevation of head of bed 30 degrees
Provide oxygen as necessary by nasal cannula, 4 to 6 liters per minute		Initiation of nothing by mouth order
		Positioning and suctioning to maintain airway
		Notification of physician
		Oxygen record for administration of oxygen by nasal

Continued.

Critical nursing management recording and reporting	Health education	Specific instruction for data retrieval

Aneurysm, intracranial, or subarachnoid hemorrhage—cont'd

Maintain nothing by mouth until further orders

Maintain adequate airway by positioning and suctioning as necessary

Notify physician within 15 minutes

cannula at 4 to 6 liters per minute

Graphic record for increase in pulse rate

Aneurysm, intracranial, or subarachnoid hemorrhage in children

Observe, record, and report the presence of decreased sensorium, bulging fontanelle in infant, headache in older child, decreased pulse and/or respiration rate, elevated temperature, increased blood pressure, projectile vomiting, irritability; and alternating periods of lethargy and restlessness	Explanation to parents; reinforcement of physician's rationale for treatment; identification of medical and nursing management	Nurse's notes for:
Notify physician immediately		Description of decrease in sensorium, bulging fontanelle in infant, headache on effort in older child, decreased pulse and/or respiratory rate, projectile vomiting, irritability, and alternating periods of lethargy and restlessness
Implement physician's orders		Notification of physician
Keep child flat in bed; do not raise head		Comparison of physician's orders with nursing actions for implementation of physician orders
Monitor vital signs and rectal temperature and implement neurological check every 15 minutes until stable		Maintenance of patient flat in bed; no head raising
Provide nonstimulating and nonstressful environment, with all care provided by nursing staff		Graphic record for monitoring vital signs and rectal temperature every 15 minutes until stable

Arrhythmias

Observe, record, and report disturbances in pulse rate (bradycardia or tachycardia) and/or rhythm	Teach patient to take own pulse correctly and to note irregularities; instruct patient to see physician if irregularities persist	Nurse's notes for:
Monitor patient via cardiac monitor, with immediate reporting to physician of the presence of warning or lethal arrhythmias; monitor continually until cardiac function returns to normal and remains normal for at least 4 consecutive days	Instruct on the purpose and duration of oxygen therapy	Description of disturbances in pulse rate (tachycardia—heart rate faster than 100 beats per minute—and/or bradycardia—heart rate slower than 60 beats per minute)
Administer appropriate drug therapy according to phy-	If patient is discharged on medications for cardiac condition, instruct on the name, purpose, dosage, frequency, side effects, action to take if side effects occur, and precautions of each	Description of disturbances in rhythm (ventricular tachycardia or ventricular fibrillation)
		Evidence of physician notification of pulse rate variations

Critical nursing management recording and reporting	Health education	Specific instruction for data retrieval
sician's orders (usually lidocaine intravenously, followed by intravenous infusion at a rate of 1 to 2 mg per minute)		Record of effectiveness of oxygen administration and of lidocaine for emergency situation and of response of patient
If ventricular fibrillation occurs, accomplish defibrillation with 30 seconds, followed by lidocaine intravenous infusion to prevent recurrence		Electrocardiogram monitor sheet for observation and/or identification of arrhythmias and for notification of physician
Administer oxygen by nasal cannula or catheter at 4 to 6 liters per minute		Oxygen record for administration of oxygen at 4 to 6 liters per minute
Provide adequate rest periods during and after nursing care		

Aspiration

Critical nursing management recording and reporting	Health education	Specific instruction for data retrieval
Observe, record, and report the presence of choking, cyanosis, pallor, or respiratory difficulty	Teach family to recognize signs of aspiration should they occur during home care	Nurse's notes for:
Suction patient frequently	Teach family to suction patient	Description of cyanosis (blueness) or pallor around mouth and/or nail beds
Position patient to aid in the drainage of secretions	Teach family method of positioning patient properly to drain secretions	Variation in rate, depth, or characteristics of respiration
Administer oxygen by nasal cannula or catheter at 4 to 6 liters per minute	Encourage family to get a small bottle of emergency oxygen for home use; teach family to use it	Patient's verbalization of difficulty in breathing or belief that something went down airway
	Instruct family in precautions of oxygen administration (for example, no smoking or flames in room where oxygen is in use)	Frequency of suctioning
		Positioning to aid in drainage of secretions
		Oxygen record for administration of oxygen at 4 to 6 liters per minute
		Graphic record for change in respiratory rate
		Instruction and return demonstration of family about signs of aspiration, suctioning methods, and safe oxygen administration

Atelectasis

Critical nursing management recording and reporting	Health education	Specific instruction for data retrieval
Observe, record, and report the presence of fever, elevated pulse rate, dyspnea or in-	Instruct patient on purpose and methods of deep breathing and coughing	Nurse's notes for: Rate, characteristics, and depth of respiration

Continued.

Critical nursing management recording and reporting	Health education	Specific instruction for data retrieval
Atelectasis—cont'd		

Atelectasis—cont'd

creased rate in respiration, apprehension, chest pain, coughing, or abnormal chest x-ray

Turn patient every hour, maintaining correct position and alignment

Assess chest physiotherapy prior to deep breathing and coughing every hour

Provide oxygen as needed at 4 to 6 liters per minute by nasal cannula

Suction as needed using blow bottle every hour

Provide adequate rest periods during and after nursing care as well as comfort measures to reduce pain that may be associated with coexisting pneumonia or pleurisy

Explain purpose and duration of oxygen

Instruct on importance and method of changing position frequently and keeping in correct position and alignment

Instruct on purpose and method of using blow bottle, humidifier mists, and/or intermittent positive pressure breathing

Encourage intake of warm fluids

Monitoring of pulse rate and notation if increased

Evaluation of patient's emotional status (presence or absence of apprehension)

Description of coughing; presence of sputum

Hourly turning and positioning of patient

Instruction of patient/family on uses of blow bottle and frequent suctioning

Discussion of comfort measures employed to reduce pain associated with coexisting conditions

Oxygen record for administration at 4 to 6 liters per minute

Atrial fibrillation

Observe, record, and report an abnormal heart rate in which the ventricular rate is rapid and the rhythm is irregular

Monitor pulse deficit

Observe and record if the intensity of the irregularity increases with exercise when the heart rate is slow

Immediately notify physician of arrhythmia

Provide emotional support to patient/family

Instruct patient/family to monitor possible arrhythmias by observing and recording apical and pulse rates

Stress the importance of regular administration of medication; help patient/family understand potential side effects, appropriate dosage and frequency, desired effects, and precautions of the medication

Nurse's notes for:

Observation of ventricular response that is irregular, ranging from 80 to 160 beats per minute

Record of pulse deficit (the difference between apical rate and pulse rate; the deficit is greater when the ventricular rate is high)

Immediate notification of physician of atrial fibrillation

Observation of effect of exercise on heart rate

Verbalization by patient/family of responses to condition and treatment

Response of patient/family to instruction about monitoring pulse and medication administration

Cardiac monitor record for

identification of arrhythmias

Bleeding, with anticoagulant therapy

Observe, record, and report the presence of hematuria, pain, tarry stools, hematemesis, epistaxis, bleeding gums, hemoptysis, subcutaneous bleeding, hematoma, joint pain, bleeding at site of incision or injection, increased menstrual flow, and medications that potentiate or retard anticoagulation	Instruct patient/family in importance of medication, including the name, dosage, frequency, purpose, side effects, and precautions	Nurse's notes for: Presence of hematuria, diarrhea, vomiting, elevated temperature, pain in joints, epistaxis, bleeding gums, or other problems
Monitor and record vital signs every 4 hours	Stress the necessity of reporting hematuria, diarrhea, vomiting, elevated temperature, pain in joints, epistaxis, or bleeding gums to physician	Inspection of puncture sites every 4 hours
Notify physician of suspected bleeding		Notification of physician about suspected bleeding
Coordinate laboratory work to avoid multiple punctures	Explain to patient the reasons for avoidance of vigorous nose blowing, vigorous brushing of teeth, water jet tooth cleaners, use of sharp-edged razors, excessive intake of alcoholic beverages, and bruises	Notation that salicylates are not to be administered to the patient
Keep protamine sulfate or phytonadione available as emergency drug	Explain importance of wearing or carrying a medical alert tag or card indicating that patient is on anticoagulant therapy	Graphic record for recording vital signs every 4 hours
		Output record for color (tarry or not tarry) and frequency of stools
		Medication record for sites of injections and for medications that potentiate anticoagulant therapy

Bleeding, recurrent, and shock

Record and report the presence of tachycardia; increased shallow respiration; cold, clammy skin; sudden drop in blood pressure or blood pressure that drops below 90/60; cyanosis; pallor; or urinary output of less than 30 ml per hour	Instruct patient/family of the need to monitor vital signs, urinary output, and drainage at incision site in order to avoid complications	Nurse's notes for: Presence of signs and symptoms of shock (tachycardia; increased shallow respiration; cold, clammy skin; sudden drop in blood pressure or blood pressure below 90/60; cyanosis; pallor; or urinary output of less than 30 ml per hour)
Notify physician of signs of shock or bleeding		Notation that antihypertensive medications were held
Hold all antihypertensive drugs until further orders		Notification of physician of signs of shock or bleeding
Avoid Trendelenburg's position; elevate lower extremities 20 degrees, keeping knees straight, trunk horizontal, and head slightly elevated		Positioning patient with

Continued.

Critical nursing management recording and reporting	Health education	Specific instruction for data retrieval

Bleeding, recurrent, and shock—cont'd

Speed up rate of intravenous infusion; keep patient warm but not overheated

Administer oxygen as needed by nasal cannula at 4 to 6 liters per minute, if not contraindicated

lower extremities elevated 20 degrees, but Trendelenburg's position not used

Intravenous infusion rate increase or, if intravenous therapy not already present, initiation

Maintenance of warmth without overheating the patient

Oxygen administration at 4 to 6 liters per minute

Instruction of patient/family about monitoring for possible complications

Output record for maintenance of urinary output at greater than 30 ml per hour

Intravenous record for increased infusion rate at time symptoms of shock were identified

Oxygen record for administration of oxygen at 4 to 6 liters per minute

Medication record for stopping of antihypertensive drugs

Graphic record for monitoring of blood pressure every 15 minutes until stable, then hourly

Blindness

Observe, record, and report difficulty in seeing, blurred or distorted vision, frequent falling or bumping into objects, or clumsiness in carrying out activities of daily living

Notify physician of failing eyesight

Maintain patient's personal items and the furniture in the same location at all times; familiarize patient with new items through sense of touch

Instruct patient/family on the importance of maintaining furniture and personal items in the same place for safety reasons

Instruct patient/family on the importance of maintaining a safe environment; explain methods to achieve this

Inform patient/family of community resources for the blind and the type of services available

Instruct family of diabetic patient on techniques of steril-

Nurse's notes for:

Evaluation of patient's eyesight (difficulty seeing, blurred or distorted vision, frequent falling or bumping into objects, or clumsiness in carrying out activities of daily living)

Notification of physician of decreasing eyesight

Referral to social services and/or appropriate community agencies

Instruction of patient/family about safety for blind peo-

Critical nursing management recording and reporting	Health education	Specific instruction for data retrieval
Refer to social services and/or appropriate community agencies for services to the blind	izing equipment, administering insulin, encouraging independence as much as possible, and what can be done safely by the patient	ple and methods by which to adapt to decreased eyesight
For diabetic patient, secure insulin syringe designed for self-administration of insulin by blind patients (preset dosage regulator and safety guard); instruct patient in its use	To the family of diabetic patient stress the importance of correct medication and adherence to diet and activity level as means of preventing further deterioration of sight and possibly other complications	Special adaptations, such as diabetic syringes for the blind, to primary diagnosis
For diabetic patient, instruct in safety measures; teach to utilize equipment for insulin injection properly, as well as to recognize correct medication by adaptive devices on labels and by touch		
Review diabetic diet instructions for patient/family		
For diabetic patient, identify responsible person to assist with meal preparation and urine testing after discharge		
Refer diabetic patient to home-nursing agency for home teaching and follow-up nursing care		

Blood urea nitrogen, rising

Observe, record, and report presence of nausea, vomiting, confused state, change in intake and output, itching skin, and urea frost on skin	Instruct patient/family in necessity of maintaining accurate intake and output records	Nurse's notes for:
		Observation of mental state; presence of nausea and/or vomiting, itching skin, and urea frost on skin, and change in intake and output
Notify physician of abnormal laboratory report of blood urea nitrogen (BUN) greater than 20 mg per 100 ml of blood		Notification of physician
Maintain accurate intake and output every 2 hours		Intake and output record for accurate monitoring every 2 hours
Monitor vital signs every 2 hours		Graphic record for monitoring of vital signs every 2 hours
		Laboratory report for blood urea nitrogen greater than 20 mg per 100 ml of blood

Continued.

Bone, pathological involvement and/or fractures of

Observe, record, and report the location, severity, and frequency of pain	Teach patient how to move to prevent pain	Nurse's notes for:
Administer analgesics as needed and ½ hour before ambulation	Teach importance of moving in spite of pain to prevent further complications	Description of pain—location, frequency, and severity
Provide careful handling and adequate support of painful body parts		Measures implemented to reduce pain
Prevent hypostatic pneumonia and skin breakdown by turning patient every 2 hours		Frequency of analgesic administration
Keep stools soft to prevent straining for bowel movements		Prevention of complications by turning every 2 hours
Monitor laboratory reports of calcium levels		Encouragement to patient to move, turn, cough, and deep breath every 2 hours
Immediately notify physician of increased calcium levels		Characteristics of stools—frequency and consistency
		Notification of physician of increased calcium levels
		Laboratory reports for calcium levels
		Flow sheet for turning and moving patient every 2 hours and for evaluation of skin condition

Bone marrow suppression

Observe, record, and report infections or bleeding	Inform patient/family of the possibilities of bone marrow suppression and of the need to avoid infections	Nurse's notes for:
Notify physician of bleeding or infections	Teach patient/family of rationale and relationship of complication to disease process and treatment	Daily evaluation of patient for signs of infection or bleeding
Protect patient from exposure to infections		Notification of physician of infection or bleeding
Monitor patient's complaints of pain in long bone areas or tenderness, especially when pressure is applied		Instruction of patient/family about avoidance of infection or injury
		Evaluation of patient's complaints about pain or tenderness in long bone areas, especially when pressure is applied
		Laboratory reports for variations in complete blood counts
		Graphic records for monitoring of temperature above 101.4° F

Critical nursing management recording and reporting	Health education	Specific instruction for data retrieval

Bowel obstruction

Observe, record, and report such symptoms as the presence of abdominal pain or distention, nausea, vomiting, loss of appetite, fever, hyperactive bowel sounds, decreased urinary output or renal shutdown, signs of dehydration, abnormal serum electrolytes, or shock	Explain reason for placing patient on nothing by mouth order	Nurse's notes for:
Maintain patient on nothing by mouth order until further orders are given	Instruct on purpose and methods of turning, coughing, and deep breathing every 2 hours; encourage patient to carry out these measures	Description of observations—such as presence of abdominal pain or distention, nausea, vomiting, loss of appetite, fever, hyperactive bowel sounds, urinary output decrease, dehydration, cold, clammy skin, or restlessness
Monitor vital signs every 10 to 15 minutes		Maintaining patient on nothing by mouth
Administer pain-reducing measures as appropriate (if paralytic ileus, avoid giving morphine); place in semi-Fowler's position		Notification of physician
Administer parenteral fluids according to rate of flow and type ordered for 24-hour period		Administration of pain-reducing measures
Notify physician of possible bowel obstruction		If paralytic ileus, no administration of morphine
		Placement in semi-Fowler's position
		Administration of parenteral fluids
		Laboratory reports for abnormal serum electrolytes
		Output record for decreased urinary output
		Temperature record for temperature above 101.4° F
		Graphic record for vital signs every 15 minutes

Cancer, complications of
Hemorrhage from blood vessels eroded by malignant tissues
Infections of tissues undergoing malignant changes
Metastatic deposition of tumor cells
Pathological fractures

Observe, record, and report the presence of pain or discomfort in body parts not involved in malignancy; signs of hemorrhage, fever and/or chills, bone pain resulting from falls or accidents	Teach patient/family about condition, possible sites of metastatic disease, prognosis, treatment plan, and symptoms to report to physician	Nurse's notes for:
Notify physician	Explain good health habits, safety, nutrition, and activity levels	Description of signs of spread of cancer, presence of hemorrhage, symptoms of infections, or signs of pathological fractures
Give emotional support; allow patient to express feelings about cancer and/or death		Notification of physician
		Emotional support to patient
		Instruction to patient/family about condition, prognosis, treatment, symptoms to report to physician, and good health habits

Continued.

Critical nursing management recording and reporting	Health education	Specific instruction for data retrieval
Cardiac arrest		
Initiate cardiopulmonary resuscitation within 3 minutes of cardiac arrest	Provide family with emotional support; inform them of emergency situation of cardiac arrest	Nurse's notes for:
Monitor vital parameters after cardiac arrest, including temperature, pulse, respiration, blood pressure, central venous pressure, urinary output, circulation, level of consciousness, and blood gases hourly until stable; discontinue reporting, recording, and monitoring for abnormal findings after 5 consecutive days of normal findings		Notation, prior to calling a cardiac arrest, of six or more premature ventricular complexes per minute Patient's responses Notification of physician of abnormalities Administration of oxygen at 4 to 6 liters per minute Comparison of time of cardiac arrest with time cardiopulmonary resuscitation was initiated—must be less than 3 minutes
Monitor for lethal or warning arrhythmias hourly until stable; discontinue after 5 consecutive days of normal findings		Graphic sheet, intensive care flow record, nurse's notes, and intake and output record for hourly monitoring of vital parameters until stable and for 5 consecutive days of normal findings
Administer oxygen as needed by nasal cannula or catheter at 4 to 6 liters per minute		Cardiac monitoring record for identification of lethal or warning arrhythmias hourly and for 5 consecutive days of normal findings
Cerebrovascular accident (CVA)		
Observe, record, and report the presence of flushed face; stertorous or Cheyne-Stokes respiration; full and slow pulse rate; one arm and/or leg flaccid; derangement of speech, thought, motion, sensation, or vision; possible alterations in consciousness; headache; dizziness, drowsiness, mental confusion; fever; vomiting; convulsions; or coma	Instruct patient/family on name, purpose, frequency, dosage, side effects, action to take if side effects occur, and precautions of each discharge medication Instruct patient on safety measures at home If a diabetic, reinforce diabetic teaching Discuss types and methods of rehabilitation appropriate for patient's residual complications, such as paralysis or speech derangement	Nurse's notes for: Observation of sudden onset of neurological complaints—flushed face; stertorous or Cheyne-Stokes respiration; one arm and/or leg flaccid; full and slow pulse; derangement of speech, thought, motion, sensations, or vision; possible alterations in level of consciousness; headache; dizziness; drowsiness; mental confusion; fever; vomiting; convulsions; or coma
Notify physician of sudden onset of neurological complaints		Notification of physician of sudden onset of neurological complaints
Monitor vital signs every 15 minutes until stable, then every 4 hours		

Critical nursing management recording and reporting	Health education	Specific instruction for data retrieval
Maintain airway with frequent suctioning Administer oxygen by nasal cannula or catheter at 4 to 6 liters per minute Evaluate level of consciousness, movement of extremities, urinary output every hour; report any changes		Evaluation of level of consciousness, movement of extremities, and urinary output every hour until stable Notation that airway was maintained and frequent suctioning was performed Instruction of patient/family about medications, safety measures, rehabilitation, and appropriate community agencies Graphic record for monitoring temperature and for reporting temperature greater than 101.4° F Output record for hourly measurement of urinary output Oxygen record for administration of oxygen at 4 to 6 liters per minute

Chemotherapy, complications of
Alopecia
Bone marrow disturbances
Gastrointestinal disturbances
  Constipation
  Diarrhea
  Muscositis
  Nausea and vomiting
Tissue breakdown
Toxicity beyond therapeutic units

Critical nursing management recording and reporting	Health education	Specific instruction for data retrieval
Observe, record, and report signs of toxicity, abrasions of mouth, nausea and vomiting, diarrhea, absence of bowel movement for 3 consecutive days, bleeding, increased temperature, decreased white blood cell count, decreased platelets, loss of hair, or skin breakdown Notify physician of signs and/or symptoms of chemotherapy complications Maintain patient's mouth clear	Instruct patient/family about possible toxic reactions and symptoms of and preventive measures used with chemotherapy Explain bowel program procedure Teach rationale for purchasing wig or hair piece before hair loss occurs Instruct in measures to maintain or improve skin integrity	Nurse's notes for: Description of side effects of chemotherapy[*] Notification of physician Instruction of patient/family about chemotherapy, toxic reactions, bowel program, use of wig, and ·measures to maintain skin integrity Intake and output record Medication record for administration of antiemetic and/or antidiarrhea medications Laboratory reports for white blood cell count less than

[*]Data analyst will require a list of individual chemotherapy agents and specific side effects.

Continued.

Critical nursing management recording and reporting	Health education	Specific instruction for data retrieval
Chemotherapy—cont'd		4,000 per ml of blood and/or platelets less than 150,000 per ml
and free from abrasions; offer nonirritating food and/or fluids		Flow sheet for skin care, positioning, and turning every 2 hours
Monitor intake and output		
Administer antiemetic medications as ordered for nausea and vomiting		
Replace fluid in event of diarrhea		
Establish bowel program, if constripation present		
Observe for evidence of bleeding		
Evaluate laboratory results; notify physician of white blood cell count less than 4,000 per ml of blood and/or platelets less than 150,000 per ml		
Assess hair loss		
Maintain skin integrity through maintenance of cleanliness, avoidance of pressure or irritation, and elimination of use of lotions if cobalt therapy ordered		
Coma, diabetic		
Observe, record, and report the presence of thirst; loss of appetite; vomiting; abdominal pain; double or blurred vision; dry, hot skin; headache; listlessness; lack of patient response, Kussmaul-Kien respiration; acetone breath; decreased blood pressure; or marked sugar and acetone spillage in the urine	Instruct patient on necessity of adhering to diet; stress diet allowances; have patient plan three separate meals, using exchange list, to determine understanding of diet; persist in instruction until patient successfully shows understanding of diet through appropriate meal planning	Nurse's notes for: Observation of symptoms and signs of diabetic coma—thirst; loss of appetite; vomiting; abdominal pain; double or blurred vision; dry, hot skin; headache; listlessness; lack of patient response; acetone breath, Kussmaul-Kien respiration, decreased blood pressure, or marked sugar and acetone spillage in the urine
Monitor urinary spillage of sugar and acetone every 2 hours; immediately report findings regarding blood glucose, carbon dioxide, pH, electrolytes, acetone, blood urea nitrogen, or hematocrit levels, when abnormal	Instruct patient on need to adhere to prescribed daily administration of hypoglycemic agent; supervise self-administration of agent accomplished properly Instruct on name, dosage, purpose, frequency, side effects, action to take if side effects	Notification of physician of possible diabetic coma or abnormal laboratory reports Instruction and return demonstration of patient/fam-

Critical nursing management recording and reporting	Health education	Specific instruction for data retrieval
Administer rapid-acting insulin according to established orders Administer parenteral fluids according to type and amount per 24 hours, as ordered; maintain strict intake and output records; if there is no Foley catheter present and there is difficulty obtaining specimens because of patient's inability to void, incontinence, or some other problem, secure order for a Foley catheter; insert it, using strict sterile technique Monitor vital signs every 2 to 4 hours, unless otherwise ordered for monitoring circulatory status	occur of each medication; if on insulin, stress importance of sterile equipment, rotating sites of injection and dosage, as well as technique of administration Instruct patient on measures, such as good skin hygiene, preventing circulatory stasis, regular dental care, and receiving proper immunizations, and importance of preventing infection and the need for prompt medical attention should one occur Instruct patient on the importance of adhering to prescribed activity levels	ily on all aspects of diabetic care Intake and output record for strict recording of intake and output per 24 hours Laboratory reports for abnormal blood glucose, carbon dioxide, pH, electrolytes, acetone, blood urea nitrogen, 4+ acetone and sugar in urine, positive urinary acetoacetic acid, elevated blood glucose, low serum carbon dioxide; serum potassium unusually elevated, serum sodium and chloride low, plasma acetone positive, nonprotein nitrogen elevated, lipemia present, and blood urea nitrogen elevated Diabetic flow sheet for monitoring urine acetone and glucose every 4 hours Diabetic insulin administration flow sheet or medication record for administration of rapid-acting insulin (not isophane insulin, protamine zinc insulin, or lente insulin) at onset of episode Intravenous infusion record for fluid replacement; while patient is unconscious infuse at about 60 drops per minute, unless contraindicated Graphic record for monitoring of vital signs every 2 to 4 hours for observation of circulatory status

Coma, diabetic, irreversible

Observe, record, and report the presence of coma state and lack of response to specific nursing measures Maintain adequate airway, suctioning, and administering oxygen by nasal cannula	Instruct family about complications of irreversible diabetic coma and rationale for treatment Defer patient teaching until patient is conscious	Nurse's notes for: Description of coma state and lack of response to specific nursing measures Maintenance of airway, through frequent suctioning

Continued.

Critical nursing management recording and reporting	Health education	Specific instruction for data retrieval
Coma, diabetic, irreversible—cont'd		
or catheter at 4 to 6 liters per minute		Notification of physician of patient's unresponsiveness and coma state
Notify physician of patient's unresponsiveness		Turning and positioning every 2 hours
Maintain safety of patient by correct positioning, use of side rails, and close observation		Emotional support and instruction to family about irreversible coma
Turn patient every 2 hours		Observation of level of consciousness every 2 hours
Monitor urinary spillage of sugar and acetone every 2 hours; immediately report findings regarding blood glucose, carbon dioxide, pH, electrolytes, acetone, blood urea nitrogen and hematocrit levels, when abnormal		Laboratory reports for changes in blood glucose, carbon dioxide, pH, electrolytes, acetone, blood urea nitrogen or hematocrit levels
Evaluate vital signs, temperature, level of consciousness, movement of extremities, and urinary output every 2 hours		Graphic sheet for vital signs and elevated or subnormal temperature
		Intake and output record sheet for urinary output at least 30 ml per hour
		Diabetic flow sheet for urine testing for glucose and acetone; insulin administration correlation with intravenous therapy for intake
		Oxygen record for administration of oxygen by nasal cannula or catheter at 4 to 6 liters per minute

Consciousness, deterioration of, with rapid correction of hyperglycemia, pH, or dehydration

Observe, record and report the presence of fluctuation of moods, indigestion or heartburn, extreme hunger, sweating, generalized weakness, rapid pulse, distorted vision, syncope, weight gain, unconsciousness, seizures, or low blood sugar	Instruct patient/family about hypoglycemic reactions and corrective and preventive measures to use	Nurse's notes for:
		Description of signs and symptoms indicating deterioration of consciousness—fluctuation of moods, indigestion or heartburn, extreme hunger, sweating, generalized weakness, rapid pulse, distorted vision, or syncope
Monitor patient for symptoms occurring 2 to 4 hours after meals	Stress the importance of strict adherence to diet	
Maintain high-protein, high-fat, low-carbohydrate diet as ordered, providing small frequent feedings (six feedings)	Teach family safety measures to employ when patient experiences deterioration of consciousness	Observation of symptoms occurring 2 to 4 hours after meals
Encourage patient not to		Notification of physician of symptoms
		Encouragement of patient to adhere to diet

Critical nursing management recording and reporting	Health education	Specific instruction for data retrieval
"cheat" on diet; discourage foods for snacking brought by visitors Provide fluid intake of 2,700 ml per 24 hours, unless contraindicated Ambulate patient at least every 4 hours, unless otherwise ordered, or unless patient is unconscious Preserve safety of patient during onset of symptoms and during unconsciousness, including maintaining adequate airway and protection from self-injury during convulsions Administer carbohydrate feeding at onset of symptoms		Response of patient to treatment plan Implementation of safety measures to protect patient during onset of symptoms Instruction for patient/family about signs and symptoms Diet sheet for meals six times daily Intake record for fluids, at least 2,700 ml per 24 hour period Laboratory report for blood sugar below 70 mg per 100 ml of blood Graphic record for daily weighing and notation of weight gain Graphic record for increase in pulse above 100

Contractures

Observe, record, and report the presence of deformity, rigidity of joints and extremities, parts of extremities being drawn toward the midline, muscle spasms, and/or decreased range of motion Notify physician of contractures beginning Implement range-of-motion exercises every 4 hours, with gentle massage of contracted muscles prior to range-of-motion exercises to reduce spasticity and rigidity Maintain proper positioning and alignment at all times, when patient is standing, sitting, lying, or walking Change patient's position every 2 hours Implement use of supportive devices, such as pillows, sandbags, footboards, slings, and trochanter rolls to prevent deformity Provide warm bath to relax tightened muscles	Teach family signs and symptoms of contractures, in the event the patient is discharged for home care and is semi-invalid Teach family range-of-motion exercises Teach family methods of obtaining proper positioning and alignment and the need for frequent changing of position Teach family use of supportive devices	Nurse's notes for: Description of deformities—inappropriate alignment of extremities, muscle tightness, paralysis, or spasticity Comparison daily of changes in joint range of motion Patient's response and ability to administer self-care Notification of physician of contractures Utilization of warm baths to relax tightened muscles and patient's response to this Observation of body alignment at all times; correction of malalignment Effect of range-of-motion exercises and response of patient to them Use of firm mattress and supportive devices, such as pillows, sandbags, footboards, and slings Instruction of patient/family

Continued.

349

Critical nursing management recording and reporting	Health education	Specific instruction for data retrieval

Contractures—cont'd

Encourage maximum patient participation in own care

about prevention and treatment of contractures

Turning flow sheet or nurse's notes for turning, positioning, and rotating supportive devices every 2 hours

Dehydration

Observe, record, and report thirst; flushed, dry skin; skin turgor; dry, coated tongue; atonic muscles; blood urea nitrogen; dyspepsia

Maintain intake and output record; schedule oral fluids so that 2,800 ml are taken in within 24 hours

Encourage intake of fluids easily tolerated, such as tea, Jell-o, ice cream, carbonated beverages, bland juices, soups, or milk

If an antiemetic has been prescribed, give it ½ hour before breakfast, lunch, supper, and late snack, if not contraindicated

If nothing by mouth ordered and on parenteral fluids, maintain rate of infusion per order; should infusion rate lag, increase rate of flow by no more than 50 to 75 ml per hour until caught up

Instruct family that only fluids taken are counted; any fluids given are to be put on intake and output record

Instruct family about the importance of fluid intake of 2,800 ml per 24 hours

Nurse's notes for:

Description of symptoms—increased thirst; flushed, dry skin; decreased skin turgor; dry, coated tongue; atonic muscles; anorexia; or dyspepsia

Scheduling of oral fluid intake to reach 2,800 ml per 24 hours

Instruction of family to record fluids taken on the intake record

Intake and output record for intake of at least 2,800 ml per 24 hours

Identification on dietary sheet of patient's preference for fluids, such as ice cream rather than bland juices

Laboratory report for increase in blood urea nitrogen

Comparison of doctors orders for parenteral fluids with intravenous infusion record for accuracy in administration

Delirium tremens (acute alcohol toxic psychosis)

Observe, record, and report restlessness, disturbed sleep, irritability, clouded consciousness, confusion, seizures, maniacal destructive behavior, terrifying hallucinations, panic fever, sweating, or increase in blood pressure or in cardiac rate

Notify physician of possible

Stress the importance of patient/family informing staff of excessive alcohol intake within previous 10 days

Reassure patient/family that observation will be provided for assessment of delirium tremens

Nurse's notes for:

Assignment of patient to an area from which observations can be made, such as a semiprivate room or intensive treatment area

Removal of self-destructive articles, such as belts, razors, glass objects, ropes, knives; and scissors

Critical nursing management recording and reporting	Health education	Specific instruction for data retrieval
delirium tremens within 30 minutes		Documentation of patient's whereabouts at 15-minute intervals during waking hours and at 30 to 60-minute intervals during sleeping hours, or as necessary
		Description of signs/and symptoms of impending delirium tremens—restlessness, disturbed sleep, irritability, clouded consciousness, confusion, seizures, maniacal destructive behavior, terrifying hallucinations, panic, fever, sweating, or increase in blood pressure or in cardiac rate
		Notification of physician of signs/symptoms of impending delirium tremens
		If hallucinations are present, a description of the frequency of distorted moving animals and figures
		Graphic record for increase in blood pressure or in temperature above 101.4° F
		Medication record for the administration of tranquilizers and/or sedatives according to physician's orders
		Nursing history and assessment form for excessive alcohol intake within the previous 10 days
Dementia		
Observe, record, and report the presence of disorientation, impairment of memory, shallowness of affect, impairment of intellectual functions, impairment of judgment, irritability, rigidity of behavior, garrulousness, and/or narrowed interest	Instruct family as to status of condition and that there is no cure	Nurse's notes for:
	Instruct family on discharge medications, such as the name, purpose, dosage, frequency side effects, action to take if side effects occur, and precautions of each	Description of patient's orientation to time and place, impairment of memory, shallowness of affect, impairment of intellectual functions, impairment of judgment, irritability, rigidity of behavior, garrulousness, and/or narrowed interest
Maintain safety as related to	Instruct family on safety measures to take	

Continued.

Critical nursing management recording and reporting	Health education	Specific instruction for data retrieval
Dementia—cont'd		
patient's behavior through supervision of smoking, use of side rails at night, and supervision of movements	Instruct family on orientation measures to implement	Safety measures related to patient's behavior
Use measures, such as clocks and calendars, to help orient patient		Description of measures used to help orient patient and their effectiveness
Digitalis toxicity°		
Observe, record, and report the presence of cardiac arrhythmias, anorexia, nausea and/or vomiting, diarrhea, palpitations, change in cardiac rate, fatigue, headache, drowsiness, insomnia, restlessness, irritability, vertigo, mood change, loss of memory, aphasia, confusion, hazy vision, or visual color disturbances	Instruct patient/family how to take pulse correctly and to note irregularities	Nurse's notes for:
	If patient is discharged taking digitalis, instruct on name of drug and its purpose, dosage, frequency, side effects, precautions, and possible toxicity	Cardiac rate above 100 or below 60 beats per minute
		Description of signs and symptoms of digitalis toxicity—cardiac arrhythmias, anorexia, nausea and/or vomiting, diarrhea, palpitations, change in cardiac rate, drowsiness, fatigue, headache, insomnia, restlessness, irritability, vertigo, mood changes, loss of memory, aphasia, confusion, hazy vision, visual color disturbances
Monitor laboratory reports for decreased potassium levels, digoxin level over 2 ng per ml, and digitoxin level over 20 ng per ml		
Provide continuous cardiac monitoring		Continuous cardiac monitoring with identification of prolonged P-R interval
Notify physician of sign and symptoms		Notification of physician of signs and symptoms
Evaluate apical pulse rate and rhythm hourly		Hourly evaluation of apical pulse and rhythm
Measure intake and output every 8 hours		Graphic record for monitoring of vital signs and respiration every 4 hours
Monitor vital signs and respiration every 4 hours		Intake and output record for maintaining intake and output at least at 2,800 ml per 24-hour period
		Laboratory reports for decreased potassium levels, digoxin level over 2 ng per ml, and digitoxin level over 20 ng per ml
		Instruction of patient/family about monitoring pulse rate, noting irregularities, and the importance of digitalis administration

°See also Arrhythmias.

Critical nursing management recording and reporting	Health education	Specific instruction for data retrieval

Discharge environment, medically suitable, absence of

Involve patient/family in discharge planning

Refer to social services and/or other appropriate community resources

Provide instruction about patient's nursing and medical care that require the support of family or friends to ensure a suitable discharge environment

Instruct patient/family about what constitutes an acceptable medical discharge environment

Evaluate patient's/family's ability to continue medical and nursing regime in the discharge environment

Provide instruction to patient/family in areas of deficiency about medical and nursing regime

Inform patient/family about available community resources, services available, and whether referrals have been initiated

Nurse's notes for:

Patient/family verbalization about involvement in discharge planning

Description of reasons for medically suitable discharge environment

Instruction and return demonstration by patient/family about medical and nursing regime required in the discharge environment

Referral to social services department or appropriate outside agency if hospital does not have a social service department

Social services' progress notes for the involvement of social services and the plan for discharge care

Discharge summary for referrals to community agencies and for transfer of pertinent patient information

Drug reaction, adverse

Observe, record, and report the presence of nausea, vomiting, urticaria, hypotension, irregularities in rate and/or rhythm of pulse, disturbances of gait and/or balance, dizziness, mental dullness, or anaphylactic shock

Withhold suspected drug until further orders

Notify physician of adverse drug reaction

In the case of shock, start intravenous therapy to aid in maintaining the pressure and to provide a rapid route for the administration of emergency drugs

Administer oxygen as needed by nasal cannula at 4 to 6 liters per minute

Instruct patient to carry a medical alert tag or bracelet with information about the name of the drug giving a reaction and, its drug classification, and the physician's name

Instruct patient to inform any physician or nurse from whom health care is being received of the drug reaction, each hospitalization, and any other pertinent information

Nurse's notes for:

Description of adverse drug reaction—nausea and/or vomiting, urticaria, hypotension, irregularities in rate and/or rhythm of pulse, disturbances in gait and/or balance, dizziness, mental dullness, or anaphylactic shock

Withholding of suspected drug

Notification of physician about signs and symptoms of possible drug reaction

Instruction of patient/family about use of medical alert tag or bracelet for information about adverse drug reaction and of the necessity of telling health per-

Continued.

Drug reaction, adverse—cont'd

Administer appropriate drugs as ordered

sonnel about previous drug reactions

Medication record for identifying drug causing adverse reaction and stopping its administration

Drug reaction, adverse, to diuretics

Observe, record, and report the presence of drowsiness, weakness, lethargy, restlessness, muscle cramps, muscle fatigue, decreased blood pressure, oliguria, tachycardia, nausea, vomiting, and itching

Withhold suspected drug until further orders

Give medication with food when nausea and vomiting occur

Review serum potassium reports, if available; report abnormalities

Give foods high in potassium

Instruct patient/family about signs and symptoms of hypokalemia and other side effects of diuretics

Encourage patient to increase foods high in potassium, such as bananas and oranges

Instruct patient to weigh daily; maintain record of weight

Nurse's notes for:

Description of side effects—excessive drowsiness, weakness, lethargy, restlessness, muscle cramps, muscle fatigue, decreased blood pressure, oliguria, tachycardia, nausea, vomiting, and itching

Suspension of medication until further medical orders

Administration of medication with food if nausea and vomiting were the only side effects

Instruction and understanding by patient/family of need to increase foods high in potassium, such as bananas and oranges

Patient/family instruction to weigh and record patient's weight daily

Graphic record of daily weight being recorded

Laboratory reports for abnormalities in serum potassium reports

Notification of physician about abnormalities in serum potassium reports

Drug reaction, adverse, or dye reaction in cardiac diagnostic testing

Observe, record, and report the presence of abnormal cardiac rates or rhythms, skin eruptions, or anaphylactic shock

Instruct patient/family about the possibility of adverse reaction to drug and/or dye and the precautions that will be utilized

Nurse's notes for:

Description of symptoms of anaphylactic shock—apprehension, paresthesia, generalized urticaria or

Critical nursing management recording and reporting	Health education	Specific instruction for data retrieval
Notify physician of possible adverse drug reaction Maintain open intravenous infusion Provide respiratory assist equipment at bedside Assure patient/family of constant surveillance of patient Monitor vital signs, respiration, response to treatment, and intake and output hourly Consult with pharmacist regarding other related substances in patient's environment	Instruct patient/family in the necessity of identifying allergic substances	edema, choking sensation, cyanosis, wheezing, coughing, incontinence, shock, fever, dilation of pupils, loss of consciousness, or convulsions Notation of patient's allergies to medications Notification of physician about abnormal observations related to adverse drug reaction Presence of respiratory assist equipment at bedside Monitoring of vital signs, respiration, response to treatment, and intake and output hourly for first 24 hours after reaction Result of consultation about related substances in patient's environment Reassurance to patient/family that constant surveillance will be maintained until condition is stable Intravenous infusion record for maintenance of patient's intravenous therapy Graphic record for hourly monitoring of vital signs, respiration, and temperature Intake and output record for hourly monitoring of intake and output for first 24 hours after onset of reaction

Drug reaction, adverse, to iron

Observe, record, and report signs of vomiting, abdominal pain, and/or diarrhea Report above to physician within 15 minutes Position patient to prevent aspiration of vomitus Prepare patient for gastric aspiration or lavage Maintain fluid and electrolyte balance Monitor and record vital signs hourly until stable, then every 4 hours	Instruct patient/family about the side effects of iron administration, including headache, loss of appetite, gastric pain, nausea, vomiting, and constipation or diarrhea During a severe reaction to iron, inform the family of patient's progress, procedures being used, and other pertinent information	Nurse's notes for: Description of signs of vomiting—such as amount, color, characteristics, and frequency; of abdominal pain—such as frequency, duration, location, and type; and of diarrhea—such as color, frequency, and consistency Notification of physician within 15 minutes of onset of side effects to iron Positioning of patient to pre-

Continued.

Drug reaction, adverse, to iron—cont'd

vent aspiration of vomitus

Instruction given to patient/family about possible side effects of iron therapy

Continued communication with family during treatment of patient for adverse reaction to iron administration

Graphic record for evidence of vital signs monitored hourly until stable, then every 4 hours

Intake and output record for evidence of fluid and electrolyte balance

Drug reaction, adverse, in neurological disorders

Observe, record, and report the presence of muscle incoordination, swelling gums, speech disturbances, weight loss, tachycardia, anorexia, drug fever, dizziness, drowsiness, bone marrow depression, urinary retention, frequent hypertension, confusion, headaches, fatigue, diplopia, peripheral pain (as in neuritis), paresthesia, tinnitus, or urticaria

Withhold suspected medication until further orders from physician

If nausea and vomiting are the only adverse reaction present, give medication with food

When anti-emetic is ordered, give it ½ hour prior to the time that the medication is to be given

In case of shock, maintain airway by positioning and suctioning; if intravenous infusion is present speed up infusion to assist circula-

Instruct about side effects of medication with which patient is discharged and appropriate action to take

Instruct about methods of reducing minor side effects such as nausea or vomiting

Nurse's notes for:

Description of observation about presence of muscle incoordination, swelling of gums, speech disturbances, weight loss, tachycardia, anorexia, drug fever, dizziness, drowsiness, bone marrow depression, urinary retention or frequency, hypertension, confusion, headaches, fatigue, diplopia, peripheral neuritis, paresthesia, tinnitus, or urticaria

Withholding of suspected medication until further medical orders

Administration of medication with food, if the only side effects were nausea and vomiting

Administration of antiemetic (if ordered) ½ hour before time for medication administration

Instruction of patient/family about side effects of medications

Critical nursing management recording and reporting	Health education	Specific instruction for data retrieval
tion; improve blood pressure, but not to a rate that will create circulatory overload; if no intravenous infusion present, initiate one for administration of emergency drugs and maintenance of blood pressure		Notification of physician about side effects Description of patient's reactions to medications Presence of shock, as evidenced by decreased or falling blood pressure; thready radial pulse; irregular or absent peripheral pulse; restlessness; anxiety; tachypnea; pale, cool, clammy, and cyanotic skin; urinary output below 30 ml per hour, electrolyte imbalance Graphic record for weight loss Temperature record for evidence of drug fever Laboratory records for bone marrow depression Output record for urinary retention and/or frequency Physician's orders for antiemetic order, for example, chlorpromazine, dimenhydrinate, or meclizine

Duct stone, common, residual, following cholecystectomy

Observe, record, and report the presence of unusual postoperative pain, jaundice, dark urine, or light colored stools Notify physician Monitor vital signs every 4 hours	Instruct patient to report dark urine or light colored stools	Nurse's notes for: Description of color of urine and stools Notification of physician Instruction of patient about reporting color of urine and stools Graphic sheet for monitoring blood pressure, temperature, pulse, and respiration every 4 hours

Edema, massive or persistent, of lower extremity

Observe, record, and report an increase in the measurement of thigh, calf, and ankle circumferences twice daily Notify physician of possible edema of lower extremity Monitor blood pressure, apical pulse, respiratory rate and	Instruct patient/family about the relationship of exercises to relief of edema Explain relationship of dietary intake to edema Encourage patient to avoid use of restrictive clothing, sitting for long periods of time,	Nurse's notes for: Measurement of thigh, calf, and ankle circumferences twice daily Fluctuations in blood pressure, apical pulse, and respiratory rate and pattern Monitoring of all available

Continued.

Critical nursing management recording and reporting	Health education	Specific instruction for data retrieval

Edema, massive or persistent, of lower extremity—cont'd

pattern; implement cardiac monitoring (especially Lead I or II electrocardiogram), CVP, and lung auscultation every 4 hours

Apply Jobst device within 1 hour of physician's order

Provide dorsiplantar flexion exercises hourly with legs elevated 4 inches

Measure intake and output every 8 hours

Monitor sodium intake

crossing legs, or in other ways restricting blood flow

Demonstrate and explain the use of Jobst device

cardiovascular parameters every 4 hours (with cardiac monitor)

Notification of physician of edema of lower extremity

Instruction of patient/family about relationship of exercises to relief of edema

Dieting restrictions, avoiding restricting blood circulation, and use of Jobst device

Dorsiplantar flexion exercises hourly with legs elevated 4 inches

Graphic record for recording of blood pressure, apical pulse, and respiratory rate

Intake and output record for evaluation every 8 hours

Comparison of physician's order for Jobst device with application in nurse's notes (within 1 hour)

Edema, pulmonary

Observe, record, and report the presence of acute anxiety, dyspnea, orthopnea, wheezing, pallor, bubbling rales, productive cough, blood tinged mucus, confusion, and/or abnormal chest x-rays

Decrease the venous return to the heart by placing patient in semi-Fowler's position or in a chair

Notify physician

Administer pain medication; for example, morphine sulfate to relieve anxiety, depress pulmonary reflexes, and induce sleep, per physician's order

Administer oxygen by mask at 6 liters per minute

Implement measures to decrease anxiety

Instruct patient/family about pulmonary edema and rationale for treatment

Nurse's notes for:

Description of presence of acute anxiety, difficulty with breathing, wheezing, skin pallor, bubbling rales, productive cough, bloody sputum, and confusion

Notifyication of physician

Placing patient in semi-Fowler's position or in a chair

Instruction of patient and/or family about condition

Implementation of measures to decrease anxiety

Medication record for administration of pain medication, for example, morphine

Oxygen record for administration of oxygen by mask at 6 liters per minute

Critical nursing management recording and reporting	Health education	Specific instruction for data retrieval
Embolism, arterial		
Observe, record, and report sudden or gradual onset of pain, numbness, coldness, and tingling	Instruct patient/family to report pain, numbness, coldness, and/or tingling of patient's limbs	Nurse's notes for: Description of symptoms (pain, numbness, coldness, or tingling of limb)
Observe, record, and report absence of pulsations in the arteries distal to the block; coldness, pallor, or mottling; hypesthesia or anesthesia; weakness or paresis of the limb; and collapse of the superficial veins	Encourage patient to avoid habits that constrict blood vessels, such as sitting, standing for long periods, wearing tight clothing, smoking, and crossing legs	Description of absence of pulsations in arteries distal to block Evaluation of skin for coldness, pallor, or mottling Patient's verbalization of weakness or paresis of limb
Notify physician immediately	Encourage patient to wear elastic stockings all day daily	Condition of superficial veins as collapsed or non-collapsed
Provide emergency care, including giving heparin sodium, 5,000 units intravenously, implementing a sympathetic block, keeping the extremity at or below the horizontal plane, not applying heat or cold, relieving pain with analgesics, and preparing patient for embolectomy within 12 hours of confirmed diagnosis of embolism	Teach patient to elevate legs slightly when lying down Do not rub affected part	Notification of physician immediately Preparation of emergency care Positioning of extremity at or below the horizontal plane Instruction of patient/family about precautions and prevention of an arterial embolism
Monitor heart rhythm with electrocardiogram		Medication record for administration of analgesics and for patient's response Cardiac monitor record for heart rate monitoring
Embolism, pulmonary		
Observe, record, and report a sudden onset of dyspnea and anxiety, with or without substernal pain; pleuritic pain, cough, hemoptysis, distended neck veins, changes in cardiac rate and rhythm, rise in temperature at onset of symptoms, rales, or pleural friction rub	Instruct patient/family about signs and symptoms of pulmonary embolism and rationale for treatment	Nurse's notes for: Description of sudden onset of dyspnea and anxiety, with or without substernal pain Observation for presence of pleuritic pain, cough, hemoptysis, distended neck veins, changes in cardiac rate and rhythm, rales, or pleural friction rub
Notify physician immediately of symptoms of pulmonary embolism		Notification of physician of sign and symptoms
Administer oxygen in high concentration by mask		Instruction of patient/family about rationale for treatment
Administer narcotics intra-		

Continued.

Critical nursing management recording and reporting	Health education	Specific instruction for data retrieval
Embolism, pulmonary—cont'd venously for severe pain (do not use intramuscular medications on heparinized patients) Observe for signs and symptoms of shock Monitor for elevated CVP		Observation for signs of shock Graphic record for systolic blood pressure above 90 mm Hg and CVP over 15 cm H_2O Temperature record for rise of temperature at onset of symptoms Medication record for intravenous administration of narcotics and for notation that intramuscular medications were not administered to heparinized patient Oxygen record for administration of high concentration of oxygen by mask

Emotional problems, feelings of suicide, or inappropriate behavior

Use therapeutic communication to help set up a trusting relationship and help patient express feelings Report pertinent information to physician Maintain suicide prevention Establish behavior modification program for inappropriate behavior	Teach measures to help patient vent feelings without exhibiting inappropriate behavior or attempting suicide	Nurse's notes for: Measures applied to develop a trusting relationship Listening to allow patient to express feelings in nonjudgmental atmosphere Notification of physician of pertinent information Instruction of patient about ways to vent feelings without engaging in inappropriate behavior Suicide prevention Establishment of behavior modification program

Endocarditis, bacterial

Observe, record, and report vital signs, elevated temperature, symptoms of septicemia, pallor, petechial hemorrhages, splenomegaly, and other superficial lesions Notify physician of fever and/or other signs and symptoms Assist with repeated blood cultures daily for 3 to 5 days before active treatment is initiated	Instruct patient/family in the necessity of monitoring temperature and inspecting skin for pallor, petechial hemorrhages or superficial lesions Explain the procedure for blood cultures and the frequency of three or more blood cultures to be taken daily for 3 to 5 days	Nurse's notes for: Inspection of patient's skin for presence of pallor, petechial hemorrhages, or superficial lesions Instruction of patient/family in observing skin for pallor, petechial hemorrhages, or superficial lesions Notation that the procedure and frequency of blood cultures was explained to patient/family

Critical nursing management recording and reporting	Health education	Specific instruction for data retrieval
		Notification of physician about fever
		Laboratory report for three blood cultures per day for 3 to 5 days
		Temperature graphic for monitoring temperature above 101.4° F

Esophageal rupture and/or perforation

Observe, record, and report the presence of dysphagia, midsternal or substernal pain, characteristics of respiration (rate and depth); difficulty in breathing; or cyanosis, swelling, or crepitus in neck	Instruct patient/family about nothing by mouth order and the necessity of recording output	Nurse's notes for:
		Observation of presence of dysphagia; midsternal or substernal pain; characteristics of respiration; difficulty in breathing; or cyanosis, swelling, or crepitus in neck
Have someone remain with patient while physician is notified		Hospital personnel remaining with patient until physician notified
Give patient nothing by mouth		Monitoring of infusion site for patency
Maintain hydration with intravenous fluids		Establishing patient on nothing by mouth
Monitor temperature every 4 hours and vital signs every 15 to 30 minutes until stable		Graphic record for monitoring temperature every 4 hours and reporting any elevations and for monitoring vital signs every 15 to 30 minutes until stable

Family and/or social support system, failure of

Reassess and build family strength by establishing and maintaining ongoing dialogue	Explain expectations and results of failure to family	Nurse's notes for:
	Continue dialogue with family, school, and patient concerning problems, emphasizing aspects of relationship with patient	Family history evaluation
Allow family or social services to use hospital for backup; may require physician evaluation, if readmission is contemplated		Patient return to hospital for length of time to specified behavior or accomplish specific goals
	Teach therapeutic techniques	Notation that family and patient were in planning conference
Clarify expectations of family or social services and results of failure to live up to expectations		Description of troublesome situation and implementation of supportive measures
Accompany and provide necessary supportive services to patient in troublesome situations in home or community;		

Continued.

Critical nursing management recording and reporting	Health education	Specific instruction for data retrieval

Family and/or social support system, failure of—cont'd
for example, refer teenager with alcoholic parent to Alateen or accompany patient to court
Continue observation, assessment, and intervention in situation

Fecal impaction

Observe, record, and report the presence of putty-like stools in the rectum, constipation or watery diarrhea, distended abdomen, palpable mass in abdomen, complaints of rectal discomfort, frequency of bowel movements
Notify physician of possible fecal impaction
Administer enemas as ordered
Encourage fluids and adequate diet with roughage
Record frequency and character of bowel movements
	Instruct patient/family about necessity of normal bowel movements and the relationship of diet, exercise, and fluids to stool consistency	Nurse's notes for:
		  Description of stool, frequency, distended abdomen, palpable mass in abdomen, and complaints of rectal discomfort
		  Notification of physician of fecal impaction
		  Encouragement of fluids and roughage in diet
		  Instruction of patient/family about normal bowel movements and avoidance of fecal impaction

Fever, persistent

Observe, record, and report fever in terms of dehydration, drug fever, or presence of infection
Force fluids as ordered
Implement fever-reducing measures, such as ice packs and fever sponges
Monitor temperature, pulse, and respiration every 4 hours until temperature returns to normal for 3 consecutive days
	Instruct patient/family on method of taking temperature and reading a thermometer and on utilization of fever-reducing measures	Nurse's notes for:
		  Description of underlying causes of elevated temperature, such as drug fever, infection, or dehydration
		  Description of fever-reducing measures
		  Teaching patient/family techniques of monitoring temperature and using fever-reducing measures
		Comparison of intake record with physician's orders for forcing fluids to amount ordered
		Graphic record for temperature above 101.4° F, increased pulse, and respiration

Critical nursing management recording and reporting	Health education	Specific instruction for data retrieval
Fistula, intestinal		
Observe, record, and report the presence of increasing abdominal distention, nausea and vomiting, abnormal stools, severe pain in upper abdomen, fever, and electrolyte imbalance	Instruct patient/family about signs and symptoms of fistula and about rationale for treatment	Nurse's notes for:
Notify physician of signs and symptoms of impending intestinal fistula	Stress importance of avoiding alcohol, spicy foods, excessive coffee intake, and large heavy meals	Daily measuring of abdominal girth, comparing from one day to the next
Obtain stool specimen for guaiac per physician's orders		Observation of clay-colored stools or blood in stools
Measure intake and output every hour; report output less than 30 ml per hour		Patient complaints of severe upper abdominal pain that may radiate to shoulder or may worsen when in supine position
Evaluate blood pressure, pulse, and respiration hourly; take rectal temperature every 2 hours		Notification of physician of signs and symptoms
Auscultate abdomen for bowel sounds every 2 hours; note decrease or absence		Instruction of patient/family about complication and rationale for treatment
		Graphic record for blood pressure, pulse, and respiration every hour and for rectal temperature above 101.4° F
Gout, gouty arthritis, or uric acid nephropathy		
Observe, record, and report acute onset of inflammation involving the metatarsophalangeal joint of the big toe or other joints of the feet, ankles, or knees; fever, headache; malaise; anorexia, or tachycardia	Explain to patient/family the rationale for treatment and signs and symptoms to report to the physician	Nurse's notes for:
Notify physician		Description of swollen and extremely tender joints, with intense pain
Measure intake and output		Presence of fever, headache, malaise, anorexia, or tachycardia (heart rate above 100)
Maintain bedrest for 24 hours after acute attack has subsided		Notification of physician
		Maintenance of bed rest during attack and for 24 hours after acute attack subsides
		Instruction of patient/family about rationale for treatment and observation of signs and symptoms
		Intake and output record for monitoring of intake and output

Continued.

Critical nursing management recording and reporting	Health education	Specific instruction for data retrieval

Heart failure, congestive

Observe, record, and report the presence of dyspnea (first on exertion and finally at rest); orthopnea; rales at the lung bases; abnormal, unexplained increase in weight; venous engorgement with increased venous pressure; dependent edema; prolonged arm-to-tongue circulation; cardiomegaly; gallop rhythm; or hepatomegaly

Notify physician within 30 minutes of respiratory distress; tachycardia with pulse greater than 100, tachpnea, respiration greater than 30, or intake exceeding output

Monitor intake and output hourly until stable

Assess vital signs hourly until stable

Provide bedrest with bedside commode

Observe for complications

Offer frequent, small, bland, low-calorie, low-residue meals with vitamin supplements

Administer digitalis and diuretics as ordered; observe for side effects

Weigh daily and note variations in weight, especially gains

Control fatigue by limiting activities

Position to facilitate respiration

Administer oxygen by nasal cannula or catheter at 4 to 6 liters per minute, for respiratory distress

Explain to patient/family symptoms, treatment, prognosis, and the possibility of congestive heart failure as a complication of an existing condition, for example, of diabetus mellitus

Teach procedure for measuring intake and output and rationale for monitoring fluids

Stress the importance of weighing daily and reporting difficulty with breathing or edema of extremities

Instruct on therapeutic and restricted activities

Instruct on medications, including the name, dosage, purpose, frequency, side effects, action to take if side effects occur, and precautions concerning each

Explain need for avoiding activities that cause circulatory stasis

Instruct about diet, may include low-sodium or diabetic diet

Reinforce diabetic teaching, if appropriate, as a means of preventing further deterioration of heart condition

Nurse's notes for:

Description of respiratory difficulty

Evaluation of amount and location of edema

Heart rate and rhythm

Notification of physician within 30 minutes of onset of respiratory distress, tachycardia with pulse greater than 100, tachpnea with respiration greater than 30, or intake exceeding output

Enforcement of bedrest

Observation of complications, including pulmonary embolization, pulmonary infections, myocardial infarction, and/or severe hypertension

Frequent, small meals

Instruction about condition, diet, medications, monitoring fluids, and weighing daily

Notation about variations in daily weight

Intake and output record for hourly monitoring

Weight record for daily weighing

Graphic record for vital signs hourly until stable and for cardiac rate and rhythm

Oxygen record for administration of oxygen at 4 to 6 liters per minute, if respiratory distress is present

Activities flow sheet or nurse's notes for control of fatigue by limiting activities and providing bedside commode

Hemorrhage complicating leukemia

Observe, record, and report the presence of petchiae and/or

Instruct patient/family about the possibility of bleeding

Nurse's notes for:

Description of location and

Critical nursing management recording and reporting	Health education	Specific instruction for data retrieval
bleeding from body orifices Notify physician of onset of bleeding Monitor laboratory reports for platelet counts below 60,000 per cubic millimeter Evaluate vital signs, pulse, and respiration every 15 minutes until stable	and the necessity of watching for petechiae and/or bleeding from body orifices	amount of bleeding or the presence of petechiae Notification of physician at onset of bleeding Instruction of patient/family about observations related to bleeding Graphic record for monitoring of vital signs, respiration, and pulse every 15 minutes until stable

Hemorrhage, gastrointestinal

Observe, record, and report the presence of sudden weakness or fainting associated with or followed by tarry stools or vomiting of blood, melena, hematemesis, pallor, or weakness Notify physician of signs and symptoms of gastrointestinal hemorrhage at onset Monitor laboratory reports for decrease in hematocrit and/or hemoglobin Evaluate blood pressure, pulse, and respiration every 15 to 60 minutes Place patient on bed rest Observe fluid intake, urine output, and temperature Provide liquid diet for first 24 hours, followed by mechanically soft diet Administer antacids every hour as ordered	Instruct on diet Teach the name, purpose, dosage, frequency, side effects, action to take if side effects occur, and precautions of each medication Explain need to avoid nicotine, alcohol, and spicy foods	Nurse's notes for: Description of sudden weakness or fainting associated with or followed by tarry stools or vomiting of blood (coffee ground vomitus), melena, hematemesis, pallor, weakness Notification of physician of signs and symptoms Observation for signs of shock (blood pressure below systolic of 70 mm Hg) Maintenance of patient on bed rest Instruction of patient/family about diet, medications, and avoidance of nicotine, alcohol, and spicy foods Maintenance on liquid diet for 24 hours after onset of symptoms Medication record for administration of antacids as ordered Intake and output record for monitoring of hydration Laboratory reports for decrease of hematocrit and/or hemoglobin

Hemorrhage, rectal

Observe, record, and report an estimate of the amount, color, and frequency of bleeding from the rectum	Instruct patient/family about reporting amount, color, and frequency of any rectal bleeding	Nurse's notes for: Description of amount, color, and frequency of rectal bleeding

Continued.

Critical nursing management recording and reporting	Health education	Specific instruction for data retrieval
Hemorrhage, rectal—cont'd Test stool for guaiac with each bowel movement Notify physician of bleeding Monitor vital signs every 2 hours or as needed Assist patient with rectal dressing changes		Results of testing each stool for guaiac Notification of physician of bleeding Assisting patient with rectal dressing changes Instruction of patient/family about reporting amount, color, and frequency of any rectal bleeding Graphic sheet for monitoring vital signs every 2 hours until stable, then as needed
Hopelessness, unrealistic feelings of Observe, record, and report attitude of hopelessness, depression, frustration, and/or helplessness Notify physician Support attempts at self-care and independence in activities of daily living Accept frustration; allow purposeful weeping Determine with patient realistic, obtainable, measurable goals Communicate patients' status with other nursing staff	Explain to patient/family actual physical limitation, usual course of disease, and measures to support individuality of patient/family needs	Nurse's notes for: Description of patient's attitude and responses Notification of physician of unrealistic hopelessness Implementation of measures to support patient's attempts at self-care Acceptance of patient's frustration and allowing purposeful weeping Explanation of goals determined by patient and staff as realistic and obtainable Teaching of patient/family about actual physical limitations, course of disease, and measures to support individuality of needs of patient/family
Hypocalcemia Observe, record, and report the presence of muscle cramps, tetany, convulsions, stridor, dyspnea, diplopia, abdominal cramps, urinary frequency, or personality changes Notify physician of signs and symptoms of hypocalcemia Offer a high-calcium, low-phosphate diet, omitting milk and cheese Monitor output	Instruct patient/family about signs of hypocalcemia to report to physician Explain the rationale for high-calcium, low-phosphate diet; encourage the avoidance of milk and cheese	Nurse's notes for: Description of tetany, muscle cramps, convulsions, stridor, dyspnea, abdominal cramps, diplopia, urinary frequency, and/or personality changes Notification of physician of possible hypocalcemia Restriction of milk and cheese intake Output record for urinary frequency

Hypoglycemia

Observe, record, and report the presence of nausea, hunger, lethargy, weakness, frequent yawning, trembling, distortion of vision, inability to concentrate, low blood pressure, slow pulse, dizziness, numbness in tongue or lips, profuse sweating, palpitations, rapid pulse, high blood pressure, convulsions, unconsciousness, changes in personality, nightmares, sleep-walking, and/or deterioration in mental functioning

Administer 4 ounces of orange juice, 2 teaspoons of sugar or candy, or other rapid-acting carbohydrate when initial symptoms appear, followed by a meal containing fat or protein, such as milk, bread, or cheese

If patient is unconscious, give glucagon according to established order; when response occurs (within 5 to 15 minutes), give patient some milk, bread, or other food high in protein or fat

Test urine for sugar and acetone every 4 hours for 48 hours following reaction, unless otherwise ordered; secure blood sugar immediately following reaction and additional blood sugars as ordered

Assess reaction in terms of precipitating causes; take appropriate actions, that is, notify physician of fever and symptoms of infection, assess activity level of patient in terms of hypoglycemia and increase of caloric needs or restriction and/or modification of activity; review

Instruct patient/family in signs and symptoms of hypoglycemic reaction and of appropriate action to take

Instruct patient on the importance of maintaining activity level at a status quo without fluctuation, as related to control of diabetics in terms of hypoglycemic agent and diet

Instruct patient on the importance of adhering to diet

Instruct on the importance of carrying or wearing a medical alert bracelet with the patient's name, diagnosis, physician's name, and hypoglycemic drug on it

Stress the importance of carrying a rapid-acting carbohydrate, such as sugar lumps or pieces of candy, at all times

Nurse's notes for:

Description of signs and symptoms of hypoglycemia, including weakness, hunger, sweating, irritability, faintness, tremors, and/or convulsions

Notification of physician of hypoglycemia

Administration of rapid-acting carbohydrate, such as orange juice or sugar or, if patient unconscious, glucagon

Monitoring of urine for abnormal sugar and/or acetone

Assessment of precipitating causes of hypoglycemia and corrective action implemented

Reinforcement of diabetic teaching

Instruction of patient/family about signs and symptoms of hypoglycemic reaction and appropriate action to take; the importance of carrying medical alert tag, and the importance of carrying a rapid-acting carbohydrate

Graphic record for temperature above 101.4° F

Diabetic flow sheet for urine testing, insulin administration, and diet consumption

Activity flow record for patient's level of activity

Continued.

Critical nursing management recording and reporting	Health education	Specific instruction for data retrieval

Hypoglycemia—cont'd

dosage of hypoglycemic agent taken by the patient; note skipping parts of meals or snacks that are on diet, which may need to be corrected through patient consultation with dietician or through "weigh backs" for portions of diet not eaten

Hypoglycemia prolonged over 30 minutes

Observe, record, and report the presence of prolonged symptoms of nausea, shakiness, hunger, lethargy, weakness, distorted vision, pallor, slow or rapid pulse, low or elevated blood pressure, dizziness, sweating, tremors, palpitations, convulsions, and unconsciousness that does not respond to administration of glucose Maintain adequate airway Notify physician immediately of prolonged hypoglycemia Prevent patient from self-injury through provision of a safe environment Assess reaction in terms of precipitating causes; take appropriate action, such as assessing fever, symptoms of infection, activity level variation, dosage of hypoglycemic agent taken by patient, skipping of meals, and need for dietician consultation or weigh backs from meals	Instruct family about prolonged hypoglycemia and prompt action required	Nurse's notes for: Description of prolonged symptoms of nausea, shakiness, hunger, lethargy, weakness, distorted vision, pallor, variations in pulse or blood pressure, dizziness, sweating, tremors, convulsions, and unconsciousness that does not respond to administration of glucose Notification of physician of prolonged hypoglycemia Implementation of measures to protect patient and provide safe environment Diabetic flow sheet for urine testing, insulin administration, and food intake

Inanition

Observe, record, and report the presence of vomiting, diarrhea, skin disorders, bradycardia, hypotension, fatigue, night blindness, extremity	Instruct patient/family on signs and symptoms and proper surveillance should inanition become a problem after discharge	Nurse's notes for: Description of vomiting, diarrhea, skin disorders, bradycardia, hypotension, fatigue, night blindness,

Critical nursing management recording and reporting	Health education	Specific instruction for data retrieval
pain, backache, sore gums, dizziness, faintness and/or paresthesia	Encourage increase in food intake	extremity pain, backache, sore gums or tongue, dizziness, faintness, and/or paresthesia
Inquire about the type and amounts of fluids and food intake over the last week; compare with patient's food preferences	Instruct on principles of good nutrition and the types of foods that should be eaten	Notification of physician of signs and symptoms
Notify physician of signs and symptoms	Instruct on importance of and procedure for good oral hygiene	Patient's response to small portions of food
Provide small portions of preferred foods that are easily chewed and swallowed (soft or pureed) at 8 a.m., 10 a.m. 12 noon, 2 p.m., 4 p.m. 6 p.m., and as requested by patient		Oral hygiene administration every 12 hours
Administer oral hygiene every 12 hours and as required; when patient is unable to swallow or chew food, a tube feeding regime or high-calorie, high-protein diet should be implemented with feedings every 2 hours, starting at 8 a.m. and ending at 8 p.m.		Instruction of patient/family about signs and symptoms, increasing food intake, principles of good nutrition, and techniques of oral hygiene
Force fluids to 3,000 ml per 24-hour period		Intake record for 3,000 ml fluids per 24 hours

Infection, brain

Observe, record, and report the presence of headache, weakness of arms or legs, diminished vision, focal epileptic seizures, fever, leukocytosis, change in mental alertness, purulent drainage from wound, odor from wound, tachycardia, or chilling	Instruct family/patient to avoid disturbing the dressing	Nurse's notes for: Description of headache, weakness in extremities, diminished vision, focal epileptic seizures, fever, leukocytosis, change in mental alertness, purulent drainage from wound, odor from wound, tachycardia, or chilling
Observe, record, and report evidence of preceding infection such as otitis media, mastoiditis, sinusitis, bronchiectasis, or pneumonia	Instruct family/patient on care of wound after discharge, if appropriate	Notification of physician of fever or infection
Notify physician of onset of fever and/or signs and symptoms of infection	Instruct family/patient, in the event of postabscess epilepsy, of actions to take in the presence of aura or seizure and safety precautions after seizure	Identification of preceding infection of ears, throat, sinuses, bronchi, or lungs
	Instruct in specifics, as related to discharge medications, including the name, purpose, dosage, frequency, side effects, action to take if side	Evaluation of signs of increased intracranial pres-

Continued.

Critical nursing management recording and reporting	Health education	Specific instruction for data retrieval

Infection, brain—cont'd

Support patient during seizures, taking proper safety precautions and actions

Evaluate every hour for signs of increased intracranial pressure, such as papilledema, headache, slowed pulse, slowed respiration, somnolence, or slowing of the mental processes

If signs present, report immediately to physician

Do not change head dressing unless specifically ordered to do so, but reinforce dressing with sterile dressing or sterile towels; if dressing change is permitted, use sterile technique; take wound specimen for culture; cleanse wound according to orders; redress, noting character and amount of drainage, and appearance of wound

effects occur, and precautions of each

In the event of neurological deficits postabscess, instruct family on rehabilitative measures, including range-of-motion exercises, transfer techniques, methods of assisting patient in carrying out activities of daily living; and methods of improving communication

sure of papilledema, slowed pulse, slowed respiration, or slowing of mental processes

Changing of head dressing, if ordered, or reinforcement of dressing

Instruction of patient/family about wound care, seizure precautions, discharge medications, and rehabilitation measures, if neurological deficits are present

Graphic record for temperature above 101.4° F, pulse below 60, and respiration below 16

Infection complicating leukemia

Observe, record, and report the presence of temperature above 101.4° F; septicemia; or infection of throat, lungs, skin, urinary tract, or anorectal areas

Notify physician of onset of fever and/or sign of infection

Monitor vital signs every 4 hours and intake and output every 8 hours

Administer mouth care with lemon and/or glycerine swabs every 2 hours, with petroleum jelly to lips, and avoiding use of toothbrush, which may injure oral mucosa and introduce infection

Provide patient with soft diet

Instruct patient/family to observe signs and symptoms of impending infection, such as fever, sore throat, cold, respiratory infection, burning on urination or frequency of urination, and to report them to physician

Stress the importance of avoiding exposure to infections and preventing possible injury to self by not using sharp objects, not constricting blood vessels with tight clothes, and avoiding large crowds

Nurse's notes for:

Observations of signs of infection in urine, throat, skin anorectal areas, or lungs

Notification of physician of fever and/or infection

Measures to prevent patient exposure to infections and/or infectious people

Oral hygiene every 2 hours

Patient's response to soft diet

Instruction of patient and/or family about infections and rationale for prevention and/or treatment

Graphic record for temperature above 101.4° F, pulse above 100, and respiration above 30

Critical nursing management recording and reporting	Health education	Specific instruction for data retrieval
to avoid mechanical irritation to oral mucosa and gums Implement measures to prevent infections, including providing reverse isolation, implementing handwashing, restricting visitors, and maintaining noninfectious environment		Intake and output record for 2,800 ml per 24 hours

Infection, overwhelming, secondary to leukopenia or anemia

Observe, record, and report the presence of elevated temperature, increased pulse, increased respiration, headache, irritability, overt infection (for example, upper respiratory infection, urinary tract infection, septicemia, or wound infection) Notify physician of signs and symptoms of impending infection Place in noninfectious environment and/or implement reverse isolation Monitor vital signs every 2 hours Record intake and output every 8 hours Stress handwashing procedure for all persons entering room and/or caring for patient Prevent exposure to infections and/or people with infections, especially upper respiratory infections Restrict visitors Evaluate stool, urine, and sputum, for bleeding	Instruct patient/family about signs and symptoms of infection; handwashing and avoiding exposure to infections; careful use of sharp objects, such as scissors, razors, or tweezers; reporting to physician signs of cold, flu, elevated temperature, reddening areas of skin, burning on urination, or frequency of urination; avoidance of constricting blood vessels with tight clothing, such as waistbands, girdles, belts, or shoes, or by sitting too long in one position	Nurse's notes for: Description of temperature elevation, increased respiration, increased pulse, headache, or overt infection Notification of physician Reverse isolation implementation Restriction of visitors and/or staff with infections Observation of stools, urine, and sputum for blood Instruction of patient/family about infections and methods to prevent and/or treat Intake and output record for minimum of 2,800 ml per 24 hours Graphic record for temperature above 101.4° F, pulse above 100, and respiration above 30

Infection, ulcers, and gangrene of toes or foot

Observe, record, and report the presence or absence of pulsations in lower extremities; color changes in the feet (reddened skin of feet); pallor on elevating feet; in-	Assure patient/family that gangrene infections are noncommunicable Stress the importance of avoiding injury to extremities with impaired circulation	Nurse's notes for: Description of pulses in lower extremities; color changes in feet; pallor of feet on elevating; increased flushing time of

Continued.

Critical nursing management recording and reporting	Health education	Specific instruction for data retrieval

Infection, ulcers, and gangrene of toes or foot—cont'd

crease in flushing time of feet; beefy redness of toes or foot on dependency; patchy cyanosis and pallor; loss of hair over toes, foot, and lower leg; skin smooth and shiny with thickened and deformed nails; sweating of feet; ulcerations; and/or infections

Notify physician of signs and symptoms

Prevent injury to extremity

Provide foot cradle

Place patient at complete bed rest with leg position horizontal or slightly depressed

Cover open or discharging lesions with light sterile gauze dressing, but not using tape on the skin

If patient is diabetic, follow routine diabetic nursing procedures

Do not give propranolol because it reduces peripheral blood flow

feet; beefy redness of toes or feet on dependency; loss of hair; smooth, shiny skin; and thickened, deformed toenails

Notification of physician of signs and symptoms

Measures to prevent injury to extremities

Patient on complete bed rest

Use of sterile dressing without tape for open or discharging lesions

Instruction of patient/family about noncommunicability of gangrene infections

Medication record for *not* administering propranolol

Intracranial pressure, increased

Observe, record, and report the presence of increased pulse rate that later becomes slow and bounding; widening pulse pressure; irregular respiration; warm, dry, pinkish red skin; unequal or unreactive pupils; decreased levels of consciousness; increased loss of motor power; headaches; vomiting; altered level of consciousness; restlessness, anxiety, or irritability; elevated blood pressure; seizure activity; or visual disturbances of diplopia or blurred vision

Notify physician immediately of signs and symptoms of increased pressure

Instruct patient/family about possibility of increased intracranial pressure and the necessity of reporting such signs as headaches, vomiting, irregular respiration, and changes in mental alertness

Teach about discharge medications including the name, purpose, dosage, frequency, side effects, action to initiate if side effects occur, and precautions of each

In the event of neurological deficits after increased intracranial pressure, instruct family on rehabilitative measures, including range-of-motion exercises, transfer techniques, methods of as-

Nurse's notes for:

Description of pulse, respiration, skin, pupils, consciousness, alterations in mental status, vomiting, elevated blood pressure, and seizures

Notification of physician

Elevation of head of bed 30 degrees

Maintenance of airway by positioning, suctioning, and administering oxygen

Nothing by mouth order

Restriction of fluids

Instruction of patient/family about signs and symptoms of increased intracranial pressure and rationale for treatment, medication, and rehabiliation, if neu-

372

Critical nursing management recording and reporting	Health education	Specific instruction for data retrieval
Elevate head of bed 30 degrees	sisting patient in completing activities of daily living, and methods of communication	rological deficit is present
Maintain airway by positioning, suctioning, and administering oxygen		Medication record to be sure that narcotics were not administered after signs of increased intracranial pressure were observed
Evaluate blood pressure, pulse, respiration, and neurological status every 30 minutes and temperature rectally every 2 to 4 hours		Diet record for nothing by mouth order
Restrict fluid intake		Intake record for restriction of fluids according to physician's orders
Monitor intake and output every hour		Graphic record for elevated blood pressure, pulse below 50, and respiration below 16 and with period of apnea
Do not administer any narcotics		
Implement nothing by mouth order		

Intracranial pressure, increased, complicating pneumocephalus, hydrocephalus, or intracranial hematoma

Observe, record, and report the presence of increased pulse rate that later becomes slow and bounding; widening pulse pressure; irregular respiration; warm, dry, pinkish red skin; unequal or unreactive pupils; increased loss of motor power; headache increasing in severity; and vomiting that may be projectile	Instruct patient/family about signs and symptoms of increased intracranial pressure and what to report	Nurse's notes for:
Notify physician of signs and symptoms of increased intracranial pressure	Teach about discharge medications, including the name, purpose, dosage, frequency, side effects, action to initiate if side effects occur, and precautions of each	Description of pulse, respiration, skin, pupils, consciousness, alterations in mental status, vomiting, elevated blood pressure, and severe headaches
Maintain airway by positioning, suctioning, and administering oxygen	In the event of neurological deficits after increased intracranial pressure, instruct family on rehabilitative measures, including range-of-motion exercises, transfer techniques, methods of assisting patient in completing activities of daily living, and methods of communication	Notification of physician of signs and symptoms of increased intracranial pressure
Implement nothing by mouth until further orders		Maintenance of airway and frequent suctioning
Do not elevate the head of the bed unless ordered by physician (practice is controversial as related to skull fractures and increased intracranial pressure)		Not elevating head of bed
		Nothing by mouth order
		Instruction of patient/family about signs and symptoms of increased intracranial pressure, and rationale for treatment, medication, and rehabilitation, if neurological deficit is present
Observe blood pressure, pulse, respiration, and neurological status every 30 minutes and		Graphic record for increased pulse rate that later becomes slow and bounding, widening pulse pressure, and irregular respiration
		Neurological check sheet for unequal or unreactive pupils

Continued.

373

Critical nursing management recording and reporting	Health education	Specific instruction for data retrieval

Intracranial pressure, increased, complicating pneumocephalus, hydrocephalus, or intracranial hematoma—cont'd

temperature rectally every 2 to 4 hours

Do not administer any narcotics

and for increased loss of motor power

Intake and output record for monitoring every 8 hours, with restricted fluid intake according to orders

Medication record to be sure that narcotics were not administered after signs and symptoms of increased intracranial pressure were observed

Diet record for nothing by mouth order

Laryngeal nerve injury

Observe, record, and report the presence of crowing respiration, retracted neck muscles, hoarseness, or respiratory obstruction

Notify physician immediately of possible injury to laryngeal nerve

Ask patient to speak as soon as recovering from anesthesia and at intervals of 30 to 60 minutes

Provide emergency tracheostomy tray in patient's room

Reassure patient that injured laryngeal nerve usually heals within a few weeks, that respiratory problems disappear, and that the patient's speaking voice will return to normal

Instruct patient/family about possible injury to laryngeal nerve and of the necessity of speaking following surgery

Nurse's notes for:

Description of sound of patient's voice following surgery, retraction of neck muscles, or signs of respiratory obstruction

Presence of tracheostomy tray in patient's room

Notification of physician about possible laryngeal nerve injury

Reassurance to patient that this injury will resolve within a few weeks

Malnutrition

Observe, record, and report the presence of diarrhea, anorexia, loss of sense of taste or smell, difficulty or inability to swallow food, pain on ingestion of food, nausea and/or vomiting, individual food eccentricities, complaints of fatigue, soreness

Should weight loss become a problem after discharge, instruct patient/family on signs and symptoms of malnutrition

Instruct patient/family on methods of increasing food intake

Instruct patient/family on the

Nurse's notes for:

Description of signs and symptoms of malnutrition, including diarrhea, anorexia, loss of sense of taste or smell, difficulty or inability to swallow food, pain on ingestion of food, nausea and/or vomiting,

Critical nursing management recording and reporting	Health education	Specific instruction for data retrieval
of tongue or gums, dizziness, faintness, skin disorders, bradycardia, hypotension, and/or paresthesia Notify physician of patient's nutritional state Review type and amounts of fluids and food taken by patient during the last 3 to 7 days; identify food preferences Provide small portions of preferred foods at frequent intervals; for example, 8 a.m., 10 a.m., 12 noon, 2 p.m., 4 p.m., 6 p.m., and 8 p.m.; choose foods that are easily chewed and swallowed (soft or pureed) Administer oral hygiene every 12 hours and as required Encourage patient to eat; feed when necessary Maintain fluid intake to at least 2,800 ml per 24 hours If patient is comatose, administer tube feedings or intravenous hyperalimentation per physician's orders Weigh daily	principles of good nutrition and the types of foods that should be included in diet Instruct patient/family on the importance of good oral hygiene as related to symptoms of inanition and appetite and how to achieve it	food eccentricities, complaints of fatigue, soreness of tongue or gums, dizziness, faintness, skin disorders, bradycardia, hypotension, and paresthesia Notification of physician of nutritional state Comparison of patient's food preferences with food intake for past 3 to 7 days Provision of small meals Oral hygiene every 12 hours or as needed Encouragement of patient to eat, with assistance provided as required Intake and output record for fluid intake at least 2,800 ml per 24 hours Graphic record for weight variations

Meningitis

Observe, record, and report the presence of high fever; nausea and/or vomiting; headache; confusion; delirium, convulsions, rigidity of neck, shoulders, and back; positive Kernig's and Brudzinski's signs, and petechial rash Observe for signs and symptoms of increased intracranial pressure; monitor for shock Notify physician of signs and symptoms of meningitis Employ measures, such as sponge baths, to decrease temperature	Defer patient teaching during acute phase Teach family about disease and rationale for treatment Instruct family and/or visitors about isolation techniques to be used during visits	Nurse's notes for: Description of signs and symptoms of meningitis, such as high fever, delirium, rigidity of neck, and presence of petechial rash Notification of physician at onset of signs and symptoms Measures to reduce high fever Implementation of isolation Graphic record for monitoring of vital signs and for neurological checks every 15 minutes until stable, then every 2 hours Intake and output record for

Continued.

Critical nursing management recording and reporting	Health education	Specific instruction for data retrieval

Meningitis—cont'd

Force fluids per physician's order

Place patient on isolation

Monitor vital signs every 2 hours; provide neurological checks every 15 minutes until stable, then every 2 hours

(Specific instruction for data retrieval) fluid intake according to physician's orders

Mesenteric vascular occlusion (bowel ischemia)

Observe, record, and report the presence of severe abdominal pain with nausea, fecal vomiting, and bloody diarrhea; severe prostration and shock; abdominal distention and tenderness; rigidity; and elevated temperature

Immediately notify physician of signs and symptoms or the absence of bowel sounds after 8 hours postoperatively

Give patient nothing by mouth

Maintain adequate blood volume; insert intravenous feeding, if not already in use

Monitor output for greater than 50 ml per hour

(Health education) Instruct patient/family on the importance of recording bowel activity, such as expelling of gas or fecal material

(Specific instruction for data retrieval) Nurse's notes for:
  Description of abdominal pain, differentiating it from incisional pain
  Description of pattern of signs and symptoms of shock, which include ashen pallor, cold and moist skin, collapse of superficial veins of the extremities, rapid and weak pulse, air hunger, thirst, and oliguria
  Notification of physician of the absence of bowel sounds or of other difficulties
  Instruction of patient/family about reporting expelling of gas or fecal material
Output record for urine output greater than 50 ml per hour
Intravenous record for maintenance of blood volume

Myocardial infarction

Observe, record, and report the sudden onset of atypical angina, or unusual "ingestion," or sudden pressing anterior chest pain, accompanied by cold sweat, weakness, apprehension, inability to lie still, lightheadedness, syncope, dyspnea, orthopnea, coughing, wheezing, nausea and vomiting, or abdominal bloating

Monitor electrocardiogram,

(Health education) Defer patient teaching during acute phase but freely respond to questions

(Specific instruction for data retrieval) Nurse's notes for:
  Description of chest pain with radiation to arms, jaws, or back plus two or more of the following: dyspnea, pallor, diaphoresis, increased systolic blood pressure 20 to 30 mm Hg, electrocardiogram changes of Q wave or ST, or variation of heart rate of less than 50 or more than 100

Critical nursing management recording and reporting	Health education	Specific instruction for data retrieval
watching for abnormal Q waves, elevated ST, and later symmetric inversion of T waves Notify physician of signs and symptoms within 30 minutes of onset Initiate medical protocol for myocardial infarction Monitor vital signs, including apical pulse, electrocardiogram strips, and heart sounds every hour until stable Administer analgesic (narcotic) per physician's orders to relieve pain Provide emotional support and/or reassurance to patient and family		Notification of physician within 30 minutes of onset Initiation of medical protocol; provision of medical protocol for myocardial infarction to data analyst for comparison of nurse's actions with protocol Description of heart sounds (first and second heart sounds are faint, often indistinguishable on auscultation and assume the so-called tic-tac quality); observation for gallop rhythm, distended neck veins, or basal rales Emotional support to patient and family Medication record for administration of analgesics for control of pain

Obesity

Observe, record, and report weight of patient; determine if patient has an increase in weight of over 10% above "normal" as the result of generalized deposition of fat in the body Discuss the relationship of obesity to primary diagnosis, such as thrombophlebitis Reinforce diet teaching; encourage patient to avoid eating snacks brought by visitors Stress to patient that in order to lose weight, it is necessary to decrease the caloric intake below the individual's caloric requirement Weigh patient daily, at same time and with same amount of clothing	Reinforce diet teaching to patient/family Educate patient/family that overeating is largely a matter of habit and that the patient must be retrained in regard to eating habits and must understand that once weight is normal it can easily become excessive again if the patient eats more than necessary Explain the relationship of obesity to the primary condition, for example, thrombophlebitis	Nurse's notes for: Determination of patient obesity Discussion of obesity and its relationship to primary condition Reinforcement of diet teaching Encouragement of patient to eat only what is provided on the diet Description of patient's understanding of overweight and its relationship to caloric intake and caloric requirement Instruction of patient/family about methods to retrain eating habits Graphic record for daily weighing at same time and with same amount of clothing

Continued.

Critical nursing management recording and reporting	Health education	Specific instruction for data retrieval

Pain, intractable

Observe, record, and report the character, location, duration, and aggravating activities of the pain

Evaluate measures that seem to provide no relief or moderate relief, the duration of the relief, and the frequency of request for pain medication; record assessments

Provide comfort measures with positive manner that relief will be achieved; use measures such as distraction, waking-imagined analgesics, and positioning to relieve pain

Encourage patient to decide measures that might relieve the pain; implement those measures if medically feasible

Provide rest periods to ensure that discomfort is not accentuated by fatigue

Notify physician of intractable pain

Health education:

Instruct patient on relaxation techniques

Stress the importance of careful description of the characteristics, nature, location, radiation, aggravating actions, and alleviating factors of the pain

Specific instruction for data retrieval:

Nurse's notes for:

Description of the character, duration, location, frequency, and aggravating activities of the pain

Measures employed to relieve the pain and their effectiveness

Patient's response to pain and patient's suggestions about relief measures

Instruction of patient about relaxation techniques and their effectiveness

Provision of rest periods to prevent fatigue

Notification of physician about intractable pain

Medication record for frequency of administration of analgesics in relationship to comfort measures to relieve pain

Pancreatitis, acute

Observe, record, and report abrupt onset of acute epigastric pain, often with radiation to back, made worse by lying supine; nausea; vomiting; constipation; severe prostration; sweating; anxiety; tender, distended abdomen, with bowel sounds absent; fever of 101° to 102° F; tachycardia; hypotension; pallor; cool, clammy skin; and/or mild jaundice

Notify physician of signs and symptoms of pancreatitis within 30 minutes of onset

Implement nothing by mouth order

Health education:

Explain to patient/family the condition and rationale for treatment

Specific instruction for data retrieval:

Nurse's notes for:

Description of pain and/or other signs and symptoms of acute pancreatitis, including nausea, vomiting, sweating, shock, tender abdomen, absent bowel sounds, pallor, and jaundice

Notification of physician within 30 minutes of onset of signs and symptoms

Nothing by mouth order

Medication record for nonadministration of opiates

Intake record for at least 2,000 ml per 24 hours

Diet record for nothing by mouth

Critical nursing management recording and reporting	Health education	Specific instruction for data retrieval
Administer medications to relieve pain; avoid use of opiates Use nasogastric suction per physician's orders Maintain fluid balance		

Panophthalmitis

Observe, record, and report the presence of tearing, ocular pain, redness, edema, or drainage from eye Irrigate eye with sterile normal saline solution every 30 minutes until orders received Notify physician of signs and symptoms Apply sterile eye patch to eye to reduce irritation	Instruct patient to avoid rubbing eye	Nurse's notes for: Description of eye irritation, ocular pain, tearing, edema, redness, or drainage from eye Notification of physician Application of eye patch Instruction of patient not to rub eye Treatment and medication record for irrigation of eye every 30 minutes until physician's orders received

Paralysis

Observe, record, and report the presence of weakness, flaccidity, or impairment of movement of extremities Maintain proper alignment with use of supportive devices to prevent footdrop, wristdrop, contractures, and/or dislocation of hip Instigate active and passive exercises at least every 8 hours if not contraindicated Maintain skin integrity	Instruct family in active and passive exercises Instruct family on maintaining proper alignment Instruct family in use of supportive devices to prevent contractures and deformities Instruct family about preventing skin breakdown	Nurse's notes for: Description of muscle weakness, flaccidity, or impairment of movement of extremities Notification of physician Proper alignment at all time with use of supportive devices, such as foot board, positioning splints, pillows, and sand bags Response of patient to active and passive exercises every 8 hours Description of skin with absence of decubitus ulcers

Paralysis, facial

Observe, record, and report the presence of drooping facial muscles and the inability to smile on one side, raise forehead, or blink Notify physician about possible facial paralysis Maintain muscle tone by gently massaging the in-	Explain to patient/family about paralysis and the possible duration Instruct patient to chew food on unaffected side to avoid biting the affected cheek or lips	Nurse's notes for: Description of drooping facial muscles and the inability to smile on one side, raise forehead, or blink Notification of physician of possible facial paralysis Application of facial sling

Continued.

379

Critical nursing management recording and reporting	Health education	Specific instruction for data retrieval

Paralysis, facial—cont'd

volved muscles upward for 5 to 10 minutes three times daily

Apply facial sling to reduce loss of muscle tone and stretching of muscles and to improve ability to eat

Provide small, frequent meals at 8 a.m., 10 a.m., 12 noon, 2 p.m., 4 p.m., 6 p.m., and 8 p.m. to reduce chances of malnutrition and weight loss resulting from eating difficulties

Provide foods that are room temperature to prevent patient from getting burned

Gentle upward massage of involved muscles for 5 to 10 minutes three times daily

Instruction of patient/family about facial paralysis and chewing food on unaffected side

Diet record for provision of small, frequent meals at room temperature

Pelvic infection, postoperative

Observe, record, and report the presence of purulent drainage from incision, elevated temperature, odor, or vaginal drainage

Notify physician of signs and symptoms of infection

Place patient in semi-Fowler's position to facilitate drainage into pelvic venous system

Provide emotional support

Monitor vital signs every 4 hours

Provice patient/family with information about symptoms and treatment of complication

Nurse's notes for:

Description of wound condition, drainage, temperature or odor

Notification of physician

Placement in semi-Fowler's position

Instruction to patient/family about complication and its treatment

Emotional support

Graphic record for temperature above 101.4° F after second day postoperatively, elevated blood pressure, and increased pulse

Peptic ulcer

Observe, record, and report the presence of melena, coffee ground vomitus, complaints of pain before meals, pallor, weakness, low hemoglobin or hematocrit, irritability, anxiety, and/or prolonged use of aspirin, adrenocorticotropic hormone (ACTH), or reserpine

Notify physician

Instruct patient/family about diet and about avoidance of nicotine, alcohol, and spicy foods.

Teach name, dosage, frequency, side effects, action to take should side effects occur, and precautions of each discharge medication

Nurse's notes for:

Description of nausea and vomiting of coffee ground vomitus

Complaints of weakness, irritability, or anxiety

Possible drug history of aspirin, adrenocorticotropic hormone, and/or reserpine

Notification of physician

Critical nursing management recording and reporting	Health education	Specific instruction for data retrieval
Monitor vital signs every 4 hours		Instruction of patient/family about diet, foods to avoid, and medications
Maintain modified bedrest until further orders		Graphic record for monitoring vital signs every 4 hours
Provide milk and cream every 2 hours unless contraindicated		Diet record for milk and cream every 2 hours
Measure intake and output every 8 hours		Intake and output record for measuring intake and output every 8 hours
Avoid administration of aspirin, adrenocorticotropic hormone, and/or reserpine		Medication record to see that aspirin, adrenocorticotropic hormone, and/or reserpine are not given

Peripheral hypoglossal nerve deficit

Observe, record, and report difficulty with swallowing and/or speech	Instruct patient and/or family about alternate means of verbal communication: for example, with a writing tablet; and about nonverbal communication	Nurse's notes for:
Notify physician		Description of difficulty with swallowing or speech
Give nothing by mouth until patient can swallow teaspoons of water without difficulty		Notification of physician
		Frequent suctioning
Suction frequently		Establishing communication other than speech, such as writing and a bell
Provide alternatives to verbal communication		Instruction of patient/family about alternate means of communicating
		Diet record for nothing by mouth order

Peritonitis, acute

Observe, record, and report vomiting; fever; prostration; malaise; nausea; abdominal rigidity and diffuse or local tenderness (often rebound), or distention; lack of peristalsis; or paralytic ileus	Explain to patient/family that generalized peritonitis is a complication of a wide variety of acute abdominal disorders	Nurse's notes for:
		Description of signs and symptoms of possible acute peritonitis, including vomiting; fever; prostration; malaise; abdominal rigidity or tenderness; and paralytic ileus
Notify physician of possible peritonitis	Stress the importance of informing staff about nausea, abdominal pain, absence of peristalsis (not passing gas or stool), and discomfort of the abdomen	Notification of physician of signs and symptoms
Place patient on bed rest in the medium Fowler's position		Placing patient in medium Fowler's position
Give nothing by mouth		Maintenance of bed rest
Maintain patency of gastric (Levin) tube or intestinal (Miller-Abbott) tube, if ordered		Identification that patient received nothing by mouth
Inspect intravenous infusion site and maintain intravenous infusions according to physician's orders		Implementation of comfort measures to ensure control of pain
		Instruction of patient/family about peritonitis

Continued.

Critical nursing management recording and reporting	Health education	Specific instruction for data retrieval
Peritonitis, acute—cont'd		
Implement comfort measures and provide rest periods for the patient		Infusion record for intravenous administration according to physician's orders
Monitor intake and output every 8 hours		
Observe for signs and symptoms of shock, such as low blood pressure; rapid pulse; shallow respiration; and cold, clammy skin		Intake and output record for hydration and elimination to 2,800 ml per 24-hour period
Provide play therapy and comfort measures to minimize depression and irritability in pediatric patients		Graphic record for vital signs, including systolic blood pressure above 70, temperature below 101.4° F, pulse less than 80 to 90, and respiration between 20 and 24
Pneumonia		
Observe, record, and report the presence of fever, cough, dyspnea, expectoration of greenish yellow sputum, chest pain, chest rales, and color of skin (cyanotic)	Explain to patient/family about condition, rationale for treatment, chest physiology measures, and measures to prevent recurrence	Nurse's notes for: Description of cough, dyspnea, purulent sputum, color of skin, chest rales, and chest pain
Notify physician		Notification of physician
Implement chest physiology measures, including postural drainage, frequent change of position, intermittent positive pressure breathing treatment, and coughing		Implementation of chest physiology measures
		Patient/family instruction about condition, rationale for treatment, chest physiology measures, and measures to prevent recurrence
Increase fluids to 3,500 ml per day, unless medically contraindicated		Provision of rest periods
Provide adequate rest periods		Graphic record for monitoring of vital signs, including low-grade, irregular temperature (100° to 101° F) or temperature above 101.4° F for pediatric patient
Monitor vital signs every 4 hours		
Administer oxygen, if cyanosis or marked dyspnea present		Oxygen record for administration of oxygen, if cyanosis or severe dyspnea present
Provide percussion and postural drainage every 2 hours and suctioning with bulb syringe for pediatric patient		Inhalation therapy record for intermittent positive pressure breathing treatments and results, as well as results of percussion and postural drainage in pediatric patient
		Intake record for fluids forced to 3,500 ml per day, unless medically contraindicated

Critical nursing management recording and reporting	Health education	Specific instruction for data retrieval

Pneumomediastinum

Observe, record, and report a sudden onset of severe retrosternal pain radiating to the neck, shoulders, and anus; mild dyspneas; crepitus on palpation of neck and chest; "crackling" or "crunching" sounds in the substernal and precordial areas synchronous with the heartbeat; and/or grotesque puffing of the neck and face

Notify physician of signs and symptoms of pneumomediastinum

Monitor vital signs every 15 minutes until stable, then every 4 hours

If patient has had esophageal surgery, explain that pneumomediastinum is a possible complication that usually has spontaneous recovery

Nurse's notes for:
Description of sudden onset of retrosternal pain that radiates, mild dyspneas, crepitus on palpation of neck and chest, crackling sounds synchronous with heartbeat, or puffing of neck and face
Notification of physician
Instruction of patient about complication and rationale for treatment
Graphic record for monitoring of vital signs every 15 minutes until stable, then every 4 hours

Polyneuritis

Observe, record, and report the presence of slowly progressing muscular weakness, paresthesia, tenderness and pain (mostly of distal portions of extremities), fatigability, sensory impairment, glossy red skin of extremities, and impairment of sweating mechanism

Implement bed rest

Place cradle over foot of bed to prevent pressure from bed covers

Administer analgesics per physician's order to control pain

Instruct patient/family about need to encourage active motion of extremities to prevent contractures

Nurse's notes for:
Description of slowly progressing muscular weakness, paresthesia, tenderness or pain in distal portions of extremities, fatigability, and impairment of sweating mechanism
Assessment of skin color as glossy red
Notification of physician
Implementation of bed rest
Use of cradle over foot of bed to prevent pressure from bed covers
Instruction of patient/family about movement and range-of-motion exercises to prevent contractures
Medication record for administration of pain medication

Postgastrectomy (dumping) syndrome

Observe, record, and report if any of the following symptoms occur within 20 minutes after meals: sweating, tachycardia, pallor, epigas-

Instruct patient/family about the signs and symptoms of "dumping" syndrome and means to counteract symptoms

Nurse's notes for:
Observation of any of the following symptoms occurring within 20 minutes after meals: sweating,

Continued.

Critical nursing management recording and reporting	Health education	Specific instruction for data retrieval

Postgastrectomy (dumping) syndrome—cont'd

tric fullness and grumbling, warmth, nausea, abdominal cramps, weakness, syncope, vomiting, and/or diarrhea

Notify physician of symptoms

Give small, frequent, equal feedings of high-protein, low-carbohydrate meals, moderately high in fat

Monitor blood sugar during attack, per physician's order

Encourage patient to eat frequent, small, equal feedings for meals, according to prescribed diet

tachycardia, pallor, epigastric fullness and grumbling, warmth, nausea, abdominal cramps, weakness, syncope, vomiting, and/or diarrhea

Notification of physician of symptoms

Patient's response to small, frequent, equal feedings

Instruction of patient/family of symptoms of "dumping" syndrome

Laboratory reports for blood sugar that is not low during an attack

Diet record for the provision of high-protein, and low-carbohydrate meals, moderately high in fat

Premature ventricular beats (PVCs)

Observe, record, and report monitoring of heart rate and rhythm while in critical care unit; on progressive unit take apical pulse every 4 hours

Notify physician within 5 minutes of contractions

Initiate medical protocol for standing physician's orders within 5 minutes of onset of condition

Defer teaching during acute phase but respond openly to all questions

Nurse's notes for:

Description of six or more PVCs per minute

Notification of physician

Implementation of medical protocol within 5 minutes; provision copy of medical protocol to data analyst for comparison of nurse's actions with protocol

Progressive deterioration

Observe, record, and report the patient's lack of response to treatment and progressive deterioration

Maintain physical comfort

Provide turning, positioning, skin care, and oral hygiene every 2 hours

Implement passive and active range-of-motion exercises to all joints every 2 hours

Encourage nutrition and fluids to at least 2,000 ml per 24 hours

Instruct patient/family on necessity of good nutrition, fluid balance, oral hygiene, and skin care

Teach family member basic nursing care and/or techniques; such as bed bath, transfer techniques, range-of-motion exercises, skin care, oral hygiene, and other appropriate care; that will enhance patient's care after discharge

Nurse's notes for:

Patient's response to treatment and/or progressive deterioration

Utilization of physical comfort measures

Range-of-motion exercises to all joints every 2 hours

Positioning and inspection of skin for reddened areas and/or decubitus ulcers every 2 hours

Administration of oral hygiene every 2 hours

Critical nursing management recording and reporting	Health education	Specific instruction for data retrieval
Provide emotional support to patient/family		Instruction of patient/family on good nutrition, fluid balance, oral hygiene, and skin care
		Instruction of family on basic components of patient care for posthospitalization care
		Intake record for intake of at least 2,000 ml per 24 hours
		Documentation about provision of emotional support to patient/family

Renal failure

Observe, record, and report the presence of sudden onset of oliguria, urine volume of 20 to 200 ml per day, proteinuria, hematuria, isosthenuria with a specific gravity of 1.010 to 1.016, anorexia, nausea and/or vomiting, lethargy, elevation of blood pressure, signs of uremia, or increased blood urea nitrogen	Explain procedures, condition, treatment, medical and nursing management, and prognosis to patient/family	Nurse's notes for:
	Instruct on procedure for measuring intake and output	Description of urine output, characteristics of urine, anorexia, nausea and/or vomiting, and lethargy
	Stress importance and rationale of limiting fluid intake and how to adhere to limit	Notification of physician within 30 minutes of urine output less than 30 ml per hour
Carefully monitor intake and output hourly for maintenance of body fluid volume, restrict fluid intake per physician's orders (usually to 400 ml per day)	Instruct on diet, stressing importance and rationale of not eating protein and of controlling renal deterioration through diet	Indwelling catheter care
		Bed rest with reverse isolation to protect from infections; oral hygiene
Notify physician	Instruct patient on importance and methods of maintaining good skin hygiene to prevent breakdown or infection	Restriction of protein from diet and of fluids per physician's orders
Implement bed rest with reverse isolation to protect patient from exposure to hospital infections, turn and position hourly; provide skin care		Instruction of patient/family about condition, treatment, procedures, and diet
Limit sources of nitrogen, potassium, phosphate, and sulfate by restricting protein intake		Inspection of skin for reddened areas; positioning and turning hourly
		Notation of signs and symptoms of uremia
Maintain indwelling catheter care		Graphic record for vital signs (blood pressure and temperature) hourly and weight daily
Weigh patient daily		Intake and output record for hourly monitoring
If uremia is present, prepare for hemodialysis or peritoneal dialysis		Laboratory reports for specific gravity of urine; for progressive increase in blood urea nitrogen, creatinine, potas-

Continued.

Critical nursing management recording and reporting	Health education	Specific instruction for data retrieval

Renal failure—cont'd

Monitor vital signs hourly until stable

Provide oral hygiene every 2 hours

sium, phosphate, and sulfate; and for decrease in sodium, calcium, and carbon dioxide

Diet record for restricted protein intake

Respiratory arrest

Establish and maintain airway

Initiate pulmonary resuscitation within 1 minute of respiratory arrest

Administer oxygen by nasal cannula or catheter at 4 to 6 liters per minute

Notify physician within 5 minutes of respiratory arrest

Administer drug therapy per physician's orders (antibiotics, drugs to stimulate respiration, sodium bicarbonate, or others)

Closely observe for respiratory distress after arrest period

Monitor vital signs, blood gases, and pulmonary function tests hourly until stable

Defer patient teaching until acute phase is resolved

Explain condition and rationale of treatment to family

Nurse's notes for:

Absence of respiration

Documentation that airway was cleared and maintained

Pulmonary resuscitation initiated within 1 minute of arrest

Notification of physician within 5 minutes of arrest

Explanation provided family members

Oxygen record for administration of oxygen by nasal cannula or catheter at 4 to 6 liters per minute

Laboratory reports for monitoring blood gases after arrest

Medication record for administration of medications per physician's orders

Respiratory failure

Observe, record, and report restlessness, headache, confusion, tachycardia, diaphoresis, impaired motor function, asterixis, cyanosis, hypotension or hypertension, coma, or change in respiration

Notify physician of possible impending respiratory failure

Notify physician of blood gas results: arterial oxygen tension (PaO_2) less than 50 mm Hg for respiratory failure or arterial carbon dioxide ($PaCO_2$) greater than 50 mm Hg for ventilatory failure

Instruct patient/family that smoking is not permitted when oxygen is in use

Explain the rationale for oxygen therapy and the method of administering oxygen

Nurse's notes for:

Presence of restlessness, headache, diaphoresis, confusion, tachycardia, impaired motor function, asterixis, cyanosis, coma, hypo- or hypertension, or changes in respiration

Notification of physician of signs and symptoms of possible respiratory failure

Instruction of patient/family about no smoking when oxygen is in use and about the rationale of oxygen therapy

Description of respiratory

Critical nursing management recording and reporting	Health education	Specific instruction for data retrieval
Administer oxygen by nasal cannula or catheter at 1 to 4 liters per minute, per physician's order		rate, character, and depth Blood pressure record for hypotension (lowered blood pressure) or hypertension (elevated blood pressure) Laboratory reports for blood gases greater or lesser than normal

Respiratory obstruction

Observe, record, and report the presence of voice changes (weak or hoarse); persistent scratchy or croupy cough; difficult or painful swallowing; positional or inspiratory dyspnea that may be accompanied by wheezing, restlessness, excitement, or apprehension; and respiratory rate and depth	Defer teaching until acute respiratory obstruction has been relieved	Nurse's notes for: Description of voice changes; persistent, scratchy or croupy cough; difficult or painful swallowing; positional or inspiratory dyspnea that may be accompanied by wheezing, restlessness, excitement, or apprehension; and respiratory rate and depth
Clear airway, if possible, by suctioning, positioning, or using an oral airway		Use of suctioning, positioning, or oral airway to clear and maintain airway
Administer oxygen, as needed, by nasal cannula at 4 to 6 liters per minute		Notification of physician Implementation of measures to reduce apprehension
Notify physician and have ready equipment necessary for respiratory assistance, including respirator, endotracheal tube, and tracheostomy tray		Oxygen record for administration of oxygen by nasal cannula at 4 to 6 liters per minute
Remain with patient and provide measures to reduce apprehension, restlessness, or excitement		
Monitor oxygen concentration for pediatric patient		

Seizures

Observe, record, and report the presence of localized or generalized muscular spasms, spasms that affect both sides of the body simultaneously, spasms that seem to spread to the entire body gradually, loss of consciousness (duration of seconds to minutes)	Instruct patient/family on significance of aura, if present, and what immediate action to take	Nurse's notes for: Description of the character, duration, and frequency of seizures
Do not restrain patient during seizure, but protect from self-injury	Instruct family what action to take to maintain patient's safety during and after a seizure	Protection of patient from self-injury through seizure precautions, such as padded side rails and padded tongue blades
	Teach medications, including the name, purpose, dosage, frequency, side effects, action to take if side effects	Maintenance of airway during seizure activity Notification of physician

Continued.

Critical nursing management recording and reporting	Health education	Specific instruction for data retrieval

Seizures—cont'd

Insert airway or tongue blade between teeth, if teeth are not clenched; maintain airway

Notify physician

Protect patient from injury, as the result of confusion, amnesia, and disorientation, after seizure

Administer oxygen, as needed, by nasal cannula at 4 to 6 liters per minute

Provide cardiopulmonary resuscitation, if necessary, in the event of an intractable seizure

occur, and precautions of each; stress the importance of constant administration of drug therapy according to prescribed dosage and frequency as related to control of seizures and side effects

Instruct on activity moderation, as means of reducing number of seizures, and avoidance of excitement and fatigue, as precipitators of seizures

Instruct in avoidance of alcohol

Inform patient/family of legal implications of having a convulsive disorder, with regard to employment, driving a car, and other activities

Instruction of patient/family about seizures, warning signals, care during and after a seizure, medication, and avoidance of alcohol

Oxygen record for administration of oxygen by nasal cannula at 4 to 6 liters per minute

Seizures associated with diabetes

Observe, record, and report the presence of sudden cry or fall, loss of consciousness, rapid breathing, jerking or twitching movements of muscles, rigidity of the body, urinary or fecal incontinence, apneic periods, and cyanosis

If teeth are not clenched, insert padded tongue blade; maintain adequate airway; give oxygen, as needed, by nasal cannula at 4 to 6 liters per minute

Protect patient from self-injury during seizure but do not restrain movement

Note character and duration of seizure; report immediately if convulsions repeat without patient returning to consciousness

Administer appropriate sedatives, anticonvulsive medication, or rapid-acting carbohydrate, as ordered

Instruct patient/family on relationship of convulsions to diabetic hypoglycemic state

Instruct patient on importance of dietary, hypoglycemic medication, and activity level adherence as means of preventing convulsions

Instruct family on safety measures to take should convulsions occur and proper action to take to correct hypoglycemia, as precipitator of convulsions

Instruct on the importance of taking snacks that are prescribed at proper times, especially if the patient is taking insulin

Nurse's notes for:

Description of fall, loss of consciousness, rigidity of body, rapid breathing, jerking or twitching movements of muscles, urinary or fecal incontinence, apneic periods, or cyanosis

Description of character and duration of seizure

Implementation of safety precautions for possible seizures

Notification of physician of seizure activity

Instruction to patient/family about convulsions, diabetic care, safety measures during seizures, and other pertinent information

Oxygen record for administration of oxygen by nasal cannula at 4 to 6 liters per minute

Critical nursing management recording and reporting	Health education	Specific instruction for data retrieval
Evaluate blood pressure, pulse, respiration, and neurological checks immediately after seizure and as indicated thereafter		

Seizures in children

Observe, record, and report the presence, frequency, duration, and characteristics of seizure activity Notify physician immediately Do not insert tongue blade, simply position on side and protect child from self-harm during convulsions Provide privacy and emotional support during and following seizure Monitor vital signs every 2 hours Provide equipment for suctioning if patient cannot handle own secretions Explain procedures to parents; provide emotional support	Defer teaching during seizure episode Explain procedures to parents	Nurse's notes for: Description of frequency, duration, and characteristics of seizure activity Notification of physician Positioning on side without use of tongue blade Emotional support to child and parents after seizure Graphic record for monitoring vital signs every 2 hours

Self-destructive or other destructive behavior

Observe, record, and report the presence of self-other-destructive behavior, such as head banging, rocking, picking or hitting self, refusal to eat, or refusal to sleep Implement immediate steps to ensure patient's physical safety Notify physician if immediate physical danger is present Participate in interdisciplinary conference for discussion and planning Maintain ongoing dialogue with family about plans and perceptions	Explain to family about exacerbation of clinical signs and symptoms	Nurse's notes for: Description of head banging, rocking, picking or hitting self, refusing to eat, or refusing to sleep Detailed notes for limiting dangerous activity, including helmet for head banger, mittens for patient picking at body, seclusion of assaultive patient, tube feeding for refusal to eat, or sedation of patient who refuses to sleep Consultation with physician within 1 hour Presentation at interdisciplinary conference for discussion and planning Dialogue with family Explanation to family about exacerbation of clinical signs and symptoms

Continued.

Critical nursing management recording and reporting	Health education	Specific instruction for data retrieval

Septicemia

Observe, record, and report the presence of chills, fever, and sweating, accompanied by backache, headache, inflammation of a skin lesion, purulent drainage from an open wound, productive coughing, tachycardia, or breathing difficulty

Notify physician

Assist in taking blood cultures during chill

Monitor temperature, pulse, and respiration every 15 minutes during chill and then every 4 hours for the next 48 hours

Administer antibiotics per physician's orders

Following chill, institute fever-reducing measures, such as administration of antipyretics, ice packs, or hypothermia blankets until temperature decreases to 101° F

Notify infection control officer; initiate isolation

Instruct patient/family on purpose, duration, and method of maintaining isolation

Explain purpose of blood culture and fever-reducing measures

Nurse's notes for:

Description of chills

Presence of backache, headache, inflammation of skin lesions, purulent drainage from an open wound, productive coughing, or breathing difficulty

Notification of physician

Assisting in taking blood culture

Implementation of fever-reducing measures following chills

Notification of infection control officer

Initiation of isolation procedures

Graphic record for temperature greater than 102° F and heart rate greater than 100

Shock as adverse reaction to x-ray contrast media

Observe, record, and report the presence of tachycardia, thready pulse, hypotension, or respiratory wheezing

Place patient in recumbent position

Hyperextend patient's neck to maintain open airway

Notify physician

Insert an intravenous tube to help maintain arterial pressure and to provide a rapid route for the administration of emergency drugs

Have the following emergency medications available: diphenhydramine, 50 mg; epinephrine, 1:1,000; hydrocortisone succinate, 250 mg

Administer oxygen, as needed,

Teach patient/family to report adverse reaction to contrast media anytime the patient is admitted to a hospital

Instruct patient to wear a medical alert tag or bracelet and to keep "allergic" information in wallet

Nurse's notes for:

Description of heart rate, thready pulse, or respiratory wheezing

Positioning of patient in recumbent position with hyperextension of neck to maintain open airway

Notification of physician

Initiation of intravenous tube

Availability of emergency drugs in room

Instruction of patient/family about reporting adverse reaction to contrast media during future hospitalizations and about the use of medical alert information

Critical nursing management recording and reporting	Health education	Specific instruction for data retrieval
by nasal cannula at 4 to 6 liters per minute		Oxygen record for administration of oxygen by nasal cannula at 4 to 6 liters per minute Graphic record for decreased blood pressure and thready pulse

Shock, hypovolemic

Observe, record, and report the presence of excessive body fluid loss from internal or external injuries, pallor, coldness, cyanosis, sweating, tachycardia, arterial hypotension, syncope, vertigo, restlessness, anxiety, tachypnea, subnormal temperature, urinary output below 30 ml per hour, central venous pressure reading below 3 cm H_2O, or diminished breath sounds Notify physician of impending shock Position patient with the head and torso in horizontal or slightly elevated position with moderate (30 degree) elevation of legs; avoid Trendelenburg's position Maintain complete bed rest Implement nothing by mouth order Initiate intravenous tube to maintain patient vein Measure intake and output hourly (output should be more than 30 ml per hour) Evaluate blood pressure, respiration, apical pulse, and femoral pulse every 15 minutes until stable Keep patient warm and dry Auscultate chest for breath sounds hourly Apply pressure to control bleeding, if necessary; for hemorrhage from a stump, apply a tourniquet	Instruct patient/family about complication and rationale for treatment	Nurse's notes for: Description of the presence of excessive body fluid loss, skin pallor, coldness, cyanosis, sweating, tachycardia, arterial hypotension (systalic blood pressure below 70), synocope, anxiety, tachypnea, subnormal temperature, or diminished breath sounds Notification of physician of impending shock Positioning of patient with lower extremities elevated moderately Implementation of strict complete bed rest Implementation of nothing by mouth order Application of pressure to control bleeding, if necessary Instruction of patient/family about rationale for treatment Intake and output record for hydration of at least 2,800 ml and hourly output of 30 ml Graphic record for decreased blood pressure, subnormal temperature (below 97° F), and weak, thready pulse

Continued.

Critical nursing management recording and reporting	Health education	Specific instruction for data retrieval

Shock, hypervolemic, drug-induced

Record and report the presence of urticaria, diaphoresis, rapid pulse, hypotension, wheezing, or cardiac arrest

Hold suspected drug

Provide cardiopulmonary resuscitation as necessary

Notify physician

Keep airway open; Give oxygen, as needed, by nasal cannula at 4 to 6 liters per minute

Insert intravenous tube to help maintain arterial pressure and to provide a rapid route for emergency drug administration

Instruct patient always to inform health personnel of allergic reaction whenever medical care is recieved

Instruct patient/family about medical alert tag

Nurse's notes for:

Description of urticaria (itching skin), diaphoresis, rapid pulse, wheezing, hypotension, or cardiac arrest

Initiation of cardiopulmonary resuscitation within 3 minutes of onset of arrest

Notification of physician

Instruction of patient/family about allergy reaction, the necessity of telling health personnel whenever medical treatment is rendered, and the use of medical alert information

Medication record for holding suspected drug

Graphic sheet for rapid pulse (greater than 100) or decreased blood pressure (below 100/80)

Intravenous record for initiation of intravenous equipment

Shunt failure in children

Observe, record, and report the presence of increased restlessness, signs of increased intracranial pressure or increased cranial circumference, axorexia, or lethargy

Notify physician

Monitor vital signs, respiration, and apical pulse hourly until stable, then every 4 hours; weigh patient daily

Measure cranial circumference daily

Provide emotional support to parents

Explain to parents the purpose of shunt, signs of shunt failure, and the rationale for treatment

Nurse's notes for:

Description of signs of increased intracranial pressure, including changes in level of consciousness, projectile vomiting, anorexia; slowed heart rate, slowed respiration, or subnormal temperature, increased restlessness, variation in measurement of cranial circumference, or lethargy

Notification of physician

Provision of emotional support to parents

Instruction of parents about signs of shunt failure and rationale of treatment

Graphic record for monitoring vital signs, respiration, and

Critical nursing management recording and reporting	Health education	Specific instruction for data retrieval
		apical pulse hourly until stable, then every 4 hours, and for monitoring daily weight

Shunt malfunction

Observe, record, and report the presence of increased restlessness, headache, vomiting, papilledema, or signs of increased intracranial pressure or increased cranial circumference Notify physician	Instruct patient/family about shunt functioning and malfunctioning	Nurse's notes for: Description of increased restlessness, headache location and severity, vomiting, papilledema, or increased intracranial pressure or cranial circumference Notification of physician Instruction of patient/family about shunts, their functioning and malfunctioning

Skin flap necrosis

Observe, record, and report the presence of drainage at both donor and recipient sites; signs of infection, such as odor, or purulent drainage; complaints of pain; or decreased circulation to recipient site Notify physician of possible skin flap necrosis Inspect wound sites daily Provide sterile wound care according to physician's orders Monitor temperature, pulse, respiration, and blood pressure every 4 hours	Instruct patient/family about skin flap care	Nurse's notes for: Description of wounds at donor and recipient sites; the presence of signs of infection, such as odor or purulent drainage; and the status of circulation to recipient site Notification of physician of possible skin flap necrosis Utilization of sterile technique at all times Instruction of patient/family about skin flap care Graphic record for temperature above 101.4° F, increased pulse rate, increased respiration, and blood pressure changes

Sleeplessness

Observe, record, and report patterns of waking, sleeping, and stressful conditions prior to sleep Implement nursing measures to induce sleep, such as giving a back rub, sitting with patient, and providing warm milk	Explain relationship of pain, fear, and stress as deterrents to sleep; teach methods to reduce pain, fear, or stress and to encourage sleep	Nurse's notes for: Description of patterns of waking, sleeping, and/or stressful conditions prior to sleep Documentation of measures implemented to induce sleep Notification of physician

Continued.

Critical nursing management recording and reporting	Health education	Specific instruction for data retrieval
Sleeplessness—cont'd		
Notify physician of sleeplessness		Evaluation of relationship of pain, stress, or fear to sleeplessness
Validate relationship of pain, stress, or fear of sleeping to sleeplessness		Instruction of patient/family about relationship of pain, fear, and stress to sleeping and about measures to reduce conditions preventing sleep
Status epilepticus		
Observe, record, and report the presence of recurrent severe seizures, with short or with no intervals between seizures	Defer teaching until acute phase has ceased	Nurse's notes for:
Notify physician immediately		Description of seizure activity, duration, and characteristics
Maintain airway; administer oxygen by nasal cannula at 4 to 6 liters per minute		Notification of physician of prolonged seizures, adequate airway, and oxygenation
Evaluate comatose patient for exhaustion and or hyperthermia		Evaluation of comatose patient for exhaustion and/or hyperthermia
Initiate intravenous fluids to maintain vein for drug administration		Seizure precautions to protect from self-injury
Protect patient from self-injury		Maintenance of nonstimulating, quiet environment
Maintain nonstimulating, quiet environment		Assessment for presence of complications of respiratory depression or hypotension
Observe for complications of respiratory depression or hypotension		Emotional support to family
Provide psychological support to family		Monitoring of vital signs hourly until stable
Monitor vital signs hourly until stable		Intravenous record for initiation of intravenous fluids
		Oxygen record for administration of oxygen by nasal cannula at 4 to 6 liters per minute
Thromboembolism in children		
Observe, record, and report the presence of pain or cramping in an extremity; swelling; fever; chills; diaphoresis, inflammation of the skin over a vein; sharp, stabbing pains in the chest; acute anxiety; cyanosis; pupillary	Instruct parents and child, at appropriate level, about condition, treatment, prognosis, and medical and nursing management	Nurse's notes for:
	Instruct child/parents in the need to avoid restrictive devices, such as straps on pros-	Description of pain or cramping in extremity, swelling, diaphoresis, inflammation of skin over a vein, anxiety, cyanosis, changes in pulse, changes in peripheral pulses

Critical nursing management recording and reporting	Health education	Specific instruction for data retrieval
dilatation; rapid, irregular pulse; or diminished or absent peripheral pulses Notify physician Administer oxygen for respiratory distress, as needed, by nasal cannula at 4 to 6 liters per minute Elevate extremity Protect affected extremity from trauma and/or cold Implement measures to relieve discomfort Provide emotional support to child/parents Provide diversional activities to help child remain quiet	thetic devices like braces, that tend to cause circulatory stasis Should the patient go home on anticoagulant therapy, teach child/parents the name, purpose, dosage, frequency, side effects, and precautions of the drug Stress the importance of exercise (within certain limits) as a means of prevention; teach appropriate exercises Instruct in the importance of frequent change of position as a means of prevention If patient should be required to use elastic stockings or Ace bandages after discharge, instruct in the proper application, the need for using them daily, and the duration of usage	Notification of physician Elevation of extremity Measures to protect extremity from trauma or cold Emotional support to child/parents Instruction of child/parents about condition, treatment, anticoagulatn therapy, exercise, changing of position, and use of elastic stockings Provision of diversional activities Graphic record for temperature above 101.4° F and for changes in pulse Oxygen record for administration of oxygen in presence of respiratory distress

Thrombophlebitis

Observe, record, and report the presence of stiffness, soreness, or edema in calf of leg; assumption of a frog-like leg position; pain in the upper posterior calf on dorsiflexion of the foot; and/or muscle ache Elevate affected extremity, if not contraindicated Protect the affected extremity from trauma or cold Notify physician	Instruct patient/family not to rub leg Instruct patient to avoid restrictive clothing, and once ambulatory to avoid sitting or standing in one position for long periods of time or crossing legs, since these activities cause circulatory statis If the patient is discharged on anticoagulant therapy, teach the dosage, frequency, side effects, action to take should side effects occur, and precautions of the medication If the patient is required to wear elastic stockings or Ace bandages at home, instruct in proper application, the need to wear them daily, and the duration of use	Nurse's notes for: Description of soreness, edema, or pain in calf of leg Elevation of affected extremity Measures to protect extremity from trauma or cold Notification of physician Instruction of patient/family about not to rubbing leg, avoiding restriction of blood flow, precautions for anticoagulant therapy, and applying elastic stockings, if ordered

Continued.

Critical nursing management recording and reporting	Health education	Specific instruction for data retrieval
Thyroid crisis or storm		
Observe, record, and report the presence of high fever, tachycardia, central nervous system irritability, and/or delirium	Defer patient teaching until acute phase controlled	Nurse's notes for:
Notify physician	Instruct family about condition, prognosis, and treatment	Description of pulse above 140, temperature about 106° F, central nervous system irritability, or delirium
Institute measures, such as hypothermia blanket or tepid sponges, to decrease temperature		Notification of physician
Monitor vital signs every 15 minutes until stable		Implementation of measures to decrease temperature
Administer fluids high in glucose		Administration of fluids high in glucose
Measure intake and output		Maintenance of dark, quiet room, with limited number of visitors
Maintain quiet, dark room, with limited number of visitors		Instruction of family about condition, prognosis, and treatment
		Graphic record for monitoring vital signs every 15 minutes, temperature about 106° F, and pulse above 140
		Intake and output record for monitoring
Transfusion reaction, hemolytic		
Observe, record, and report the presence of chills; fever; pain in back, chest, or abdomen; or anxiety, apprehension, or headache	Instruct patient/family about signs and symptoms of transfusion reaction and necessity of notifying staff if reaction occurs	Nurse's notes for:
Discontinue administration of blood transfusion		Presence of chills; fever; pain in back, chest, or abdomen; or anxiety, apprehension, or headache during a blood transfusion
Notify physician		Discontinuation of transfusion when reaction occurs
Send transfusion equipment to laboratory; complete transfusion reaction record		Notification of physician
Collect first urine specimen after transfusion for laboratory analysis		Completion of blood reaction procedure, usually including sending transfusion equipment to laboratory with a completed transfusion reaction record
		Instruction of patient/family about transfusion reactions and reporting of reactions
		Collection of first urine specimen after transfusion for laboratory analysis

Critical nursing management recording and reporting	Health education	Specific instruction for data retrieval
		Graphic sheet for temperature above 101.4° F

Urinary obstruction or retention

Observe, record, and report the presence of dribbling, anuria, bladder distention, bladder pain, oliguria, or inability to void	Instruct patient/family on purpose of increased fluid intake and the necessity that all intake and output be measured	Nurse's notes for:
Encourage voiding in upright position out of bed	Explain methods to increase intra-abdominal pressure to aid in micturation, if medically permitted	Description of dribbling, anuria, bladder distention, bladder pain, oliguria, or inability to void
Monitor temperature every 4 hours		Encouragement of voiding out of bed
Record output, frequency, color, and difficulty of urinating		Record of urinary color, frequency, and difficulty of urination
Review intake record; force fluids to at least 3,500 ml per day, unless medically contraindicated		Notification of physician
Notify physician		Application of methods to increase intra-abdominal pressure to aid in micturition, if permitted
Apply methods to increase intra-abdominal pressure to aid in micturition, if permitted, or use measures to encourage voiding, such as pouring warm water over genital area, running water, and offering fluids before voiding is attempted		Explanation of nursing measures to assist with voiding, such as pouring warm water over genital area, running water, and offering fluids
Catheterize as ordered, using strict sterile technique; if Foley catheter is inserted, provide catheter care every 6 hours		Instruction of patient/family about rationale for increased fluid intake, measurement of intake and output, and methods to aid micturition
		Intake and output record for fluids greater than 3,500 ml per day
		Graphic record for temperature greater than 101.4° F

Urinary tract infection, acute

Observe, record, and report sudden onset of chills and fever, tachycardia, flank pain, hesitancy, urgency, oliguria, frequency, dysuria, foul-smelling urine, cloudy urine, urine with large amounts of debris, elevated white blood cells, headache, prostration, or nausea and vomiting	Instruct patient/family about purpose of large oral intake of fluids, and necessity of measuring all intake, signs and symptoms of urinary tract infections, and rationale for treatment	Nurse's notes for:
Notify physician	If female patient, instruct in genitourinary hygiene (always cleansing or wiping from front to back)	Description of chills, fever, tachycardia, flank pain, difficulty with urination, headache, prostration, or nausea and vomiting
		Notification of physician
		Forcing of fluids, offering 8 ounces of cranberry juice three times daily
		Maintenance of bed rest
		Provision of rest periods

Continued.

397

Critical nursing management recording and reporting	Health education	Specific instruction for data retrieval
Urinary tract infection, acute—cont'd		
Force fluids		during and after nursing care
Measure intake and output		Instruction of patient/family about forcing fluids, treating urinary tract infection, and maintaining personal genitourinary hygiene
Place patient at bed rest		
Offer 8 ounces of cranberry juice three times daily		
Provide rest periods during and after nursing care		Intake and output record for fluids forced to at least 3,500 ml per day
		Graphic record for temperature greater than 101.4° F and pulse greater than 100
		Laboratory report for elevated white blood cells
Vascular bed, changes in size of		
Observe, record, and report episodes of hypotension, lightheadedness, marked changes in vascular bed size occuring less than 8 hours postoperatively	Stress the importance of accurate monitoring of intake and output both pre and postoperatively	Nurse's notes for:
		Description of episodes of hypotension, lightheadedness, and marked changes in vascular bed size
Notify physician of suspected changes in vascular bed sizes		Notification of physician of changes in vascular bed size
Maintain accurate pre- and postoperative intake and output record		Intake and output record for pre- and postoperative monitoring of intake and output
Monitor blood pressure		Graphic record for blood pressure monitoring for decreases in blood pressure
Wound infection, hematoma, and dehiscence		
Observe, record, and report presence of odor, purulent drainage from dressing, fever, or elevated white blood cell count, and condition of wound	Instruct patient/family on purpose of forcing fluids, desired amount per 24 hours, and method of obtaining goal	Nurse's notes for:
		Description of characteristics of wound, drainage, and odor
Do not change dressing unless ordered, but reinforce with sterile dressings or towels until physician evaluates wound	Teach patient/family care of incision after discharge, if any is necessary	Reinforcement of dressing until dressing change ordered by physician
	Explain purpose, duration, and method of maintaining isolation or wound precautions	Notification of physician of possible wound infection
Notify physician		Obtaining wound culture
Change dressings and cleanse wound per physician's orders, with notation of wound		Forcing fluids to 3,000 ml per day
		Initiation of isolation and notification of infection control officer

Critical nursing management recording and reporting	Health education	Specific instruction for data retrieval
condition, healing, and amount of drainage Obtain wound culture specimen Force fluids to 3,000 ml per day, unless medically contraindicated, to reduce fever Isolate patient; notify infection control officer		Instruction of patient/family about forcing fluids, discharge wound care, and rationale for isolation Graphic record for temperature above 101.4° F Laboratory report for positive culture and sensitive results of wound culture

APPENDIX A

BIBLIOGRAPHY

Alpers, Bernard, and Mancall, Elliott: Clinical neurology, ed. 6, Philadelphia, 1971, F. A. Davis Co.

American Cancer Association: Prostatic Ca, pamphlet, 1974.

Ancowitz, Arthur: Strokes and their prevention, New York, 1975, Van Nostrand Reinhold Co.

Arena, Jay: Poisoning—toxicology—symptoms—treatments, ed. 3, Springfield, Ill., 1974, Charles C Thomas, Publisher.

Arnold, Helen M.: Elderly diabetic amputees, Am. J. Nurs. 69(12):2646, 1969.

Balt, Linda H.: Working with dyphasic patients, Am. J. Nurs. 74(7):1320, 1974.

Bame, Kathleen B.: Halo traction, Am. J. Nurs. 69(9):1933, 1969.

Barckley, Virginia: Crisis in cancer, Am. J. Nurs. 67(2):278-280, 1967.

Barley, Joseph A., II: Traction, suspensions and ringless splints, Am. J. Nurs. 70(8):1724, 1970.

Barnard, Jan: What we know today about multiple sclerosis, RN 29(7):39-45, 1966.

Barnett, Henry, editor: Pediatrics, ed. 15, New York, 1972, Appleton-Century-Crofts.

Barney, Marie L.: The child with hydrocephalus, Am. J. Nurs. 73(5):828-831, 1973.

Beck, Rosemary: The diabetic alcoholic, RN 37(7):35, 1974.

Bennage, Barbara A., and Cummings, Marjorie E.: Nursing the patient undergoing total hip arthroplasty, Nurs. Clin. North Am. 8(3):107, 1973.

Blackwell, Ardith K., and Blackwell, William: Relieving gas pains, Am. J. Nurs. 75(1):66, 1975.

Boigli, Emily, and Steele, Mary S.: Scoliosis spinal instrumentation and fusion, Am. J. Nurs. 68(11):2399, 1968.

Boshanko, Lydia A.: Immediate postoperative prosthesis, Am. J. Nurs. 71(2):280, 1971.

Brawer, Phyllis, and Hicks, Dorothy: Muscle maintaining muscle function in patients on bedrest, Am. J. Nurs. 72(7):1250, 1972.

Brunner, Lillian, S. and others: Textbook of medical-surgical nursing, Philadelphia, 1975, J. B. Lippincott Co.

Brunner, Lillian S., and Suddarth, Doris S.: The Lippincott manual of nursing practice, Philadelphia, 1974, J. B. Lippincott Co.

Bryde, Mae, Mitchell, Cyril, and Blacklow, Stanley R.: Signs, and symptoms, ed. 5, Philadelphia, 1970, J. B. Lippincott Co.

Buergin, Pat, and others: Ravages of rheumatoid arthritis, Nursing 75 5(6):44, 1975.

Burrell, Zeb L., and Burrell, Lenette O.: Critical care, ed. 3, St. Louis, 1977, The C. V. Mosby Co.

Burt, Margaret N.: Perceptual deficits in hemiplegia, Am. J. Nurs. 70(5):1026, 1970.

Bushnell, Sharon S.: Respiratory intensive care nursing, Boston, 1973, Little, Brown and Co.

Cadoret, Remi J., and King, Lucy J.: Psychiatry in primary care, St. Louis, 1974, The C. V. Mosby Co.

Carini, Esta, and Owens, Guy: Neurological and neurosurgical nursing, ed. 6, St. Louis, 1974, The C. V. Mosby Co.

Carroll, Bettie: Fingers to toes, Am. J. Nurs. 71(3):550, 1971.

Cassidy, Freida M.: Adult hydrocephalus, Am. J. Nurs. 72(3):494, 1972.

Chinn, Peggy: Child health maintenance, St. Louis, 1974, The C. V. Mosby Co.

Chrismann, Marilyn: Dyspnea, Am. J. Nurs. 74(4):643, 1974.

Chusid, Joseph G.: Correlative neuroanatomy and functional neurology, ed. 14, Los Altos,

Calif., 1970, Lange Medical Publications.

Collart, Marie E., and Brenneman, Janice K.: Preventing postoperative atelectasis, Am. J. Nurs. 71(10):1982, 1971.

Comarr, Estin A., and others.: Sexual function in traumatic paraplegia and quadriplegia, Am. J. Nurs. 75(2):250, 1972.

Compton, Carol Y.: War injury: identity crisis for young men, Nurs. Clin. North Am. 8(1):53, 1973.

Conners, Melba: Ostomy care: a personal approach, Am. J. Nurs. 74(8):1422, 1974.

Cosgrove, Barbara D.: I have multiple sclerosis, RN 29(7):35, 1966.

Cosper, Bonnie: Physiological colostomy, Am. J. Nurs. 75(11):2014, 1975.

Cowell, Henry R.: Genetic aspects of orthopedic disease, Am. J. Nurs. 70(4):763, 1970.

Coyle, Norma R., and Miller, Barbara: Guillain-Barre syndrome nursing care, Am. J. Nurs. 66(10):2224, 1966.

Craven, Ruth F. Anaphylactic shock, Am. J. Nurs. 72(4):718, 1972.

Crigler, Lee: Sexual concerns of the spinal cord injured, Nurs. Clin. North Am. 9(4):703, 1974.

Dalessio, Donald: Mechanisms and biochemistry of headaches, Nurs. Dig. 3(3):30-32, 1975.

Davidson, Sharon V., editor: PSRO: utilization and audit in patient care, St. Louis, 1976, The C. V. Mosby Co.

Dayoff, Nancy: Re-thinking stroke—soft or hard devices to position hands, Am. J. Nurs. 75(7):1142-1144, 1975.

Devney, Ann Marie, and Kingsbury, Barbara A.: Hypothermia in fact and fantasy, Am. J. Nurs. 72(8):1424, 1972.

Dillon, Anne M.: Nursing care of the patient with multiple sclerosis, Nurs. Clin. North Am. 8(4):653-664, 1974.

Dolan, Marion B.: Re-thinking stroke—autumn months, autumn years, Am. J. Nurs. 75(7):45-47, 1975.

Downs, Florence S.: Bedrest and sensory disturbances, Am. J. Nurs. 74(3):434, 1974.

Drain, Cecil B.: The athletic knee injury, Am. J. Nurs. 71(3):536, 1971.

Durham, Nancy: Look out for complications of abdominal surgery, Nursing 75 5(2):24, 1975.

Eliasson, Sven G., and others: Neurological pathophysiology, New York, 1974, Oxford University Press.

Edmonds, Ruth E.: The hazards of immobility—effects on motor function, Am. J. Nurs. 67(4):788, 1967.

Ellis, Rosemary: Sitting problems after stroke, Am. J. Nurs. 73(11):1898, 1973.

Erb, Elizabeth: Improving speech in Parkinson's disease, Am. J. Nurs. 73(11):1910, 1973.

Eyre, Mary K.: Total hip replacement, Am. J. Nurs. 71(7):1384, 1971.

Fulton, Mary, and others: Helping diabetics adapt to failing vision, Am. J. Nurs. 74(1):54, 1974.

Fangman, Anne, and O'Malley, William E.: L-dopa and the patient with Parkinson's disease, Am. J. Nurs. 69(7):1455, 1969.

Fitzpatrick, Genevieve: Gynecologic nursing, New York, 1965, The Macmillian Co.

Flint, Thomas, and Caine, Harvey D.: Emergency treatment and management, Philadelphia, 1970, W. B. Saunders Co.

Forster, Francis M.: Clinical neurology, ed. 3, St. Louis, 1973, The C. V. Mosby Co.

Fowler, Roy S., Jr., and Fordyce, Wilbert E.: Adapting care for the brain-damaged patient, Am. J. Nurs. 72(10):1832, 1972.

Frankel, Esther C.: I spoke with the dead, Am. J. Nurs. 69(1):105, 1969.

Gaffney, Terry W. and Campbell, Rosemary P.: Feeding techniques for dysphagic patients, Am. J. Nurs. 74(12):2194, 1974.

Gardner, M. Arlene M.: Responsiveness as a measure of consciousness, Am. J. Nurs. 68(5):1034, 1968.

Gibbs, Gertrude E.: Perineal care of the incapacitated patient, Am. J. Nurs. 69(1):124, 1969.

Gibbs, Gertrude E., and White, Marilyn: Stoma care, Am. J. Nurs. 72(2):268, 1972

Given, Barbara, and Simmons, Sandra: Care of the patient with a gastric ulcer, Am. J. Nurs. 70(7):1472, 1970.

Given, Barbara A., and Simmons, Sandra J.: Gastroenterology in clinical nursing, ed. 2, St. Louis, 1975, The C. V. Mosby Co.

Govani, Laura E., and Hayes, Janice E.: Drugs and their nursing implications, Des Moines, 1971, Meredith Corporation.

Grey, Howard A.: The aphasic patient—and how you can help him, RN 33(7):46-48, 1970.

Gutch, C. F., and Stoner, Martha H.: Mosby's comprehensive, review series: review of hemodialysis for nurses and dialysis personnel, ed. 2, St. Louis, 1975, The C. V. Mosby Co.

Guthrie, Diana: Debbie got attention the hard way, Nursing '75 **5**(11):52, 1975.

Gutowski, Frances: Ostomy procedures: nursing care before and after, Am. J. Nurs. **72**(2):262, 1972.

Hafey, Lucille, and Keane, Barbara A.: Patients with acute insult to the central nervous system: an observation tool, Nurs. Clin. North Am. **8**(4):743, 1973.

Hanlon, Kathryn: Maintaining sexuality after spinal cord injury, Nursing '75 **5**(5):58, 1975.

Harkness, Laurale: Bringing epilepsy out of the closet, Am. J. Nurs. **74**(5):875, 1974.

Haymaker, Webb: Bing's local diagnosis in neurological diseases, ed. 15, St. Louis, 1969, The C. V. Mosby Co.

Hayter, Jean: Patient's who have alzheimer's disease, Am. J. Nurs. **74**(8):1460, 1974.

Hentgen, Janice H.: Dressing activities for disabled persons, Nurs. Clin. North Am. **1**(3):483, 1966.

Hinkhouse, Ann: Craniocerebral trauma, Am. J. Nurs. **73**(10):1719, 1973.

Homburger, Freddy, and Bonner, Charles D.: Medical care and rehabilitation of the aged and chronically ill, ed. 2, Boston, 1964, Little, Brown and Co.

Hoskins, Lois M.: Vascular and tension headaches, Am. J. Nurs. **74**(5):846-851, 1974.

Hughes, James: Synopsis of pediatrics, ed 4, St. Louis, 1975, The C. V. Mosby Co.

Isler, Charlotte: Compression—promising new treatment for hydrocephalus, RN **37**(7):44, 1974.

Jackson, Bettie S.: Ulcerative colitis from an etiological perspective, Am. J. Nurs. **73**(2):258, 1973.

Jacobansky, Ann M.: Stroke, Am. J. Nurs. **72**(7):1260, 1972.

Johnson, Bonnie J.: The hazards of immobility effects on gastrointestinal function, Am. J. Nurs. **67**(4):785, 1964.

Johnson, Colleen F., and Convery, Richard F.: Preventing emboli after total hip replacement, Am. J. Nurs. **75**(5):804, 1975.

Jones, Susan J.: Orthopedic injuries: II illness as deviance, Am. J. Nurs. **75**(11):2030, 1975.

Jontz, Donna L.: Prescription for living with M.S., Am. J. Nurs. **73**(5):817, 1973.

Kamenetz, Herman L.: Selecting a wheelchair, Am. J. Nurs. **72**(1):100, 1972.

Karhnelian, John G., and Sanders, Virgina: Urologic nursing, New York, 1970, The Macmillan Co.

Kelly, Mary H.: Exercises for bedfast patients, Am. J. Nurs. **66**(10):2209, 1966.

Kinnard, Leah S.: Preserving skeletal muscle tone in inactive patients, Am. J. Nurs. **69**(12):2662, 1969.

Kirkpatrick, Sandra: Battle casualty: amputee, Am. J. Nurs. **68**(5):998, 1968.

Klagsbrun, Samuel: Communications in the treatment of cancer, Am. J. Nurs. **71**(5):944-948, 1971.

Krupp, Marcus A., and Chatton, Milton J.: Current diagnosis and treatment, Los Altos, Calif., 1977, Lange Medical Publications.

Laird, Mona: Techniques for teaching preoperative and post-operative patients, Am. J. Nurs. **75**(8):1338, 1975.

Langford, Teddy O.: Nursing problem: bacteriuria and the indwelling catheter, Am. J. Nurs. **72**(1):113, 1972.

Langrehr, Audrey L.: Social stimulation, Am. J. Nurs. **74**(7):1300, 1974.

Larsen, George: Optokinetic nystagmus, Am. J. Nurs. **73**(11):1897, 1973.

Larson, Caroll B., and Gould, Marjorie: Orthopedic nursing, ed. 8, St. Louis, 1974, The C. V. Mosby Co.

Law, Jane: The fat embolism syndrome, Nurs. Clin. North Am. **8**:191, 1973.

Lee, Cata A., and others: Extracellular volume imbalance, Am. J. Nurs. **74**(5):888, 1974.

Lippincott manual of nursing practice, Philadelphia, 1974, J. B. Lippincott Co.

Lister, Jo Ann: Nursing intervention in anaphylactic shock, Am. J. Nurs. **72**(4):720, 1972.

Loxley, Alice K.: The emotional toll of crippling deformity, Am. J. Nurs. **72**(10):1839, 1972.

Luckmann, Joan, and Soresen, Karen C. Medical-surgical nursing: a psychophysiologic approach, Philadelphia, 1974, W. B. Saunders Co.

MacBryde, Cyril M., and Blacklow, Robert S.: Signs and symptoms, ed. 5, Philadelphia, 1970, J. B. Lippincott Co.

MacRae, Isabel: Arthritis, Nurs. Clin. North Am. **8**(4):643, 1973.

Maddox, Marjorie: Subarachnoid hemorrhage, Am. J. Nurs. **74**(12):2199, 1974.

Marginniss, Oscia: Rheumatoid arthritis—my tutor, Am. J. Nurs. **68**(8):1699, 1968.

Marlowe, Dorothy: Textbook of pediatric nursing, ed. 4, Philadelphia, 1973, W. B. Saunders Co.

Martin, Arlene M.: Care of a patient with cerebral aneurysm, Am. J. Nurs. **65**(4):90, 1965.

Martin, Marguerite M.: Insulin reactions, Am. J. Nurs. **67**(2):328, 1967.

Masters, Frank W., and Lewis, John R.: Symposium on aesthetic surgery of the face, eyelid, and breast, vol. 4, St. Louis, 1972, The C. V. Mosby Co.

Masters, Frank W., and Lewis, John R.: Symposium on asthetic surgery of the nose, ear, and chin, vol. 6, St. Louis, 1973, The C. V. Mosby Co.

McCaffery, Margo: Nursing management of the patient with pain, Philadelphia, 1972, J. B. Lippincott Co.

McCarthy, Joyce A.: The hazards of immobility—effects on respiratory function, Am. J. Nurs. **67**(4):783, 1967.

McCartney, Virginia: Rehabilitation and dignity for the stroke patient, Nurs. Clin. North Am. **9**(4):693-703, 1974.

McFarlane, Judith, and Nickerson, Donna: Two-drop and one-drop test for glycosuria, Am. J. Nurs. **72**(5):939, 1972.

McHenry, Lawrence: Essentials of stroke diagnosis and management, Philadelphia, 1969, Smith, Kline, and French laboratory.

Mervyn, Frances: Plight of dying patients in hospitals, Am. J. Nurs. **71**(10):1988-1990, 1971.

Methany, Ruth V.: Cerebrovascular accident and personality organization, Nurs. Clin. North Am. **1**(3):433, 1966.

Mihalov, Thelma R.: Bowel and bladder management of children with myelomeningocele, Nurs. Clin. North Am. **1**(3):459, 1966.

Monteiro, Lois A.: Hip fracture, a sociologist's viewpoints, Am. J. Nurs. **67**(6):1207, 1967.

Murray, Ruth L. E.: Principles of nursing intervention for the adult patient with body images changes, Nurs. Clin. North Am. **7**(4):697-707, 1972.

Musser, Ruth D., and Shubkagel, Betty L.: Pharmacology and therapeutics, ed. 3, New York, 1965, The Macmillian Co.

Myers, M. Bert: Sutures and wound healing, Am. J. Nurs. **71**(7):1725, 1971.

Narrow, Barbara W.: Rest is . . . , Am. J. Nurs. **67**(8):1646, 1967.

Nelson, Waldo, editor: Textbook of pediatrics, ed. 10, Philadelphia, 1975, W. B. Saunders Co.

Nett, Louise M., and Petty, Thomas L.: Acute respiratory failure, principles of care, Am. J. Nurs. **67**(9):1847, 1967.

Nickerson, Donna: Teaching the hospital diabetic, Am. J. Nurs. **72**(5):939, 1972.

Norsworthy, Edith: Nursing rehabilitation after severe head trauma, Am. J. Nurs. **74**(7):1246, 1974.

O'Dell, Arois: Hot packs for morning joint stiffness, Am. J. Nurs. **75**(6):986, 1975.

Passo, Sherrilyn D.: Positioning infants with myelomeningocele, Am. J. Nurs. **74**(9):1658, 1974.

Patterson, Patricia A.: Services offered by the National Multiple Sclerosis Society, Am. J. Nurs. **68**(10):2164, 1968.

Pendleton, Thelma, and Grossman, Burton J.: Rehabilitating children with inflammatory joint disease, Am. J. Nurs. **74**(12):2223, 1974.

Peszczynski, Mieczyslaw: Why old people fall, Am. J. Nurs. **65**(5):86, 1965.

Petrilo, Madeline, and Sanger, Sirgay: Emotional care of hospitalized children, Philadelphia, 1972, J. B. Lippincott Co.

Pfaudler, Marjorie: Afterstroke–motor skill rehabilitation for hemiplegics, Am. J. Nurs. **73**(11):1892, 1973.

Plummer, Elizabeth: The M.S. patient, Am. J. Nurs. **68**(10):2161, 1968.

Purintun, Lynn R., and Nelson, Louella: Ulcer patient, emotional emergency, Am. J. Nurs. **68**(9):1930, 1968.

Raynolds, Nancy: Teaching parents home care after surgery for scoliosis, Am. J. Nurs. **74**(6):1090, 1974.

Reif, Rita: Managing a life with chronic disease, Am. J. Nurs. **73**(2):261, 1973.

Robb, Susanne: Bunion surgery, Am. J. Nurs. **74**(12):2181, 1974.

Robbins, Stanley L.: Pathologic basis of disease, Philadelphia, 1974, W. B. Saunders Co.

Robinson, Marilyn B.: Levadopa and parkinsonism, Am. J. Nurs. **74**(4):656, 1974.

Rodman, Theodore: Management of tracheobronchial secretions, Am. J. Nurs. **66**(11):2474, 1966.

Rusk, Howard A.: Rehabilitation medicine, ed. 4, St. Louis, 1977, The C. V. Mosby Co.

Ryan, John: Compression in bone healing, Am. J. Nurs. **74**(11):1998-1999, 1974.

Sasahara, Arthur A., and Foster, Vivienne L.: Pulmonary embolism: recognition and treatment, Am. J. Nurs. **67**(8):1634, 1967.

Schauder, Marilyn R.: Ostomy care: cone irrigations, Am. J. Nurs. **74**(8):1424, 1974.

Schroeder, Lois M.: The hazards of immobility, Am. J. Nurs. **67**(4):779, 1967.

Schultz, Lucie C.: Nursing care of the stroke patient, Nurs. Clin. North Am. 8(4):633-641, 1973.

Scipien, Gladys, and others: Comprehensive pediatric nursing, New York, 1975, McGraw-Hill Book Co.

Shafer, Kathleen N., Sawyer, Janet R., Mc-Cluskey, Audrey M., and others: Medical-surgical nursing, ed. 6, St. Louis, 1975, The C. V. Mosby Co.

Sharer, Jo Ellen: Reviewing acid-base balance, Am. J. Nurs. 75(6):980, 1975.

Shaw, Bernice: Revolution in stroke care, RN 33(1):56-61, 1970.

Shearer, Donald, and others: Preparing a patient for EEG, Am. J. Nurs. 75(1):63, 1975.

Shoemaker, Rebecca R.: Total knee replacement, Nurs. Clin. North Am. 8(1):167, 1973.

Shope, Jean T.: The clinical specialist in epilepsy, Nurs. Clin. North Am. 9(4):761-772, 1974.

Skelly, Madge: Re-thinking stroke—aphasic patients talk back, Am. J. Nurs. 75(7):1140-1142, 1975.

Smith, Dorothy, and Germain, Carol P. H.: Care of the adult patient, ed. 4, Philadelphia, 1975, J. B. Lippincott Co.

Snyder, Mariah, and Baum, Rebecca: Assessing station and gait, Am. J. Nurs. 74(7):1256, 1974.

Souie, Margaret D., and Israel, Jacob S.: Use of the cuffed tracheostomy tube, Am. J. Nurs. 67(9):1854, 1967.

Sowes, Betty J.: Thalidomide victims in a rehabilitation center, Am. J. Nurs. 66(9):2023, 1966.

Sproul, Carmen W., and Mullanney, Patrick J.: Emergency care—assessment and intervention, St. Louis, 1974, The C. V. Mosby Co.

Stanton, Judith H., and others: Care of the patient with infectious neuronitis, Nurs. Clin. North Am. 1(3):603, 1966.

Staudt, Annamay R.: Femur replacement, Am. J. Nurs. 75(8):1346, 1975.

Stephens, Given J.: A delicate balance: managing chronic airway obstruction in a neurosurgical patient, Am. J. Nurs. 75(9):1492, 1975.

Stone, Marlene H.: Normal pressure—hydrocephalus, Nurs. Clin. North Am. 9(4):667, 1974.

Storlie, Frances, and others: Principles of instensive nursing, care, New York, 1969, Appleton-Century-Crofts.

Stuart, Sarah: Day to day living with diabetes, Am. J. Nurs. 71(8):1548, 1971.

Sun, Rhoda L. Trendelenburg's position in hypovolemic shock, Am. J. Nurs. 71(9):1758, 1971.

Taren, James A.: Cerebral aneurysm, Am. J. Nurs. 65(4):88, 1965.

Taylor, Ann G.: Autonomic dysreflexia in spinal cord injury, Nurs. Clin. North Am. 9(4):717, 1974.

Tinker, John H., and Wehner, Robert: The nurse and the ventilator, Am. J. Nurs. 74(7):1276, 1974.

Townley, Charles, and Hill, Leslie: Total knee replacement, Am. J. Nurs. 74(6):1612, 1974.

Tucker, Susan M., Breeding, Mary Ann, Canobbio, Mary M., and others: Patient care standards, St. Louis, 1975, The C. V. Mosby Co.

Tweed, C. Gilbert: Guillain Barré syndrome—the illness, Am. J. Nurs. 66(10):2222, 1966.

Ungvarski, Peter: Mechanical stimulation of coughing, Am. J. Nurs. 71(12):2358, 1971.

Wade, Jacqueline J.: Respiratory nursing care, physiology and technique, ed. 2, St. Louis, 1977, The C. V. Mosby Co.

Wade, Mildred: Hazards of immobility—effects on metabolic equilibrium, Am. J. Nurs. 67(4):793, 1967.

Watkins, Julia D., and Moss, Fay T.: Confusion in the management of diabetes, Am. J. Nurs. 69(3):521, 1969.

Watson, Jeannette E.: Medical-surgical nursing and related physiology, Philadelphia, 1972, W. B. Saunders Co.

Webb, Kenneth J.: Early assessment of orthopedic injuries, Am. J. Nurs. 74(6):1048, 1974.

Wells, Robin W.: Huntington's chorea—seeing beyond the disease, Am. J. Nurs. 72(5):954-956, 1972.

Whitehead, Delores J.: Emergency care in orthopedic injuries, Nurs. Clin. North Am. 8(3):435, 1973.

Whitehead, Sylvia: Nursing care of the adult urology patient, New York, 1970, Appleton-Century-Crofts.

Williams, Anne: Classification and diagnosis of epilepsy, Nurs. Clin. North Am. 9(4):747, 1974.

Williams, Donald H.: Sleep and disease, Am. J. Nurs. 71(12):2321, 1971.

Williams, Lester F.: An acute abdomen, Am. J. Nurs. 71(2):299, 1971.

Zalewski, Nancy, and others: Hemipelvectomy: the triumph of Ms. A, Am. J. Nurs. 73(12):2073, 1973.

Zieman, Hazel F.: The neurologically handicapped child, Am. J. Nurs. 69(12):2621, 1969.

APPENDIX B

PERFORMANCE EVALUATION PROCEDURE (PEP) FORMS DEVELOPED BY JOINT COMMISSION ON ACCREDITATION OF HOSPITALS*

The Joint Commission on Accreditation of Hospitals offers a seminar on the JCAH Performance Evaluation Procedure for auditing and improving patient care. This course explains in detail the utilization of the forms and the methodology for retrospective review of patient care. A book called the *Pep Primer* is available for seminar participants.

Health care providers may reproduce the worksheets for use in conducting patient care audit and evaluation activities in their own institutions. All other rights are reserved.

*Forms reproduced with permission of Joint Commission on Accreditation of Hospitals, Chicago, Ill.

406

GLOSSARY

accountability The state of being answerable; responsibility for justifying an action or other results to the public, peers, or employers

activity outcome The expected level of physical and/or mental action at the time of discharge

analysis A separation of a whole into its components; separation of variations (whole) into the subclassifications of justifiable or deficient (parts)

assessment Critical appraisal of the patient in order to determine nursing care needs

assurance The state of being sure or certain

audit A methodical examination and review; the final report of an examination of accountability

complications A disease or accident superimposed on another, affecting or modifying the prognosis of the original disease

concurrent Operating at the same time as care is being given

criteria Predetermined, measurable elements of health care, on which judgments about quality of care are made

criterion A measure on which a judgment or decision may be based

critical management To control or treat the turning point of that which modified the prognosis of the disease (complications)

deficiency Lacking in some necessary quality or element; not up to normal standards; defective

discharge status The state of the patient as a result of the care; condition at termination of care

elements Values on which conclusions are based; factors determining the outcome of a process

expected The ideal occurrence for each of the elements; it would be expected to occur "all" or "none" of the time

exceptions The art of excluding; taking or leaving out; those to be excluded

health outcome The desired level of freedom from disease as a result of care

knowledge outcome The desired patient education at the termination of care

management The control or treatment of a condition or disease

norms Average or median of observed performance, stated in numerical or statistical terms

Nursing Professional Standards Review Organization (NPSRO) A group of nurses that examine the total nursing care delivered in a specific setting

Developed by Ellen Vasey, and Mary Reilly, R.N., as an educational resource of the Western Pennsylvania Regional Medical Program, Quality Assurance: Peer Review for Nursing.

outcome A final result of care

peer An equal; like groups of individuals

peer review The process by which registered nurses, actively engaged in the practice of nursing, appraise the quality of nursing care in a given situation in accordance with established standards of practice

process Gradual changes leading to a particular result; the assessment and management of care leading to the outcome

Professional Standards Review Organization (PSRO) A group of health care professionals concerned with the quality of health care in specified regions; federally legislated programs concerned with patient care for those receiving Medicare, Medicaid, and Maternal and Child Health

quality Having the characteristics of excellence

quality assurance A commitment to excellence of care; an estimation of the degree of excellence in the alteration of health status of consumers attained through nursing performance

retrospective To look back after care has been given to screen for deviations from the established standards or criteria

standard Something established by general consent as a model or example; a rule for the measure of quality

structure The environment within which care is given including staffing, physical facilities, and equipment

variations Deviations from the predetermined criteria that have not been determined as justifiable deviations or deficiencies

INDEX

Anemia—cont'd
  hemolytic, acquired, 61-62
  iron deficiency, 62
  leukopenia or, overwhelming infection secondary
    to, 371
  pernicious, 63-64
  sickle cell, 60-61
  of undetermined origin, 60-61
Aneurysm
  aortic, abdominal, 64-65
  intracranial, or subarachnoid hemorrhage, 335-
    336
    in children, 336
Ankle
  and foot, amputation of
    acquired, 38-39
    traumatic, 39-41
  fracture of, 153-154
Anorectal abscess, 34-35, 331
Anticoagulant therapy, bleeding with, 339
Anxiety neurosis, 249
Aorta, abdominal, thrombosis of, acute, 304
Aortic aneurysm, abdominal, 64-65
Aortoiliac arterial occlusive disease, chronic, 66-67
Aplastic anemia, 58-59
Appendectomy, 33-34
Appendicitis in children, 65-66
Arrest
  cardiac, 344
  respiratory, 386
Arrhythmias, 336-337
  cardiac, in children, 90-91
Arterial embolism, 359
Arterial occlusive disease
  aortoiliac, chronic, 66-67
  extracranial, 67-68
  peripheral, of lower extremity, chronic, 68-69
Arteries of lower extremities, thrombosis of, acute,
  304
Arteriosclerotic heart disease, 181-182
Arthritis, 260-261
  gouty, 363
  of knee, degenerative, 69-70
  rheumatoid, 71-72
  of spine, degenerative, 72-74
Aspiration, 337
Asthma, acute, 74-75
Ataxia, 94-95
Atelectasis, 337-338
Atresia
  biliary, in children, 212
  esophageal, in children, 149
Atrial fibrillation, 75-76, 338
Atypical facial pain, 310-311
Audit
  behavioral outcome, 7
  nursing
    concurrent, 6-7
    retrospective, 6, 7-8
  procedural checklist for, 27
  process, 7
  structure, 7

B

Back pain, low, 258-259
  including arthritis and disc pathology, 260-261

Bacterial endocarditis, 360-361
Bacterial meningitis, 219-221
Bacterial pneumonia, 268-269
Behavior
  destructive or self-destructive, 389
  inappropriate, emotional problems, or feelings of
    suicide, 360
Behavioral disorders of childhood or adolescence,
  76-77
Behavioral outcome audit, 7
Benign tumors of spinal cord, 320-321
Biliary atresia in children, 212
Bimalleolus, fracture of, 153-154
Bleeding
  with anticoagulant therapy, 339
  recurrent, and shock, 339-340
Blindness, 340-341
Blood urea nitrogen, rising, 341
Blood vessels eroded by malignant tissues, hem-
  orrhage from, 343
Bone, pathological involvement and/or fractures of,
  342; see also Fractures
Bone marrow
  disturbances of, 345-346
  suppression of, 342
Bowel
  ischemia of, 376
  obstruction of, 343
Brain
  abscess of, 35-36, 331
  infection of, 369-370
  tumors of
    medically treated, 313-314
    with surgical intervention, 314-316
Breast
  carcinoma of, with metastasis, 79
  mass in, with mastectomy, 217-218
Bronchial foreign body in children, 307
Bronchitis in children, 290-291
Bunion, 77-78
Bureau of Quality Assurance, 3, 9

C

Cancer, complications of, 343
Carcinoma
  of breast with metastasis, 79
  of cervix, clinically invasive
    with radiation and/or chemotherapy, 80-81
    with surgical intervention, 82-83
  of colon with metastasis, 83-84
  of lung with metastasis, 84-85
  of ovary with metastasis, 85
  of pancreas with metastasis, 86
  of prostate with metastasis, 87
  of stomach with metastasis, 88
  of uterus with metastasis, 89
Carcinomatosis, 90
Cardiac arrest, 344
Cardiac arrhythmias in children, 90-91
Cardiac diagnostic testing, 91-92
  adverse drug reaction or dye reaction in, 354-355
Care
  medical, retrospective review of, development of,
    8
  nursing; see Nursing care
Cataract, 92-93

411

Disease—cont'd
  spinal cord
    cervical, with quadriplegia, 296-297
    dorsal or lumbar, with paraplegia, 298-299
    vascular, peripheral, as complication of diabetes
      mellitus, 129-130
Dislocation, recurrent
  of patella, 135-136
  of shoulder, 137-138
Disorders
  behavioral, of childhood or adolescence, 76-77
  convulsive, 110-111
    in children, 112
  neurological, adverse drug reaction in, 356-357
  personality, and certain other nonpsychotic men-
    tal disorders of childhood or adolescence,
    266-267
  psychophysiological, of childhood or adoles-
    cence, 279-280
Disturbances
  bone marrow, 345-346
  coordination, and multiple sclerosis, 235-236
  gastrointestinal, 345-346
  situational, transient, 308
    in children, 309-310
Diuretics, adverse drug reaction to, 354
Diverticular disease
  of colon, 138-139
  with surgical intervention, 173-175
Dorsal spinal cord injury or disease with paraplegia,
  298-299
Dorsal vertebra, fracture of, 155-157
Drug abuse, 140
Drug reaction, adverse, 353-354
  in cardiac diagnostic testing, 354-355
  to diuretics, 354
  to iron, 355-356
  in neurological disorders, 356-357
Drug-induced hypovolemic shock, 392
Duct stone, common, residual, following cholecys-
  tectomy, 357
Duodenal ulcer, 263-264
  with surgical intervention, 173-175
Dye reaction in cardiac diagnostic testing, 354-355
Dysrhythmias, 141
Dystrophy, muscular, 236-238

E
Edema
  massive or persistent, of lower extremity, 357-
    358
  pulmonary, 358
Education, continuing, 6
Elbow, fracture of, 169-171
Elective female surgical sterilization for family
  planning, 299-300
Electrolyte and fluid imbalance in children, 152-
  153
Embolism
  arterial, 359
  pulmonary, 359-360
Emotional problems, feelings of suicide, or inappro-
  priate behavior, 360
Encephalitis, 142-143
Encephalocele, 143-145
Encephalopathy, toxic-metabolic, 145-146

Endocarditis, bacterial, 360-361
Enteritis, chronic, in children, 146-147
Environment, discharge, medically suitable, absence of, 353
Epilepsy, 147-148
Esophageal surgery, esophageal disease with, 173-
  175
Esophagus
  anastomotic leak or stricture of, 335
  atresia of, in children, 149
  chemical injury to, 103-104
  disease of, with esophageal surgery, 173-175
  rupture and/or perforation of, 361
Evaluation, nursing care; see Nursing care evaluation; Nursing Care Evaluation studies
Exploratory celiotomy, abdominal pain, etiology
  unknown, with, 33-34
Extracranial arterial occlusive disease, 67-68
Extremity
  lower; see also Leg(s)
    amputation of, for diabetes, 334
    arteries of, abdominal aorta and/or thrombosis
      of, acute, 304
    massive or persistent edema of, 357-358
  upper, fractures of, 169-171

F
Facelift, surgical, 150-151
Facial pain, atypical, 310-311
Facial paralysis, 379-380
Failure
  of family and/or social support system, 361-
    362
  heart, congestive, 185, 364
  renal, 385-386
    in children, 289-290
  respiratory, 386-387
  shunt, in children, 392-393
  to thrive in children, 151-152
Family planning, elective surgical female steriliza-
  tion for, 299-300
Family and/or social support system, failure of, 361-
  362
Fecal impaction, 362
Feelings
  of hopelessness, unrealistic, 366
  of suicide, emotional problems, or inappropriate
    behavior, 360
Female sterilization, surgical, for family planning,
  elective, 299-300
Femoral neck of hip, fracture of, 157-159
Femur, fracture of, proximal, 159-160
Fever
  persistent, 362
  rheumatic, acute, in children, 292-293
Fibrillation, atrial, 75-76, 338
Fibrosis, cystic, 115-116
Fibula and/or tibia, fracture of shaft of, 165-166
Fingers, traumatic amputation of, 53
Fissure-in-ano, 173-175
Fistula
  intestinal, 363
  tracheoesophageal, in children, 149
Fistula-in-ano, 173-175
Fluid and electrolyte imbalance in children, 152-
  153

Foot
  and ankle, amputation of
    acquired, 38-39
    traumatic, 39-41
  toes or, gangrene, infection, and ulcers of, 371-372
Foreign body, tracheal or bronchial, in children, 307
Foreskin, redundant, circumcision of, 104
Form for nursing care evaluation, 24
  completed, 14-19
  modified, 12-13
Fracture(s)
  of ankle, 153-154
  of bimalleolus, 153-154
  of bone, pathological involvement and/or, 342
  of cervical vertebra, 155-157
  of dorsal vertebra, 155-157
  of elbow, 169-171
  of femoral neck of hip, 157-159
  of femur, proximal, 159-160
  of hip, intertrochanteric, open reduction of, 160-162
  of lateral malleolus, 153-154
  of lumbar vertebra, 155-157
  of medial malleolus, 153-154
  pathological, 343
  of pelvis, 162-164
  of shaft of humerus, 169-171
  of shaft of tibia and/or fibula, 165-166
  of skull, 167-168
  of trimalleolus, 153-154
  of upper extremity, group, 169-171
Fracture-subluxation of cervical spine, 171-172
Fungal meningitis, 222-223

G

Gangrene
  as chronic complication of diabetes mellitus, 129-130
  of toes or foot, 371-372
Gastric ulcer, 263-264
  with surgical intervention, 173-175
Gastroenteritis in children, 172-173
Gastrointestinal disturbances, 345-346
Gastrointestinal hemorrhage, 365
Gastrointestinal tract surgeries, 173-175
Gastroschisis in children, 253-254
Gout, 363
Gouty arthritis, 363
Guillain-Barré syndrome, 175-176

H

Hand, traumatic amputation of, 53
Head trauma, 177-178
  in children, 179-180
Headache, 180-181
Health care practitioners, non-physician, activities of, 4
Heart disease
  arteriosclerotic, 181-182
  congenital, in children, 182-183
  valvular, 184
Heart failure, congestive, 185, 364
Hematoma, 398-399
  hypertensive intracerebral, spontaneous, 186-187

Hematoma—cont'd
  intracranial, increased intracranial pressure complicating, 373-374
  subdural, 177-178
Hemolytic anemia, acquired, 61-62
Hemolytic transfusion reaction, 396
Hemorrhage
  from blood vessels eroded by malignant tissues, 343
  complicating leukemia, 364-365
  gastrointestinal, 365
  rectal, 365-366
  subarachnoid, or intracranial aneurysm, 335-336
    in children, 336
Hemorrhoids, 173-175
Hepatitis, viral, group, 187-188
Hernia
  hiatal, 173-175
  inguinal, in children, 189
  umbilical, in children, 190
  ventral, 173-175
Herniated cervical disc, 132-133
Herniated lumbar disc, 134-135
  radiculopathies and, 288-299
Herpes zoster, 191
Hiatal hernia, 173-175
Hip
  femoral neck of, fracture of, 157-159
  intertrochanteric, fracture of, open reduction of, 160-162
Hodgkin's disease, 192
Hopelessness, unrealistic feelings of, 366
Hospital Adoption of International Classification of Disease, 8
Humerus, fracture of, 169-171
Huntington's chorea, 193-194
Hyaline membrane disease, 194-195
Hydrocarbon poisoning, volatile, in children, 273-274
Hydrocele in children, 189
Hydrocephalus, 196-197
  in children, 197-199
  increased intracranial pressure complicating, 373-374
Hyperglycemia, deterioration of consciousness with rapid correction of, 348-349
Hypertension, 200-201
  in children, 201
Hypertensive hematoma, intracerebral, spontaneous, 186-187
Hyperthyroidism with surgical intervention, 202-203
Hypertrophic pyloric stenosis, congenital, 287
Hypocalcemia, 366
Hypochloremic alkalosis, 333-334
Hypoglossal nerve deficit, peripheral, 381
Hypoglycemia, 367-368
  in diabetes, 203-204
  prolonged over 30 minutes, 368
Hypospadias in children, 205-206
Hypovolemic shock, 391
  drug-induced, 392

I

Idiopathic seizures in children, 112
Illness, manic-depressive, 216-217

Imbalance, fluid and electrolyte, in children, 152-153
Impaction, fecal, 362
Inanition, 368-369
Inappropriate behavior, emotional problems, or feelings of suicide, 360
Increased intracranial pressure, 372-373
  complicating pneumocephalus, hydrocephalus, or intracranial hematoma, 373-374
Infarction, myocardial, 376-377
  acute, 241-242
Infection
  brain, 369-370
  complicating leukemia, 370-371
  overwhelming, secondary to leukopenia or anemia, 371
  pelvic, postoperative, 380
  respiratory, in children, 290-291
  of tissues undergoing malignant changes, 343
  of toes or foot, 371-372
  urinary tract
    acute, 397-398
    in children, 325-326
  wound, 398-399
Infectious hepatitis, 187-188
Inflammatory polyarthritis, 274-275
Inguinal hernia in children, 189
Injuries
  chemical, to esophagus, 103-104
  nerve
    laryngeal, 374
    peripheral, 246-247
  spinal cord
    cervical, with quadriplegia, 296-297
    dorsal or lumbar, with paraplegia, 298-299
  tendon, 300-302
Interface, PSRO, 29-30
International Classification of Diseases Adapted for Use, 8
Intertrochanteric fracture of hip, open reduction of, 160-162
Intestinal fistula, 363
Intestinal obstruction in children, 209
Intracerebral hypertensive hematoma, spontaneous, 186-187
Intracranial aneurysm or subarachnoid hemorrhage, 335-336
  in children, 336
Intracranial hematoma, increased intracranial pressure complicating, 373-374
Intracranial pressure, increased, 372-373
  complicating pneumocephalus, hydrocephalus, or intracranial hematoma, 373-374
Intractable pain, 378
Intraperitoneal abscess, 332
Intussusception in children, 210-211
Iron, adverse drug reaction to, 355-356
Iron deficiency anemia, 62
Irreversible coma, diabetic, 347-348
Ischemia, bowel, 376
Ischemic chest pain, 211

J

Jaundice, obstructive, in children, 212
JCAH; see Joint Commission on Accreditation of Hospitals

Joint
  major, periarthritis of, 265
  pain and swelling of, 257-258
Joint Commission on Accreditation of Hospitals
  retrospective review methodology of, 8
  revision of standards on accreditation by, 3
Juvenile diabetes mellitus, 14-19

K

Knee
  amputation of leg above, traumatic, 41-43
  amputation of leg below
    acquired, 45-46
    traumatic, 46-48
  degenerative arthritis of, 69-70

L

Laryngeal nerve injury, 374
Lateral malleolus, fracture of, 153-154
Lateral sclerosis, amyotrophic, 57-58
Lead poisoning in children, 270-271
Leak, anastomotic, or stricture of esophagus, 335
Leg(s); see also Lower extremity
  amputation of
    acquired, 43-44, 50-51
    congenital, 48-49
    above knee, traumatic, 41-43
    below knee
      acquired, 45-46
      traumatic, 46-48
    traumatic, 51-52
  peripheral arterial occlusive disease of, chronic, 68-69
Leukemia, 213-214
  acute, in children, 214-215
  hemorrhage complicating, 364-365
  infection complicating, 370-371
Leukopenia or anemia, overwhelming infection secondary to, 371
Low back pain, 258-259
  including arthritis and disc pathology, 260-261
Lower extremity; see also Leg(s)
  amputation of, for diabetes, 334
  arteries of, thrombosis of, acute, 304
  massive or persistent edema of, 357-358
Lumbar disc, herniated, 134-135
  radiculopathies and, 288-289
Lumbar spinal cord injury or disease with paraplegia, 298-299
Lumbar vertebra, fracture of, 155-157
Lung, carcinoma of, with metastasis, 84-85
Lymphoma, malignant, 215-216

M

Malfunction, shunt, 393
Malignant changes, infections of tissues undergoing, 343
Malignant lymphoma, 215-216
Malignant neoplasm
  of colon and rectum with surgical intervention, 243-244
  of stomach with surgical intervention, 173-175
Malignant tissues, hemorrhage from blood vessels eroded by, 343
Malignant tumors of spinal cord, 322-323
Malleolus, medial or lateral, fracture of, 153-154

415

Simple varicose veins, 326-327
Situational disturbances, transient, 308
  in children, 309-310
Skin, tumors of, with surgical intervention, 319
Skin flap necrosis, 393
Skin ulceration, nonhealing, as chronic complication of diabetes mellitus, 129-130
Skull, fracture of, 167-168
Sleeplessness, 393-394
Social support system and/or family, failure of, 361-362
Soft tissue, tumors of, with surgical intervention, 319
Sores, pressure, 278
Special symptoms of childhood or adolescence, 295-296
Spina bifida, 230-232
Spinal cord
  cervical, injury or disease of, with quadriplegia, 296-297
  compression of, 156
  dorsal or lumbar, injury or disease of, with paraplegia, 298-299
  tumors of
    benign, 320-321
    malignant, 322-323
Spine
  cervical, fracture-subluxation or subluxation of, 171-172
  degenerative arthritis of, 72-74
  fractures of, 155-157
Spondylosis, cervical, 132-133
Spontaneous hypertensive intracerebral hematoma, 186-187
Standards
  for accreditation, 3
  definition of, 5
  of practice, setting, 11
Status epilepticus, 394
Stenosis, pyloric, congenital hypertrophic, 287
Sterilization, female, surgical, for family planning, elective, 299-300
Stomach
  carcinoma of, with metastasis, 88
  malignant neoplasm of, with surgical intervention, 173-175
Stone, common duct, residual, following cholecystectomy, 357
Storm, thyroid, 396
Stricture of esophagus, 335
Stroke; see Cerebrovascular accident
Structure audit, 7
Study abstract sheet for nursing care evaluation, 24
Study format for nursing care evaluation, 22
Study summary for nursing care evaluation, 28
Stupor, 108-109
Subarachnoid hemorrhage or intracranial aneurysm, 335-336
  in children, 336
Subdural hematoma, 177-178
Subluxation of cervical spine, 171-172
Suicide, feelings of, 360
Suitable discharge environment, absence of, 353
Support system, social, and/or family, failure of, 361-362
Suppression, bone marrow, 342

Surgery; see also Surgical intervention
  esophageal, esophageal disease with, 173-175
  of gastrointestinal tract, 173-175
Surgical conditions of abdomen, 33-34
Surgical facelift, 150-151
Surgical intervention; see also Surgery
  abdominal trauma with, 33-34
  brain tumors with, 314-316
  chronic nonspecific ulcerative colitis with, 105-106
  clinically invasive carcinoma of cervix with, 82-83
  diverticular disease with, 173-175
  gastric or duodenal ulcer with, 173-175
  hyperthyroidism with, 202-203
  for malignant neoplasm
    of colon and rectum, 243-244
    of stomach, 173-175
  tumors of skin or soft tissue with, 319
Surgical sterilization, female, for family planning, elective, 299-300
Swelling, joint pain and, 257-258
Sympathetic nervous system, tumors of, 324-325
Symptoms, special, of childhood or adolescence, 295-296
Syndrome
  cervical pain, 102-103
  Guillain-Barré, 175-176
  Meniere's, 218-219
  nephrotic, 123-125
  organic brain, 116-117
    psychosis associated with, 280-281
    of childhood or adolescence, 281-282
  postgastrectomy (dumping), 383-384
Syphilitic meningitis
  acute, 224-225
  chronic, 225-227

T

Tendon injuries, 300-302
Testicle, undescended, orchiopexy for, 302-303
Testing, diagnostic, cardiac, 91-92
  adverse drug reaction or dye reaction in, 354-355
Therapeutic units, toxicity beyond, 345-346
Therapy, anticoagulant, bleeding with, 339
Thrive, failure to, in children, 151-152
Thrombocytopenic purpura, 285-286
Thromboembolism in children, 394-395
Thrombophlebitis, 303, 395
Thrombosis of abdominal aorta and/or arteries of lower extremities, acute, 304
Thumb, traumatic amputation of, 53
Thyroid crisis or storm, 396
Tibia and/or fibula, fracture of shaft of, 165-166
Tissue
  breakdown of, 345-346
  malignant, hemorrhage from blood vessels eroded by, 343
  soft, tumors of, with surgical intervention, 319
  undergoing malignant changes, infections of, 343
Toes
  amputation of
    acquired, 54-55
    traumatic, 55-56
  or foot, gangrene of, infection, ulcers, and, 371-372